Progress in Epileptic Disorders
Volume 7

Drug-resistant epilepsies

Progress in Epileptic Disorders
International Advisory Board

Aicardi Jean, *France*
Arzimanoglou Alexis, *France*
Baumgartner Christoph, *Austria*
Brodie Martin, *UK*
Cross Helen, *UK*
Duchowny Michael, *USA*
Elger Christian, *Germany*
French Jacqueline, *USA*
Glauser Tracy, *USA*
Gobbi Giuseppe, *Italy*
Guerrini Renzo, *Italy*
Hirsch Edouard, *France*
Kahane Philippe, *France*
Luders Hans, *USA*
Meador Kimford, *USA*
Moshé Solomon L., *USA*
Noachtar Soheyl, *Germany*
Noebels Jeffrey, *USA*
Palmini André, *Brazil*
Perucca Emilio, *Italy*
Pitkanen Asla, *Finland*
Ryvlin Philippe, *France*
Scheffer Ingrid, *Australia*
Schmitz Bettina, *Germany*
Schmidt Dieter, *Germany*
Serratosa José, *Spain*
Shorvon Simon, *UK*
Tinuper Paolo, *Italy*
Thomas Pierre, *France*
Tuxhorn Ingrid, *USA*
Wolf Peter, *Denmark*

Progress in Epileptic Disorders
Volume 7

Drug-resistant epilepsies

Philippe Kahane
Anne Berg
Wolfgang Löscher
Doug Nordli
Emilio Perucca

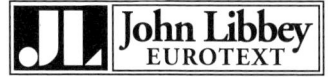

ISBN: 978-2-74200713-4
ISSN: 1777-4284
Vol. 7.

Published by
Éditions John Libbey Eurotext
127, avenue de la République, 92120 Montrouge, France
Tél. : 01 46 73 06 60
Site internet : http://www.jle.com

John Libbey Eurotext
42-46 High Street
Esher, Surrey
KT10 9KY
United Kingdom

© 2008, John Libbey Eurotext. All rights reserved.

Unauthorized duplication contravenes applicable laws.
Il est interdit de reproduire intégralement ou partiellement le présent ouvrage sans autorisation de l'éditeur ou du Centre Français d'Exploitation du Droit de Copie, 20, rue des Grands-Augustins, 75006 Paris.

Contents

Towards a clinically meaningful definition of drug-resistance
  A. Arzimanoglou, P. Ryvlin 1

The risk, correlates and temporal patterns of intractable epilepsy
  A.T. Berg 7

Are drug-resistant and drug-sensitive patients the same? Observations from the Glasgow database
  M.J. Brodie 17

Refractory versus non-refractory status epilepticus: frequency, differentiating clinical features, and outcome
  A. Neligan, S. Shorvon 29

Current knowledge on basic mechanisms of drug-resistance
  W. Löscher 47

What should the characteristics be of a pertinent model to identify new treatments for drug resistant epilepsy?
  E.H. Bertram 63

Pertinent approaches for a genetic identification of resistance to antiepileptic drugs
  S. Sisodiya 75

Molecular targets of antiepileptic drugs
  G. Sills 85

Antiepileptic drugs in development with a real potential
  E. Perucca 107

How many patients with drug-resistant epilepsy become seizure-free *because* of surgery?
  D. Schmidt 141

Neurostimulation for epilepsy: myth or reality?
   P. Kahane, S. Saillet, L. Minotti, L. Vercueil, S. Chabardès, A. Depaulis 153

Beyond seizure reduction
   F.G. Gilliam, P. Perucca 171

Early identification of drug-resistant patients
   D.R. Nordli 187

Epileptic encephalopathies *versus* "garden variety" focal epilepsies: can they be considered together?
   J.H. Cross, C. Eltze 199

Workshop on
"Drug-Resistant Epilepsies"
Sitges, april 2008

Scientific Committee:
Alexis Arzimanoglou (France), Anne Berg (USA), Edouard Hirsch (France), Philippe Kahane (France), Wolfgang Loscher (Germany), Doug Nordli (USA), Emilio Perucca (Italy), Philippe Ryvlin (France)

Editors:
Philippe Kahane, Anne Berg, Wolfgang Löscher, Doug Nordli, Emilio Perucca

List of Participants

Arzimanoglou Alexis, Assoc. Professor of Neurology-Child Neurology, Institute for children and adolescents with epilepsy-IDEE, University Hospital of Lyon, France
alexis.arzimanoglou@chu-lyon.fr

Beghi Ettore, Laboratorio Malattie Neurologiche, Istituto "Mario Negri",
Via La Masa 19, 20156 Milano, Italy
beghi@marionegri.it

Berg Anne, Research Professor, Department of Biology, Northern Illinois University,
429 Montgomery Hall, DeKalb, Illinois 60115, USA
t80atb1@wpo.cso.niu.edu

Bertram Ed, Department of Neurology, University of Virginia,
P.O. Box 800394, Charlottesville, VA 22908-0394, USA
ehb2z@virginia.edu

Brodie Martin, Director, Epilepsy Unit, Western Infirmary, Glasgow, G11 6NT, Scotland
martin.j.brodie@clinmed.gla.ac.uk

Carreno Mar, Director, Epilepsy Unit, Hospital Clínic, c/Villarroel 170, 08036 Barcelona, Spain
mcarreno@clinic.ub.es

Cole Andy, MD, FRCPC, Director, MGH Epilepsy Service, Associate Professor of Neurology, Harvard Medical School, WAC 739 L, Fruit Street, Boston, Massachusetts 02114, USA
cole.andrew@mgh.harvard.edu

Depaulis Antoine, INSERM JE-MRNT "Contrôle des réseaux synchrones épileptiques", Université Joseph Fournier, UFR Biologie – Bâtiment B, 2280 rue de la Piscine,
38000 Grenoble, France
antoine.depaulis@ujf-grenoble.fr

Eltze Christin, Child Neurologist, Institute of Child Health, University College London,
London WC1N 2AP, United Kingdom
c.eltze@ich.ucl.ac.uk

Francione Stefano, Centro per la Chirurgia dell'Epilessia "Claudio Munari", Dipartimento di Scienze Neurologiche, Ospedale Niguarda Ca' Granda, Piazza Ospedale Maggiore 3, 20162 Milano, Italy
stefano.francione@ospedaleniguarda.it

French Jacqueline, NYU Comprehensive Epilepsy Center, 403 East 34th Street, 4th floor, New York, NY 10016, USA
jacqueline.french@nyumc.org

Gaillard William, Dept of Neurology, Children's National Medical Center, 111 Michigan Ave NW, Washington, 20010 DC, USA
wgaillar@cnmc.org

Gilliam Franck, The Neurological Institute, 7th Floor, Columbia University, 710 West 168th Street, New York, NY 10032, USA
fgilliam@neuro.columbia.edu

Gil-Nagel Antonio, Programa de Epilepsia, Servicio de Neurologia, Hospital Ruber International, La Maso 38, Mirasierra, 28034 Madrid, Spain
agnagel@ruberinternacional.es

Halasz Peter, Professor, Pázmány Catholic University, Faculty of Information and Technology, 1026 Lotz K.u. 18, Budapest, Hungary
halasz@opni.hu

Hammers Alexander, Senior Lecturer, MRC Clinician Scientist Fellow, Department of Clinical and Experimental Epilepsy, National Hospital for Neurology and Neurosurgery/Institute of Neurology, UCL, 33 Queen Square, London WC1N 3BG, United Kingdom
alexander.hammers@csc.mrc.ac.uk

Hesdorffer Dale, Ph.D., Assistant Professor of Epidemiology, Columbia University, GH Sergievsky Center, 630 W 168th, P & S Unit 16, New York, NY 10032, USA
dch5@columbia.edu

Hirsch Edouard, Professor of Neurology, University Hospitals of Strasbourg and CRTS-IDEE, Strasbourg, France
edouard.hirsch@chru-strasbourg.fr

Kahane Philippe, MD, Ph.D., Professor of Neurolphysiology, Epilepsy Unit, Neurology Department and INSERM U704, CRTS-IDEE, University Hospital, 38043 Grenoble, France
philippe.kahane@ujf-grenoble.fr

Kälviainen Reetta, MD, Ph.D., Neurologist, Director Kuopio Epilepsy Center, Kuopio University Hospital, POB 1777, 70211 Kuopio, Finland
reetta.kalviainen@kuh.fi

Kimiskidis Vasilios, Department of Neurology III, Aristolte University of Thessaloniki, G. Papanikolaou Hospital, Exokhi, 57010 Thessaloniki, Greece
kimiskid@med.auth.gr

Kramer Günter, Medical Director SchweizEpilepsie-Zentrum, Swiss Epilepsy Center, Bleulerstr. 60, 8008 Zürich, Switzerland
g.kraemer@swissepi.ch

Krauss Gregory, Associate Professor of Neurology, Johns Hopkins University, Meyer 2-147, 600 N.Wolfe St., Baltimore, MD 21287, USA
gkrauss@jhmi.edu

Kwan Patrick, Associate Consultant and Hon Associate Professor, Division of Neurology, Department of Medicine & Therapeutics, The Chinese University of Hong Kong, Prince of Wales Hospital, Hong Kong
patrickkwan@cuhk.edu.hk

Leppik Ilio, MINCEP Epilepsy Care, 7-101 Weaver – Densford Hall, 308 Harvard St S.E., Minneapolis, MN 55455, USA
leppi001@umn.edu

Löscher Wolfgang, Prof. Dr, Head, Department of Pharmacology, Toxicology, and Pharmacy, University of Veterinary Medicine Hannover, and Head, Center for Systems Neuroscience Hannover, Buenteweg 17, D-30559 Hannover, Germany
wolfgang.loescher@tiho-hannover.de

Mares Pavel, Professor of Pathophysiology, Department of Developmental Epileptology, Institute of Physiology, Academy of Sciences of the Czech Republic, Videnska 1083, CZ-14220 Prague 4, Czech Republic
maresp@biomed.cas.cz

Mathern Gary, Associate Professor, Neurosurgical Director, Pediatric Epilepsy Surgery Program, David Geffen School of Medicine, University of California Los Angeles, 710 Westwood Plz, Los Angeles, CA 90095-1769, USA
gmathern@ucla.edu

Nordli Douglas, Jr., MD, Children's Memorial Hospital and Feinberg School of Medicine, Northwestern University, 2300 Children's Plaza, no. 29, Chicago, IL 60614, USA
DNordli@childrensmemorial.org

Perucca Emilio, Professor of Clinical Pharmacology Unit, University of Pavia, Piazza Botta, 10, 27100 Pavia, Italy
perucca@unipv.it

Picot Marie-Christine, Unit of Clinical Research and Epidemiology, Department of Medical Information, University Hospital of Montpellier, 34295 Montpellier Cedex 5, France
mc-picot@chu-montpellier.fr

Ryvlin Philippe, Professor of Neurology, Department of Functional Neurology and Epileptology, Neurology University Hospital, and CRTS-IDEE, HCL, Lyon France
ryvlin@cermep.fr

Sallaz Monique, Neurobiologiste, Chef de projet IDÉE, Directrice de la Fondation IDÉE, 89 rue Bellecombe, 69003 Lyon, France
monique.sallaz@fondation-idee.fr

Sander Josemir, Professor, UCL Institute of Neurology, Queen Square, London WC1N 3BG, United Kingdom
lsander@ion.ucl.ac.uk

Schmidt Bernd, MD, Ph.D., Neurology and Psychiatry Outpts Clinic, Hasenbuckweg 14, Wittnau, Germany
drs.schmidt.wittnau@t-online.de

Schmidt Dieter, Emeritus Professor of Neurology, Free University of Berlin, Epilepsy Research Group, Geothe Strasse 5, 14163 Berlin, Germany
dbschmidt@t-online.de

Semah Franck, Laboratoire de Médecine Nucléaire et de Recherche BioMédicale, Service Hospitalier Frédéric Joliot, Commissariat à l'Énergie Atomique, 4, place du Général Leclerc, 91400 Orsay Cedex, France
franck.semah@cea.fr

Serratosa José, Unidad de Epilepsia, Servicio de Neurologia, Fundacion Jimenez Diaz, Universidad Autonoma de Madrid, Avda Reyes Catolicos, 2, 28040 Madrid, Spain
serratosa@telefonica.net

Shorvon Simon, National Hospital for Neurology and Neurosurgery, UCL Institute of Neurology Clinical and Experimental Epilepsy, Queen Square, London, WC1N 3BG, UK
s.shorvon@ion.ucl.ac.uk

Sills Graeme, Division of Neurological Science, University of Liverpool, Clinical Sciences Centre for Research & Education, Walton Centre for Neurology & Neurosurgery,
Lower Lane, Liverpool L9 7LJ, United Kingdom
g.sills@liv.ac.uk

Sisodiya Sanjay, Department of Clinical and Experimental Epilepsy, National Hospital for Neurology and Neurosurgery, Queen Square, London, UK
sisodiya@ion.ucl.ac.uk

Spreafico Roberto, Division of experimental neurophysiology and epileptology, Istituto Nazionale Neurologico "C. Besta", Via Celoria, 11, 20133 Milano, Italy
spreafico@istituto-besta.it

Trinka Eugen, Head of Epilepsy Service and EEG Laboratory, University Hospital Innsbruck, Anichstrasse 35, 6020 Innsbruck, Austria
eugen.trinka@uklibk.ac.at

Van Nieuwenhuizen Onno, Wilhelmina Children's Hospital,
Lundlaan 6, 3584 EA Utrecht, The Netherlands
o.vannieuwenhuizen@umcutrecht.nl

Walker Matthew, Institute of Neurology, UCL, Queen Square, London WC1N 3BG, UK
m.walker@ion.ucl.ac.uk

Wiebe Samuel, MD, MSc, FRCPC, Professor and Head, Division of Neurology, University of Calgary, Rm C-1224, Foothills Medical Centre,
1403 – 29 St NW, Calgary, Alberta, Canada T2N 2T9
swiebe@ucalgary.ca

Workshop supported by an unrestricted educational grant from UCB.

Towards a clinically meaningful definition of drug-resistance

Alexis Arzimanoglou, Philippe Ryvlin

Epilepsy, Sleep and Pediatric Neurophysiology Dept. and CTRS-IDEE (Institute for Children and Adolescents with Epilepsy), Hospices Civils de Lyon, France

Nearly 30% of patients with epilepsy are not controlled by currently available antiepileptic drugs and/or surgical procedures. Consequently, it is not surprising that terms like "drug-resistant seizures or epilepsy", "pharmaco-resistant epilepsy", "refractory epilepsy" or "intractable epilepsy" are abundantly used in the epilepsy literature. What is surprising is that very often terms used are not defined or that the definitions used differ considerably. Despite obvious etymological differences, these terms are used indifferently in a number of different settings: as a criterion for selection of patients eligible for new antiepileptic drug (AED) trials, for the selection of surgical candidates, for teaching purposes (how long a patient can be kept on the same drug, etc.), for the design of epidemiological studies, for the design of studies on quality-of-life (QOL), for the definition of the epileptic encephalopathies (in comparison to more benign epilepsy syndromes), to mention but a few. Such phrases are also used when describing the prognosis of various epilepsy syndromes, despite the fact that these epilepsy syndromes and epilepsies represent different disorders in terms of age at onset, electroclinical expression, underlying etiology or pathophysiological mechanisms. The same terms are also used in basic research studies, using criteria not necessarily relevant for human pathology (resistance to a single AED such as phenytoin or barbiturates). As a result of either the absence or the abundance of definitions, available studies in the field are usually not comparable, thus limiting the value of the conclusions drawn.

The following three phrases are examples of such definitions: "*Persistence of true epileptic seizures with a sufficient frequency or severity in a compliant patient despite optimal therapy for a minimum of two years* (Jallon 1997)"; "*When satisfactory seizure control could not be achieved with any of the potentially effective AEDs, alone or in combination, at subtoxic doses or levels* (Bourgeois 2001)"; "*The patient does not become seizure-free with even the highest dosage of antiepileptic drug tolerated without unacceptable side effects* (Wolf, 1994)". These definitions will be commented upon in turn in order to highlight the diversity of issues they introduce and comments will subsequently serve as the basis for proposing a "clinically meaningful definition", within the limits of current knowledge and aims.

- **"Persistence of true epileptic seizures with a sufficient frequency or severity in a compliant patient despite optimal therapy for a minimum of two years" (Jallon 1997)**

This definition, although apparently elusive, underscores a number of issues that one needs to address before being able to characterize a given patient with epilepsy as drug-resistant:

– the need to ascertain the diagnosis of epilepsy and to rule out the possibility of pseudo-seizures;
– the need to ensure that the patient is "compliant" with the treatment prescribed;
– the need for "optimal therapy". This term can be interpreted in more than one way, however, it can be assumed that it refers to the appropriate choice of AEDs (based on current knowledge of indicated and contra-indicated AEDs per epilepsy syndrome; the use of the maximally tolerated dosage when necessary independent of drug plasma levels, the proper evaluation for eventual adverse events, etc.).

Other terms used have, in our view, disadvantages:

– By introducing the concept of *"sufficient frequency or severity"* one accepts the notion that active epilepsy might not necessarily have an impact on quality of life. This assertion might well be true in some individual patients, but in general, and in agreement with all related studies, total seizure freedom is the key factor to restore quality of life in patients with epilepsy. Considering the major subjectivity underlying the evaluation of seizure severity (for example, are repeated and prolonged episodes of ascending epigastric sensation with aphasia more or less severe than repeated episodes of brief alteration of consciousness followed by jargonophasia?), as well as the difference between the patients and physicians perspective on this issue, there is a risk of wrongly assuming the "benign" nature of an epileptic disorder using the above terms.

– By introducing a timeframe of "a minimum of two years" of "optimal therapy", this definition is clearly not appropriate in rapidly deteriorating conditions such as infantile spasms.

In summary, this definition, although sufficiently general to cover a number of major issues related to AED resistance could be misinterpreted by a non-specialist who will defer referral to the epilepsy specialist until he/she considers the disorder to be severe enough. This undue delay might have serious consequences on the optimal early care and related long-term prognosis of various epilepsy syndromes, such Lennox-Gastaut syndrome (LGS), or surgically remediable epilepsies.

- **"When satisfactory seizure control could not be achieved with any of the potentially effective AEDs, alone or in combination, at subtoxic doses or levels" (Bourgeois 2001)**

This statement is even more general, most probably in an effort to avoid the pitfalls of a precise definition when dealing with a vast spectrum of disorders, such as epilepsies. The term *"satisfactory"* is not defined, increasing the risk of a variety of interpretations, similar to those described above. The suggestion that *"any of the potentially effective AEDs, alone or in combination"* is necessary before characterizing a given epilepsy as drug-resistant might be considered as pertinent by those working on mechanisms that explain resistance to

AEDs, however, it is certainly not applicable as an eligibility criterion for entering a new drug trial or for selecting candidates for pre-surgical evaluation. By introducing the notion of *"combination"* of AEDs used, this definition correctly underscores the importance of considering the combination as well as the choice of AEDs prescribed, when evaluating a patient with persistent seizures (for example the combined effect of sodium valproate or lamotrigine may not have the same effect when used alone or in the presence of an enzyme inducer). However, with nearly 20 AEDs available, an entire lifetime would not be sufficient to try all possible combinations and dosages. Misinterpreting such an approach could again lead to unacceptable delays in referral to surgery or to an epilepsy specialist.

■ "The patient does not become seizure free with even the highest dosage of antiepileptic drug tolerated without unacceptable side effects" (Wolf, 1994)

This definition has the merit of clearly introducing the notion of *seizure freedom*, the most important parameter from the patient's perspective. It also integrates current knowledge on how to use AEDs, i.e. not being afraid to increase the dose administered provided that tolerability is also taken into account. However, it introduces the notion of *unacceptable side effects*, suggesting that some adverse events might be acceptable. As for the notion of *seizure severity* discussed above, there is no doubt that some individual patients suffer benign and well tolerated side effects that do not interfere with their daily living. But this notion also carries the risk of ignoring the devastating long term impact of insidious cognitive adverse events, such as those encountered with barbiturates. What is also lacking from such a definition, are issues relating to the number of AEDs to be tried before considering a patient as drug-resistant and the expected minimum duration of seizure freedom.

In our view, all three examples of definitions, briefly discussed above, represent important steps for a better understanding of "drug-resistant epilepsy" and largely contributed to shaping today's "best clinical practices". Their limitations primarily reflect the complexity of the issue concerned; to provide a single and simple definition, that is applicable to a great variety of clinical situations and research studies. This is particularly relevant if the impact of epilepsy on the patient's quality of life and social functioning is also to be taken into account. In accordance with the important progresses made in the field during the last decade, it appears timely for the epilepsy community to forge a clearer, up-to-date, and easy-to-use definition of drug-resistance that will serve as a common basis for future practice and research.

What should be and what cannot be part of the definition

To be operational, a definition of "drug-resistant epilepsy"[1] needs to be generic. The reason for this is based on the fact that the term "epilepsy" refers to a number of symptoms (various types of seizures, occurring alone or in all possible combinations) and to a variety of disorders (age-dependent syndromes; as a major or minor symptom of a great variety of neurological diseases; etc.). Consequently, it must be agreed that the core definition should not intend to cover all possible issues related to drug-resistance, and in particular prognosis. Prognosis can only be discussed for each epilepsy syndrome taken separately.

---

1. The issue of "resistance to surgery" is slightly, although not completely, different and merits a separate discussion that is beyond the scope of this introductory chapter.

The issues of *seizure frequency* and *duration of active epilepsy* should not be part of the definition. Similarly, no reference should be made to an *acceptable number of persisting seizures*. These issues constitute part of the definitions for each specific epilepsy syndrome. The number of persisting seizures may be extremely variable as it is also closely related to the epilepsy syndrome. The only measurable and comparable parameter that should be emphasized in a patient-centered definition is *full control of seizures*, i.e. seizure freedom.

The *"number of AEDs to be tried"* before concluding on pharmaco-resistance appears instrumental, primarily to avoid an undue delay in establishing the diagnosis and referring the patient to an epilepsy specialist. All available studies, in both children and adults treated with old and new generation AEDs, have shown that the percentage of patients that can achieve seizure freedom after the failure of two or three AEDs diminishes dramatically, regardless of the type of epilepsy. Based on these data, it appears reasonable to consider that the failure of 2-3 appropriately chosen AEDs, used at optimal dosage[2], is a sufficient proof of drug-resistance. This applies to all forms of epilepsies regardless of seizure frequency. What will vary according to the epilepsy syndrome is the time needed to reach such a conclusion: for a partial epilepsy, this may take up to a few years, whereas this should only take a few weeks in infantile spasms or in Lennox-Gastaut syndrome.

A meaningful definition of "drug-resistance" should also include *a time reference* for the minimum period of clinically relevant seizure freedom. At this point, it should be clarified that this does not imply a cure for epilepsy (this is again referred to in the definition of each epilepsy syndrome), or of the underlying neurological disorder. The decision on what could be a "clinically meaningful" period without seizures will unavoidably be arbitrary. Two years is certainly better than one year, which in turn is better than 6 months. By convention, we could accept a minimum period of 12 months seizure freedom. Twelve months of seizure freedom in a case of severe epilepsy, like a Lennox-Gastaut syndrome or a MTLE, allows a certain degree of confidence that the appropriate drug was used. For epilepsy syndromes characterized by a low frequency of seizures, i.e. a Rolandic epilepsy, 12 months may be short, although clinical experience suggests that drug-resistant patients with this syndrome usually have more than one or two seizures per year.

In conclusion, we suggest that in order to be operational, a core (generic) definition of "drug-resistant epilepsy" should:

– Include as a main parameter the only common element between all forms of epilepsy: *seizures*.

– Incorporate what is clinically meaningful to the patient: *seizure freedom*.

– Integrate current knowledge of the response of the majority of patients to AEDs: *2-3 AEDs*.

– "Arbitrarily" fix the minimum requested period of seizure freedom to consider the result obtained as meaningful: *12 months*.

All other issues (syndrome, etiology, predictors etc.) should not be part of the core definition, but variables to be added on the basis of the context and current knowledge.

---

2. We are fully aware that the terms *"appropriate"* and *"optimal"* may be source of misinterpretations. However, they cannot be further defined within the definition of "drug-resistance epilepsies" as they are supposed to reflect current knowledge on the most appropriate AEDs to be used per epilepsy syndrome. They also presuppose a good knowledge of titration guidelines and maximal doses of each AED. If this is not the case, the physician will not be apt to judge if his patient is resistant to AEDs and he has the moral obligation to refer his patient to a specialist.

Who will use this definition and how

It should be expected that a core definition will serve all possible users: general practitioners, neurologists and child neurologists, neurologists specialized in epilepsy, pharmacologists, geneticists, basic research scientists, industry, health authorities, lay associations...

Current knowledge on epilepsy syndromes, the availability of more than 20 AEDs, the progresses of surgical treatments, the need for further research on the underlying mechanisms of epileptogenesis and on the response or resistance to drugs complicates the everyday diagnosis and care of epilepsy that benefits the patient. However, the vast majority of new-onset epilepsies is first seen by a general practitioner or, at best, in an emergency or general neurology department. Late referral to an epilepsy specialist may have dramatic consequences.

A clear-cut definition of drug-resistance based on current knowledge, as suggested above, will facilitate early identification of drug-resistant patients by a non-specialist and, hopefully, early referral. It will also support the efforts of lay associations and of the epilepsy scientific societies *vis-à-vis* the health authorities in order to obtain the appropriate means, both in terms of epilepsy experts and technical means, to allow prompt investigation.

This new approach, if validated by the epileptological community, will also influence inclusion criteria for drug trials, for the benefit of the patient. Indeed, today's practice is to include patients that have already failed a large numbers of, if not all, AEDs, thus representing a minority of drug-resistant patients and where the chance to achieve seizure freedom is very limited. In many instances, it might be more relevant to test new AEDs in the early course of pharmaco-resistance. This would be particularly interesting in patients with severe epilepsy syndromes (ex. Lennox-Gastaut) where an effective new treatment might not only help to control existing seizures but also to prevent the development of an epileptic encephalopathy. The definition of drug-resistance suggested above would allow inclusion of patients with less severe forms of refractory epilepsy and would better inform us on the potential usefulness of new AEDs in clinical practice.

The use of a common definition will also facilitate comparison of results from epidemiological studies regarding the time course of illness, as well as predictors of remission or relapse etc.

Earlier recognition of drug-resistance should also promote earlier referral for pre-surgical evaluation and result in better surgical outcome[3].

What remains to be discussed is the potential utility of the core (generic) definition suggested above for basic research, pharmacogenomic and molecular biology studies. We believe that such a definition is useful in offering a first selection step, understanding that additional criteria might be needed according to the issue under consideration (i.e. resistance to one specific AED versus refractoriness to all available drugs).

The first three chapters of this book discuss what we know today about the natural history of drug-resistant epilepsy (Anne Berg), the basis of how valuable clinical data challenge the issue of drug-resistant versus drug-sensitive patients (Martin Brodie) and the specific

---

3. Resistance to AEDs is not the only criterion for the selection of surgical candidates. Other criteria, such as the absence or presence of a lesion, the topography of the epileptogenic zone, the age of the patient, the impact of an active epilepsy on cognitive development are of primary importance.

issue of response to drugs in cases of status epilepticus (Aidan Neligan and Simon Shorvon). The basic science section critically reviews current knowledge of the mechanisms of drug-resistance (Wolfgang Löscher), of the genetic identification of refractory patients (Sanjay Sisodiya) and offers some suggestions on what should be the most relevant animal models to further investigate these issues (Ed Bertram). Present and future molecular targets (Graeme Sills) as well as a critical evaluation of AEDs in development with real potential (Emilio Perucca) introduce the next section on treatment issues. The fourth section discusses two challenging aspects relating to surgical treatment: does surgery really suppress drug-resistance and how (Dieter Schmidt)? Are innovative surgical treatments, such as deep brain stimulation, really useful (Phillippe Kahane *et al.*)? The last section of this book underscores the importance of an approach *beyond seizure reduction* (Franck Gilliam and Piero Perucca) and discusses early identification of drug-resistant patients (Doug Nordli) and differences between those epilepsies considered today by definition as epileptic encephalopathies and focal non-idiopathic epilepsies (Helen Cross and Christine Eltze).

At present, the definition proposed above can only be considered as a basis for further discussion. A consensus of the epilepsy community is desperately needed and will then be challenged by everyday clinical practice and research to either survive the proof of time or to be modified on the basis of newly acquired knowledge.

The risk, correlates and temporal patterns of intractable epilepsy

Anne T. Berg

Dept. Biology, Northern Illinois University, DeKalb, IL 60115, USA

Early characterizations of epilepsy described the disorder as an inexorably intractable, progressive disease (Gowers WR, 1881). In 1979, the first population-based epidemiological study of the seizure outcomes of epilepsy changed our understanding of the course of disorder by showing that most people became seizure-free and nearly half became seizure-free and no longer needed drugs (Annegers JF et al., 1979). A tacit assumption set in, that not being in remission was the complement to being intractable; that by studying remission, one was in essence studying intractability. In fact, for reasons discussed below, seizure outcomes are far more dynamic and complex, and intractability is an outcome that must be defined and studied in its own right.

Relatively few studies have examined the risk of developing intractable epilepsy or predictors of the condition. The frequency in the population of intractable epilepsy and the factors most associated with it are important in that they provide the context and some starting clues for more detailed intensive studies of mechanisms and treatments.

■ Frequency and risk of intractability

A recent study estimated the prevalence of intractable epilepsy in a defined population in France (Picot MC et al., 2008). The overall prevalence of epilepsy was 5.4/1000. Intractable epilepsy was present in approximately 16% of all prevalent cases meaning nearly 1 person per 1,000 in the general population has intractable epilepsy. This is the single best estimate available of the prevalence of intractable epilepsy for a developed country.

Several cohort studies of individuals with newly diagnosed epilepsy have also examined the risk and correlates of developing intractable seizures *(Table I)*. The proportion of patients who become intractable varies considerably from 6% (Arts WFM et al., 2004) to 69% (Spooner CG et al., 2006). There are several reasons for this linked to the type of population studied (general, pediatric only, selected type of epilepsy) and methods of ascertainment (prospective surveillance *versus* retrospective chart review). There is also tremendous variability in how intractability has been defined for research purposes. While

Table I. Selected definitions of intractability used in the published literature

Author (ref)	Study methods*	Drug failures	Other criteria
Huttenlocher (Huttenlocher & Hapke, 1990)	Retrospective cohort, chart review	2	1 seizure/month for ≥ 2 years
Berg (Berg AT et al., 1996); Casetta (Casetta I et al., 1999)	Retrospective case-control, chart review (Berg); Nested case-control study in prospective cohort (Casetta)	3	1 seizure/month for ≥ 2 years
Arts (Arts WFM et al., 2004)	Prospective, chart review	2	< 3 months seizure-free during 5th year of follow-up
Dlugos (Dlugos et al., 2001)	Retrospective, chart review	2	Any seizure during months 19-24 after initial diagnosis and treatment
Camfield (Camfield P & Camfield C, 2003)	Prospective, chart review	3	1 seizure every 2 months in last year of follow-up
Berg (Berg AT et al., 2006)	Prospective, direct patient contact & chart review	2	Average ≥ 1 sz/month for 18 months, no more than 3 months seizure-free
Berg (Berg AT et al., 2006), Spooner (Spooner CG et al., 2006)	Spooner: Prospective, chart review.	2	No specific seizure frequency requirements
Kwan (Kwan P & Brodie MJ, 2000)	Retrospective, chart review	No specific number required	Any seizures in the previous year

* Summaries of methods are based on the descriptions in the individual reports. If prospective was not specified, the study was assumed to be retrospective. If no mention of direct patient contact for the purposes of the study is mentioned, the study was assumed to be based on chart review.

there is moderate to good agreement among these definitions for classifying patients as intractable or not intractable [kappas ranged from 0.45 to 0.79 (Berg AT & Kelly MM, 2006)], there is still a sizeable number of cases for whom these definitions disagree.

In a Dutch study, intractability was defined at five years (Arts WFM et al., 2004). A subject could have been seizure-free for no more than 3 months during the fifth year of observation and had to have failed reasonable trials of two appropriate AEDs. Only 6% of the cohort was intractable by those criteria. In the US study, 14% met a stringent study definition of intractability *(Table I)* and 23% failed at least two drugs (Berg AT et al., 2006). In a study of a mixed age population with a median age at onset of 25 years, 37% of patients had failed an unspecified number of drugs and were not seizure-free for at least a year at last contact. Finally, in two pediatric series limited to temporal lobe epilepsy, 37% (Dlugos et al., 2001) and 69% (Spooner CG et al., 2006) of the patients were considered intractable. In both studies, patients had to have failed trials of at least two AEDs. Other details are provided in the table.

Correlates and predictors of intractability

Most studies that examine seizure outcomes focus on remission which is much easier to define than intractability. In studies of remission, the single most important predictors identified in these studies is the presence or absence of a "symptomatic" cause (Annegers JF et al., 1979; Lindsten H et al., 2001), although, not all studies report this finding (Cockerell O et al., 1997; Collaborative Group for the Study of Epilepsy, 1992) A "symptomatic" cause of epilepsy is a separate condition, acquired or congenital, that affects (damages) the brain ultimately resulting in a substantially increased risk of epilepsy (Commission on Epidemiology and Prognosis and International League Against Epilepsy, 1993). These epidemiological studies are quite powerful and provide information about broad patterns in a population. From the perspective of epileptology, they are quite crude. Furthermore, they do not explicitly address the question of intractability.

Of the studies to examine predictors and correlates of intractability, perhaps the single most powerful predictor of intractability is the type of epilepsy. Different investigators take somewhat different approaches to this issue, but the basic findings are consistent. The Canadian investigators reported that overall, 12.4% of the cohort was intractable (Camfield P & Camfield C, 2003) and included 7.9% of those with focal and generalized tonic-clonic seizures, 8% for absence seizures, and 54% for "secondary generalized" epilepsies. The Dutch study found a surprisingly low prevalence of intractability at 5 years with relatively little variation by type of epilepsy, 4% in idiopathic syndromes and 10% in the cryptogenic and symptomatic generalized syndromes (Arts WFM et al., 2004). The Scottish study reported a lower occurrence of intractability for patients with idiopathic (26%) *versus* all other forms of epilepsy (40%) (Kwan P & Brodie MJ, 2000).

In the US study, three broad groups were defined: 1) One containing the epileptic encephalopathies, and other secondary generalized syndromes. 2) The age-dependent idiopathic localization-related and generalized epilepsies. 3) The other focal and undetermined epilepsies (Berg AT et al., 2006). In the first group 50% or more, depending on the definition, met criteria for intractability. Within this group, Lennox-Gastaut is almost always intractable. West syndrome has considerably greater variability with as much as 40-50% eventually becoming seizure-free. The idiopathic syndromes rarely became intractable and are generally known for being highly responsive to AED treatment. Even when these epilepsies do not respond to AEDs initially, the epilepsy itself often completely resolves eventually and no longer requires treatment. It is not a matter of the drugs starting to work; there is simply no longer a need for them.

The third group is perhaps the most important to consider as the majority of epilepsies in adults and roughly half of all epilepsies in children are either undetermined (unclassified) epilepsies or other focal epilepsies (Berg AT et al., 2006; Callenbach et al., 1998; Jallon P et al., 2001). They are described based on their localization and are further designated as "symptomatic" if associated with a known lesion or other condition and "cryptogenic" when the cause is unknown. Both the cryptogenic and the symptomatic focal epilepsies contain a heterogeneous mix of disorders. The cryptogenic epilepsies compromise forms that are sometimes demonstrated to have a causative lesion later in their course. Others will likely be found to represent as yet unrecognized genetic forms of epilepsy. This was the case for autosomal dominant nocturnal frontal lobe epilepsy or ADNFLE (Scheffer IE et al., 1995), autosomal dominant partial epilepsy with auditory features or ADPEAF (Ottman R et al., 1999), and genetic (formerly generalized) epilepsy with febrile seizures plus, GEFS+ (Scheffer IE & Berkovic SF, 1997). Concerted effort is needed to identify specific, homogeneous forms (genetic or otherwise) of epilepsy within this broad category. The symptomatic epilepsies occur secondary to a broad range of disorders such as hypoxic-ischemic encephalopathy, stroke, neurocutaneous syndromes, malformations of cortical development, tumors, and intracranial infections. Damage occurs at different stages of brain development and ranges from very discrete and focal to quite diffuse.

The presence or absence of a symptomatic cause is an important prognostic factor for remission. Most studies (both case-control and cohort) of intractability find it to be an important prognostic factor as well (Berg AT et al., 1996; Casetta I et al., 1999; Ohtsuka Y et al., 2001; Dlugos et al., 2001; Spooner CG et al., 2006).

Pre-treatment seizure frequency (Berg AT et al., 2001; Casetta I et al., 1999; Ohtsuka Y et al., 2001) is also predictive of subsequent intractability. This association was particularly striking within the focal epilepsies and persisted even in patients who were diagnosed after only two seizures (Berg AT et al., 2001). The interval between those two seizures was shorter in those who went on to become intractable than in those who did not. To a certain extent, intractability is easier to identify in cases with high seizure frequency, but this does not seem to be the only explanation for this findings.

Factors such as age at onset, status epilepticus, and a history of febrile seizure have been looked at with varying results (Berg AT et al., 1996; Berg AT et al., 2001; Casetta I et al., 1999; Ohtsuka Y et al., 2001). They deserve further consideration, especially given the variation in definitions of intractability and the possibility that these potential prognostic factors identify different subtypes of epilepsy.

■ Recognizing intractable epilepsy

Most of what we know about intractable epilepsy in the clinical setting has been gleaned from studies of people who are already clearly in trouble. These include surgical outcome studies or randomized clinical trials of new drugs. Studies in such patients provide insights into the risk factors of severe intractability and, depending on the study, may provide some hints about the course of intractable epilepsy. The typical patient who has resective epilepsy surgery, however, has had refractory epilepsy for many years and has failed multiple AEDs. The question in these circumstances is not whether the seizures are intractable as they clearly are. Studies in these patients tell us little about how to detect intractability reliably and as early as possible in its course. To do this, we need one or possibly more reasonable and robust definitions of intractability.

The different large-scale studies presented earlier developed reasonable, realistic criteria for identifying intractability to be applied in large research studies. With the exception of two studies (Berg AT et al., 2006; Spooner CG et al., 2006) these definitions were applied in such a way that they only captured that proportion in a population having difficulty at a given point in time without reference to their seizure control prior to or after that time. Their broader use from the perspective of studying the presentation and course of intractable epilepsy is limited as they are based on a common assumption that intractability is apparent from beginning to end of the disorder and follows a relentless course. This proposition can be broken into two parts, the onset of intractability and its stability over time.

Onset of intractability

There is a tacit assumption that intractable epilepsy is intractable from the very start. Certainly a good deal is. Some of the most dramatic forms of intractable epilepsy, the epileptic encephalopathies, present immediately with multiple daily seizures. They leave little doubt about their nature right from the outset. Not all forms of epilepsy are so accommodating, however. There has long been the impression in the surgical literature that mesial temporal lobe epilepsy was often of childhood-onset and that it followed a rather quiescent course during childhood and adolescence (Engel, 1987). This impression is supported by the findings in a series of 67 patients with temporal lobe epilepsy evaluated for surgery (French JA et al., 1993). Twenty-two percent had a previous period of at least 1 year seizure-free (average length of remission, 5.9 years), at some time after the onset of epilepsy. In a large multicenter study of resective epilepsy surgery, this was formally examined (Berg AT et al., 2003). The median age at surgery was in the fourth decade of life. The median age at onset of epilepsy, however, was in the mid-teens, leaving a 20 year gap between onset of epilepsy and surgery. During that 20 year gap, a quarter of patients reported being seizure free for a year or more. This was particularly pronounced in those with onset in young childhood (< 5 years), where almost half reported having significant period of remission (> 1 year). In addition, the median time to failure of a second drug (the marker of intractability used in that particular study) was nine years overall. It was greatest (~ 15 years) in those with onset in early childhood.

Two prospective studies have since examined and confirmed these impressions and retrospective observations. In the first, a quarter to a third (depending on definition) of cases with focal epilepsy who were considered intractable over the course of 10 years met criteria for intractability more than three years after initial diagnosis of epilepsy (considered late intractability) (Berg AT et al., 2006). Intractability became evident as late as ten years after initial onset of epilepsy. The Australian study, which focused on temporal lobe epilepsy reported similar patterns with onset of intractability often not occurring until years after initial diagnosis (Spooner CG et al., 2006).

Stability over time

The second part of the assumption is that seizure outcomes are stable over time. That outcomes measured at one point in time reflect those that occur at any other point in time. One study described a control group that was assembled as a comparison for surgical patients (Ojemann LM & Dodrill CB, 1992). None of the controls become seizure-free with several additional years of observation. In the Western Ontario randomized trial of temporal lobectomy, of 40 patients randomized to delayed surgery, only one was completely seizure-free for an entire year after randomization (Wiebe S et al., 2001). In both cases, the study subjects were culled from among the most relentlessly intractable; they had epilepsy for many years standing and had all failed multiple different drugs.

Followed from its initial onset, intractability is not necessarily as relentless a process. In an older retrospective study, a series of children who were considered to have intractable epilepsy (> 1 seizure a month for two years and failed at least two appropriate AEDs) were followed for as long as 20 years (Huttenlocher and Hapke, 1990). Over time, many became seizure-free (defined as less than 1 seizure per year). Of those with normal IQ, most became seizure-free *versus* only about 30% of those with mental retardation. The recent wave of new AEDs had not yet begun, so greater efficacy of newer drugs was not an explanation for the findings, and children who had surgery were not included. Another chart-review study examined the course of 99 children with refractory epilepsy (Takenaka J *et al.*, 2000). Ten percent experienced temporary remissions ranging in duration from 1 to 14 years. All relapsed and their intractability resumed.

In the prospective Dutch study of epilepsy, the investigators noted that outcomes after two years typically tended to improve by five years and that "intractability" was often a temporary phenomenon (Arts WFM *et al.*, 2004). The US study considered variability over 10 year period (Berg AT *et al.*, 2006). Twenty-one percent of cases who met the stringent criteria for intractability (average of 1 seizure per month, failure of 2 AEDs, etc.) went on to have a period of at least one year seizure-free although a third then relapsed again. Of those who failed two drugs, 48% experienced a subsequent remission although a third relapsed again. The Australian collaborators also reported temporary remission followed by relapse in a quarter of their series. *A better understanding of the typical course of epilepsy in general and intractability in particular is required to develop meaningful definitions and determine the time period needed to make that determination prospectively as a patient is followed from visit to visit.*

■ Considerations for Mechanistic investigations

Different general and specific mechanisms have been considered including drug efflux transporter mechanisms (Loescher W, 2007; Siddiqui A *et al.*, 2003) and target desensitization (Loescher W & Schmidt D, 2006; Remy S *et al.*, 2003). While it is fairly clear that, at the molecular level, intractability does not arise from a single mechanism (Remy S & Beck H, 2006), this realization does not filter down much into clinical research.

Given the diversity in epilepsy, it seems natural that investigations of mechanisms should first be restricted to specific forms of clinical epilepsy. In pediatric epilepsy where there is a tremendous diversity in the types of epilepsy, this tends to be the rule rather than the exception. Randomized trials and often treatment guidelines are directed to specific forms of epilepsy and sometimes to specific etiologies (Glauser T *et al.*, 2006). Three examples of possible inroads made in the treatment of intractable epilepsies deserve mention. Expert opinion in Europe and the US is squarely in favor of vigabatrin for the first line treatment of West syndrome secondary to tuberous sclerosis (Wheless JW *et al.*, 2007; Wheless JW *et al.*, 2005). This is based on a series of small trials which, when data were combined, yielded a 91% success rate for the drug in this very specific setting (McKay MT *et al.*, 2004). The response rate is about twice as good as that for West syndrome overall treated with either vigabatrin or with cortico-steroids (Lux AL *et al.*, 2004). Epilepsy secondary to GLUT1 deficiency is another case in which a highly specific cause of epilepsy has implications for the use of a specific treatment, the ketogenic diet (Klepper J, 2007). Finally, the cautious but building enthusiasm over the potential benefit of stiripentol for the treatment of Dravet syndrome may be another example of a very specific syndrome, most of which is linked to errors in a gene coding for a part of the neuronal sodium channel [SCN1A, (Harkin *et al.*, 2007)] (Chiron C, 2007; Chiron C *et al.*, 2000). These three syndromes traditionally have constituted highly intractable epileptic encephalopathies with half to virtually 100% of cases being relentlessly refractory. There is good reason to hope that progress is being made toward efficacious treatments that might change their dire reputation. These (potential) successes have been made possible by being very specific about the phenotype of the epilepsy investigated.

For the focal epilepsies, we currently do not have great specificity in epilepsy phenotype. Randomized trials are typically of all-comers and assume that all patients in the trials are essentially the same, that drug responsiveness is a stochastic phenomenon (Brodie MJ et al., 2007; Marson AG et al., 2007; Privitera MD et al., 2003). There is currently no major consensus over which of perhaps half a dozen different drugs is preferable for seizure-control in focal epilepsy. The randomized trial data may provide evidence for a small relative benefit of one drug over another, sometimes because of different side-effect profiles more than seizure control. Ultimately, treatment decisions for focal epilepsy tend to rest on ease of dosing, cost, and side-effect profiles and not on clear evidence of one drug's superiority over others for controlling seizures.

■ Phenotypic features for focal epilepsies

The current approach of describing focal epilepsies as a function of presence or absence of a known lesion (symptomatic/cryptogenic) and lobe of the brain from which seizures arise (occipital, temporal parietal, frontal) is inadequate. There is considerable heterogeneity within the focal epilepsies some of which could determine drug responsiveness in general or to specific drugs. Factors to consider include specific causes, seizure types, seizure frequency, clustering of seizures, susceptibility to breakthrough seizures with various stressors, diurnal pattern of occurrence, seizure duration *(status epilepticus)*, and the specific drugs to which the epilepsy does not respond. EEG patterns are the best reflection of the underlying neurophysiological processes that can be obtained noninvasively and could conceivably provide markers that may be of use. Age at onset is a critical feature in the developmental syndromes. We do not know enough about the focal epilepsies to identify age-related phenomena within this group, but given its importance in the electro-clinical syndromes of infancy, childhood and adolescence, it is hard to understand why we ignore this feature in focal epilepsies.

■ Phenotypic features of intractability itself?

The patterns of intractability have already been alluded to. There are epilepsies, not always epileptic encephalopathies, which start with a thunder clap and never stop. Others may take a more indolent course. Is it possible (likely?) that mechanisms underlying intractability with immediate onset differ from those in which the intractability does not appear for several years after onset of epilepsy?

■ Implications for developing definitions of intractability

Clinically, one would want to be very sure about the future course of a patient's epilepsy before making a strong recommendation for surgery. At the same time, waiting until intractable epilepsy has wrought irrevocable harm, which can include developmental, cognitive and social dysfunction as well as mortality, is being overly cautious to the detriment of the patient. Factors such as severity of epilepsy, consequences to the individual and the patient's needs and preferences come into play and guide treatment decisions as much as the binary determination of whether seizures are intractable.

In mechanistic work, the ability to detect associations is enhanced when the groups being compared are clearly distinct and within group homogeneity is high. Consequently, cases (intractable epilepsy) must be truly intractable. While this is relatively straightforward in individuals with multiple daily seizures, it is not in patients with an occasional cluster of breakthrough seizures or occasional prolonged periods seizure-free.

Summary

Intractable epilepsy affects a significant proportion of people with epilepsy. Estimates of the risk of intractability depend on the study population, study design, the definition of intractability and how it is applied. Complex temporal patterns, especially in the focal epilepsies, require further consideration in order to develop meaningful, reliable definitions that can be used for early detection of intractability. While one can critique the different definitions used in the research to date, this is a difficult area for researchers. There is no single agreed upon definition of intractability in epilepsy. All of these efforts are reasonable attempts to develop a research definition. Most of the work so far must be viewed as paving the way toward consensus definitions for this field.

Epidemiology is a powerful tool for providing an overview of the forest of intractability. To make advances, however, we need to study the trees, specific forms of epilepsy and specific mechanisms of intractability. Different forms of epilepsy carry different risks for intractability. Consideration of the phenotypes, especially within the focal epilepsies, may be a next important step toward progress in identifying intractability clinically and uncovering the mechanisms of drug failure.

References

Annegers JF, Hauser WA, Elveback LR. Remission of seizures and relapse in patients with epilepsy. *Epilepsia* 1979; 20: 729-37.

Arts WFM, Brouwer OF, Peters ACB, *et al*. Course and prognosis of childhood epilepsy: 5-year follow-up of the Dutch study of epilepsy in childhood. *Brain* 2004; 127: 1774-84.

Berg AT, Kelly MM. Defining intractability: Comparisons among published definitions. *Epilepsia* 2006; 47: 431-6.

Berg AT, Langfitt J, Shinnar S, *et al*. How long does it take for partial epilepsy to become intractable? *Neurology* 2003; 60: 186-90.

Berg AT, Levy SR, Novotny EJ, Shinnar S. Predictors of intractable epilepsy in childhood: a case-control study. *Epilepsia* 1996; 37: 24-30.

Berg AT, Shinnar S, Levy SR, Testa F, Smith-Rapaport S, Beckerman B. Early development of intractable epilepsy in children: a prospective study. *Neurology* 2001; 56: 1445-52.

Berg AT, Vickrey BG, Testa FM, Levy SR, Shinnar S, DiMario F, *et al*. How long does it take epilepsy to become intractable? A prospective investigation. *Ann Neurol* 2006; 60: 73-9.

Brodie MJ, Perucca E, Ryvlin P, Ben-Menachem E, H-J M. Comparison of levetiracetam and controlled-release carbamazepine in newly diagnosed epilepsy. *Neurology* 2007; 68: 402-8.

Callenbach PM, Geerts AT, Arts WF, *et al*. Familial occurrence of epilepsy in children with newly diagnosed multiple seizures: Dutch Study of Epilepsy in Childhood. *Epilepsia* 1998; 39: 331-6.

Camfield P, Camfield C. Nova Scotia pediatric epilepsy study. In: Jallon P, Berg A, Dulac O & Hauser A (eds). *Prognosis of epilepsies*. Montrouge (France): John Libbey Eurotext, 2003: 113-26.

Casetta I, Granieri E, Monetti VC, *et al*. Early predictors of intractability in childhood epilepsy: a community-based case-control study in Copparo Italy. *Acta Neurol Scand* 1999; 99: 329-33.

Chiron C. Stiripentol. **Title to be completed**. *Neurotherapeutics* 2007; 4: 123-25.

Chiron C, Marchand MC, Tran A, d'Athis P, Vincent J, Dulac O. Stiripentol in severe myoclonic epilepsy in infancy: a randomised placebo-controlled syndrome-dedicated trial. STICLO study group. *Lancet* 2000; 356: 1638-42.

Cockerell O, Johnson A, Sander J, Shorvon S. Prognosis of epilepsy: A review and further analysis of the first nine years of the British National General Practice Study of Epilepsy, a prospective population-based study. *Epilepsia* 1997; 38: 31-46.

Collaborative Group for the Study of Epilepsy. Prognosis of epilepsy in newly referred patients: A multicenter prospective study of the effects of monotherapy on the long-term course of epilepsy. *Epilepsia* 1992; 33: 45-51.

Commission on Epidemiology and Prognosis, International League Against Epilepsy. Guidelines for epidemiologic studies on epilepsy. *Epilepsia* 1993; 34: 592-6.

Dlugos D, Sammel M, Strom B, Farrar J. Response to first drug trial predicts outcome in childhood temporal lobe epilepsy. *Neurology* 2001; 57: 2259-64.

Engel J. Update on surgical treatment of the epilepsies. In: Engel J (ed). *Surgical Treatment of Epilepsies*. New York: Raven Press, 1987: 32-48.

French JA, Williamson PD, Thadani VM, *et al*. Characteristics of medial temporal lobe epilepsy: I. results of history and physical examination. *Ann Neurol* 1993; 34: 774-80.

Glauser T, Ben-Menachem E, Bourgeois B, *et al*. ILAE treatment guidelines: evidence-based analysis of antiepileptic drug efficacy and effectiveness as initial monotherapy for epileptic seizures and syndromes. *Epilepsia* 2006; 47: 1094-120.

Gowers WR. *Epilepsy and other chronic convulsive disorders: Their causes symptoms and treatment.* London: J&A Churchill, 1881.

Harkin LA, McMahon JM, Iona X, *et al*. The spectrum of SCN1A-related infantile epileptic encephalopathies. *Brain* 2007; 130: 843-52.

Huttenlocher PR, Hapke RJ. A follow-up study of intractable seizures in childhood. *Ann Neurol* 1990; 28: 699-705.

Jallon P, Loiseau P, Loiseau J. Newly diagnosed unprovoked epileptic seizures: presentation at diagnosis in CAROLE study. *Epilepsia* 2001; 42: 464-75.

Klepper J. GLUT1 deficiency syndrome – 2007 update. *Dev Med Child Neurol* 2007; 49: 707-16.

Kwan P, Brodie MJ. Early identification of refractory epilepsy. *N Engl J Med* 2000; 3: 314-9.

Lindsten H, Stenlund H, Forsgren L. Remission of seizures in a population-based adult cohort with a newly diagnosed unprovoked epileptic seizure. *Epilepsia* 2001; 42: 1025-30.

Loescher W. Drug transporters in the epileptic brain. *Epilepsia* 2007; 48 (suppl 1): 8-13.

Loescher W, Schmidt D. Experimental and clinical evidence for loss of effect (tolerance) during prolonged traetment with antiepileptic drugs. *Epilepsia* 2006; 47: 1253-84.

Lux AL, Edwards SW, Hancock E, *et al*. The United Kingdom Infantile Spasms Study comparing vigabatrin with prednisolone or tetracosactide at 14 days: a multicentre, randomised controlled trial. *Lancet* 2004; 364: 1773-8.

Marson AG, Al-Kharusi AM, Alwaidh M, *et al*. The SANAD study of effectiveness of carbamazepine, gabapentin, lamotrigine, oxcarbazepine, or topiramate for treatment of partial epilepsy: an unblinded randomised controlled trial. *Lancet* 2007; 369: 1000-15.

McKay MT, Weiss SK, Adams-Webber T, *et al*. Practice parameter: medical treatment of infantile spasms. *Neurology* 2004; 62: 1668-81.

Ohtsuka Y, Yoshinaga H, Kobayashi K, Murakami N, Yamatogi Y, Oka E, *et al*. Predictors of and underlying causes of medically intractable localization-related epilepsy in childhood. *Pediatr Neurol* 2001; 24: 209-13.

Ojemann LM, Dodrill CB. Natural history of drug resistant epilepsy. *Epilepsy Res* 1992; 5 (suppl): 13-7.

Ottman R, Barker-Cummings C, Lee JH, Ranta S. Genetics of autosomal dominant partial epilepsy with auditory features. In: Berkovic SF, Genton P, Hirsch E and Picard F (eds). *Genetics of focal epilepsies*. London: John Libbey&Co Ltd, 1999: 95-102.

Picot MC, Baldy-Moulinier M, Daurest J-P, Dujols P, Crespel A. The prevalence of epilepsy and pharmacoresistant epilepsy in adults: a population-based study in a Western European country. *Epilepsia* 2008.

Privitera MD, Brodie MJ, Mattson RH, Chadwick DW, Neto W, Wang S. Topiramate, carbamazepine and valproate monotherapy: double-blind comparison in newly diagnosed epilepsy. *Acta Neurologica Scandinavica* 2003; 107: 165-75.

Remy S, Beck H. Molecular and cellular mechanisms of pharmacoresistance in epilepsy. *Brain* 2006; 129: 18-35.

Remy S, Gabriel S, Urban BW, et al. A novel mechanism underlying drug resistance in chronic epilepsy. *Ann Neurol* 2003; 53: 469-79.

Scheffer IE, Berkovic SF. Generalized epilepsy with febrile seizures plus a genetic disorder with heterogeneous clinical phenotypes. *Brain* 1997; 120: 479-90.

Scheffer IE, Bhatia KP, Lopes-Cendes I, et al. Autosomal dominant nocturnal frontal lobe epilepsy: A distinctive clinical disorder. *Brain* 1995; 118: 61-73.

Siddiqui A, Kerb R, Weale ME, et al. Association of multidrug resistence in epilepsy with a polymorphism in the drug transporter gene ABCB1. *Neurology* 2003; 348: 1442-8.

Spooner CG, Berkovic SF, Mitchell LA, Wrennall JA, Harvey AS. New onset temporal lobe epilepsy in children: lesion on MRI predicts poor seizure outcome. *Neurology* 2006; 67: 2147-53.

Takenaka J, Kosaburo A, Watanabe K, Okumura A, Negoro T. Transient seizure remission in intractable localization-related epilepsy. *Pediatr Neurol* 2000; 23: 328-31.

Wheless JW, Clarke DF, Arzimanoglou A, Carpenter D. Treatment of pediatric epilepsy: European expert opinion, 2007. *Epileptic Disord* 2007; 9: 353-412.

Wheless JW, Clarke DF, Carpenter D. Treatment of pediatric epilepsy: expert opinion, 2005. *J Child Neurol* 2005; 20: S1-S56.

Wiebe S, Blume WT, Girvin JP, Eliasziw M. A randomized controlled trial of surgery for temporal-lobe epilepsy. *N Eng J Med* 2001; 345: 311-8.

Are drug-resistant and drug-sensitive patients the same? Observations from the Glasgow database

Martin J. Brodie

Epilepsy Unit, Western Infirmary, Glasgow, Scotland

Around 5-10% of people will have a seizure at some time in their lives, 30% of whom will go on later to develop epilepsy. Thus 1% of the world's population will have epilepsy at any given point in time, amounting to a total of around 40 million people. Of these, 30-40% of adults will remain refractory to pharmacotherapy despite the availability of an increasingly wide range of established and newer drugs (Annegers *et al.*, 1979; Cockerell *et al.*, 1995; Kwan & Brodie, 2000a; Fosgren *et al.*, 2005). Uncontrolled epilepsy can be associated with cognitive deterioration, psychosocial dysfunction and increased morbidity and mortality (Devinsky, 1999, Kwan & Brodie, 2002). Refractory epilepsy represents a socioeconomic burden at the individual, family, societal and political level in all countries across the globe (Pugliatti *et al.*, 2007).

■ Background

The Epilepsy Unit at the Western Infirmary, Glasgow, in Scotland, was set up in 1982. From the outset all referred patients, including those with newly diagnosed epilepsy, were entered in a database. The majority of untreated patients came by direct referral from local general practitioners. From 1990 onwards, following a survey of patients reviewed at the Accident and Emergency Department, all patients presenting there with untreated seizures were reviewed rapidly at the first seizure clinic (McKee *et al.*, 1990). Patients with a single seizure were given an emergency number to call should they have another event. This programme has allowed the gradual accumulation of more than 1,000 patients, who were diagnosed and started on their first ever antiepileptic drug (AED) under our supervision. This database continues to provide a number of insights in the natural history of treated epilepsy in adolescents and adults.

Patients

Most patients with first seizures or untreated epilepsy were reviewed within two weeks of referral, often a day or two after receipt of a faxed letter or telephone call. The current policy is to see urgent cases daily at the Epilepsy Unit rather than allow a waiting time to develop at the clinic. Data are collected manually *via* a structured questionnaire and later inserted into an electronic database. Routine investigations, including electroencephalography and brain imaging, are undertaken with minimal delay. Classification of seizure types and epilepsy syndromes takes place throughout the follow-up process. For publication purposes, each patient is reviewed again at the time of analysis when as much clinical information as possible has been accumulated.

Monotherapy was employed initially in all patients. Treatment schedules were modified as necessary based on clinical response and drug tolerability. Patients developing idiosyncratic reactions, such as rash, or experiencing intolerable side effects, such as sedation, at "low" AED doses (*e.g.* carbamazepine 600 mg daily or less, valproate 1,000 mg daily or less, lamotrigine 150 mg daily or less) were deemed to have failed treatment because of adverse effects. Those who continued to experience seizures despite tolerating "higher" doses of medication (*e.g.* carbamazepine 600 mg daily, valproate 1,000 mg daily or lamotrigine 150 mg) daily were designated as treatment failure due to lack of efficacy. This judgement was often made from the narrative in the letter sent to the general practitioner by the doctor reviewing the patient. Patients not tolerating their first AED were prescribed an alternative. Those failing treatment because of lack of efficacy either had the original drug substituted or were offered combination therapy depending on the clinical status of the patient and their personal preference. The extent of seizure control was assessed at the time of the patient's last clinic visit.

Patients have been categorised into 5 outcome groups (Mohanraj & Brodie, 2006). Responders to treatment required to be seizure free for at least 12 months. If they did not report any further seizures, they were regarded as having attained remission. Patients having no further seizures after taking their first AED dose were categorised as immediate responders. Relapse was defined as complete seizure control for at least 12 months followed by the subsequent development of uncontrolled epilepsy. Non responders to AED therapy never documented any 12 month seizure-free period from the outset.

Outcomes

The original observations in the first 470 untreated patients with newly diagnosed epilepsy were published in three papers (Kwan & Brodie, 2000a & b, 2001). More recent outcome data have focused on a total of 780 individuals with a median age of 29 years followed up between July 1982 & May 2001 [median duration of treatment 6.6 years (range 2-21 years)] (Mohanraj & Brodie, 2006). Overall 59.2% of patients achieved remission, 53% of whom were categorised as immediate responders. Non-responders accounted for 35.4% of the complete population, whereas 5.4% (8.4% of responders) relapsed and never again achieved good seizure control.

There were no significant differences in outcome between the cryptogenic (n = 314, 56% remission) and symptomatic (n = 244, 57% remission) patient populations, although patients with idiopathic generalised epilepsy syndromes tended to do a little better (n = 222, 66% remission). Patients with underlying cortical atrophy (n = 42, 71%

remission; p < 0.05) or cerebrovascular disease (n = 63, 70% remission; p < 0.01) fared better, while those with diffuse brain injury due to trauma (n = 65, 35% remission; p < 0.001) did worse than the remainder of the symptomatic group. Remission rates in patients with underlying cortical dysplasia (n = 15, 60%), hippocampal atrophy (n = 14, 50%) and primary brain tumour (n = 25, 52%) appeared no different from those with other symptomatic epilepsies. Overall, 20-40% patients with each epilepsy syndrome reported no further seizures after starting AED treatment including 21% with hippocampal atrophy and 33% with cortical dysplasia.

Figure 1 compares the prognostic categories from (a) the complete population with those in (b) patients with juvenile myoclonic epilepsy (JME) and (c) those with mesial temporal lobe epilepsy and hippocampal atrophy. Thus, some patients with a potentially benign epilepsy syndrome, *i.e.* JME, did not respond to AED therapy (Mohanraj & Brodie, 2007), whereas other individuals with localization-related epilepsy on a background of hippocampal sclerosis never had another seizure after taking the first AED dose (Mohanraj & Brodie, 2005a). Outcomes in patients with newly diagnosed localization-related epilepsy and concomitant cortical dysplasia also showed a wide variety of drug responses with 60% attaining remission and 33% not responding to treatment from the outset (Monhanraj & Brodie, 2005a). There follows two short illustrative cases with different prognoses despite apparently similar clinical pictures.

Case 1

This 38 year old man presented at the age of 15 years in October 1984 having had eight secondary generalised tonic-clonic seizures over the previous nine months. Each was ushered in by a short-lived numb feeling over the palate with tingling down the right side. This was followed by loss of consciousness with right sided jerking accompanied by forward and backward head movements. Brain magnetic resonance imaging revealed heterotopic grey matter in the left temporal and parietal lobes. There was no family history of epilepsy. He was commenced on carbamazepine and has remained seizures free on 200 mg twice daily (trough concentration 6.2 mg/L) since then. He works as a travelling salesman and is married with 3 children.

Case 2

This 45 years old lady presented in 1995 at the age of 33 years following 10 seizures in rapid succession over the previous three months. Prior to each event, she noted a feeling of excitement accompanied by a rising epigastric sensation. Her face then became expressionless, her limbs jerked and her eyes rolled up. On two occasions, she experienced a secondary generalised tonic-clonic seizure lasting a few minutes. Magnetic resonance imaging demonstrated an area of cortical dysplasia in the right temporal lobe. There was no history of birth injury or febrile convulsions. However, she has a daughter with well-controlled idiopathic generalised epilepsy. Treatment with maximally tolerated doses of carbamazepine, vigabatrin, gabapentin, valproate, topiramate, levetiracetam and zonisamide did not produce seizure freedom. Despite taking three AEDs at high dosage, she continues to report an average of four partial complex seizures each month. She has given up her job as a primary school teacher due to the embarrassment of suffering seizures in class.

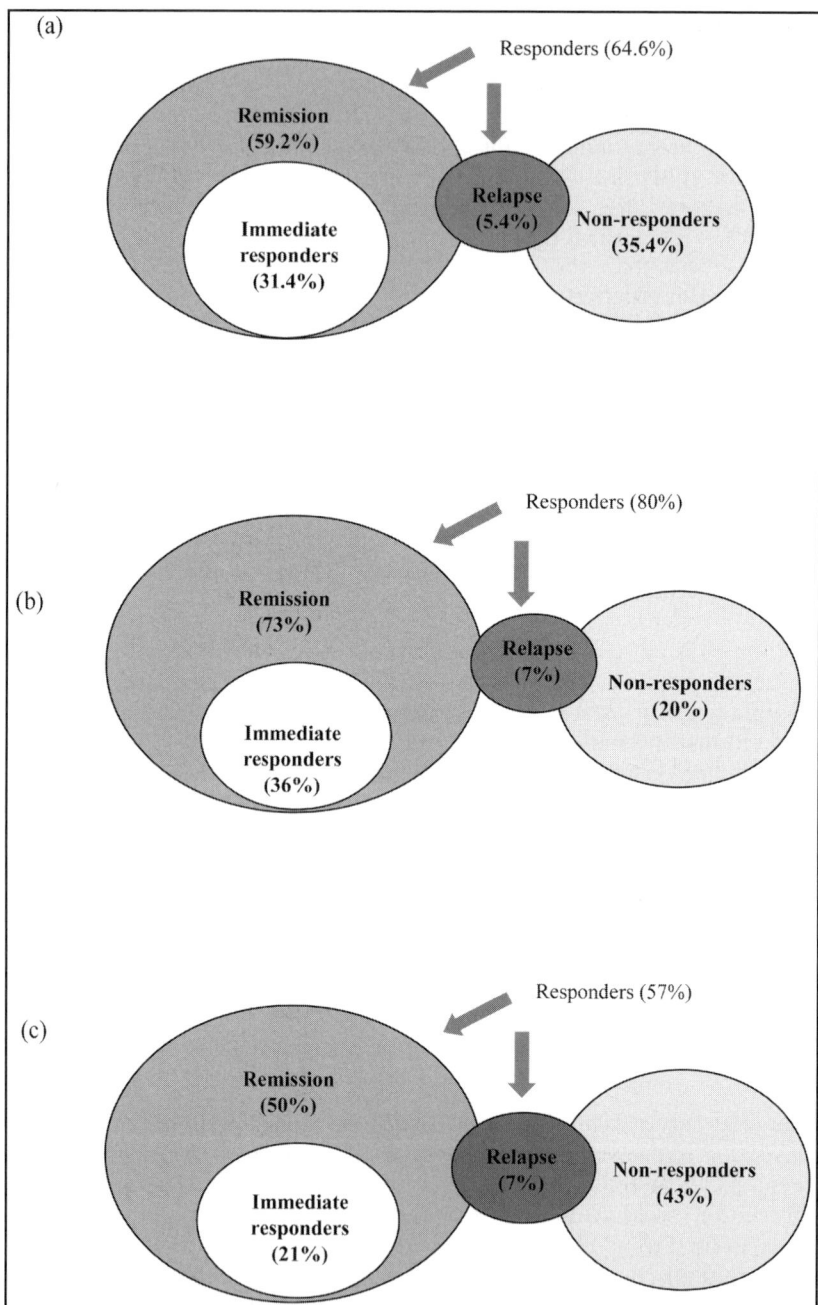

Figure 1. Outcomes in (a) all patients with newly diagnosed epilepsy (n = 780), (b) those with juvenile myoclonic epilepsies (n = 55) and (c) those with mesial temporal lobe epilepsy with hippocampal atrophy (n = 14). Data taken from Mohanraj and Brodie, 2005b, 2006 & 2007. Categories in patients with newly diagnosed epilepsies include: responder – seizure-free for a minimum of 12 months; immediate responder – no further seizures after starting treatment; remission – no relapse after responding for at least 1 year; relapse – controlled for at least 1 year and then refractory; non-responder – never seizure-free for any 12 month period.

Predictive factors

A number of studies in adolescents and adults have explored predictors of pharmacoresistant epilepsy among the common seizure types (Annegers et al., 1979; Cockerell et al., 1995; Hitiris et al., 2007). High numbers of pre-treatment seizures have been associated with poorer outcomes in a number of studies (Collaborative Group for the Study of Epilepsy, 1992; Sillanpaa 1993; Leschiner et al., 2006). We have recently added to this the observation that high seizure density within a few months of starting AED therapy (*Figure 2*) was a better predictor of subsequent pharmacoresistance than overall pre-treatment seizures numbers (Mohanraj & Brodie, 2006). The parallel observation that duration of untreated epilepsy did not predict outcome supports the suggestion that responders to AED therapy may represent a different population from non-responders. These observations may help explain the poorer overall prognosis in some active localisation-related epilepsy syndromes, such as those with hippocampal atrophy and cortical dysplasias, where pre-treatment seizure frequency and density is often high (Semah et al., 1998; Stephen et al., 2001). However, as discussed above, some patients with these syndromes have a more benign course (Andrade-Valenca et al., 2003; Kobayashi et al., 2003; Mohranraj & Brodie, 2005b).

Other predictive factors for poor outcome in patients attending our service have included family history of epilepsy, prior febrile convulsions, traumatic brain injury as a cause of the epilepsy, intermittent recreational drug use, and prior or concurrent psychiatric comorbidity, particularly depression (Hititis et al. 2007). Interestingly, Kanner and coworkers (2006) reported recently that a lifetime history of depression was the sole predictor of disabling seizures in patients failing temporal lobectomy. These two concordant observations from very different patient populations suggest that the deleterious neurobiological processes that underpin depression and perhaps other psychiatric disorders interact with those producing seizures to increase the extent of brain dysfunction and thereby the likelihood of developing pharmacoresistant epilepsy (Jobe, 2003). Elderly patients, on the other hand, tended to have a better prognosis (Mohanraj & Brodie, 2006), with 79% (n = 117) attaining remission overall, perhaps reflecting lower epileptogenicity and genetic predisposition in this population (Stephen et al., 2006).

Antiepileptic drugs

Large scale observational studies and randomised controlled trials have demonstrated that around 50% of people with newly diagnosed epilepsy will control on their first ever AED, often at modest or moderate doses (Kwan & Brodie, 2001; Mohanraj and Brodie, 2005b, Marson et al., 2007a & b; Brodie et al., 2007). The strongly predictive value of response to first AED as a measure of subsequent longterm outcome has been confirmed in other studies (Dlugos et al., 2001). Substitution for or combination with the first AED produced seizure freedom in 32% and 27% of our patients (Mohanraj & Brodie, 2005b). The remission rate after failing a first drug due to adverse effects (42%) was better than that following failure due to lack of efficacy (21%). Fewer patients in all syndromic categories did well, however, after failing 2 or 3 drugs schedules for any reason (Mohanraj & Brodie, 2006). Overall remission rates for the first, second and third treatment schedules as a proportion of the complete population were 50.4, 10.7 and 2.3% respectively, with just 6 (0.8%) patients responding well to further drug trials (*Table I*). Only 5% of these patients achieved remission with more than one AED (37 duotherapy, one each on 3 or 4 drugs).

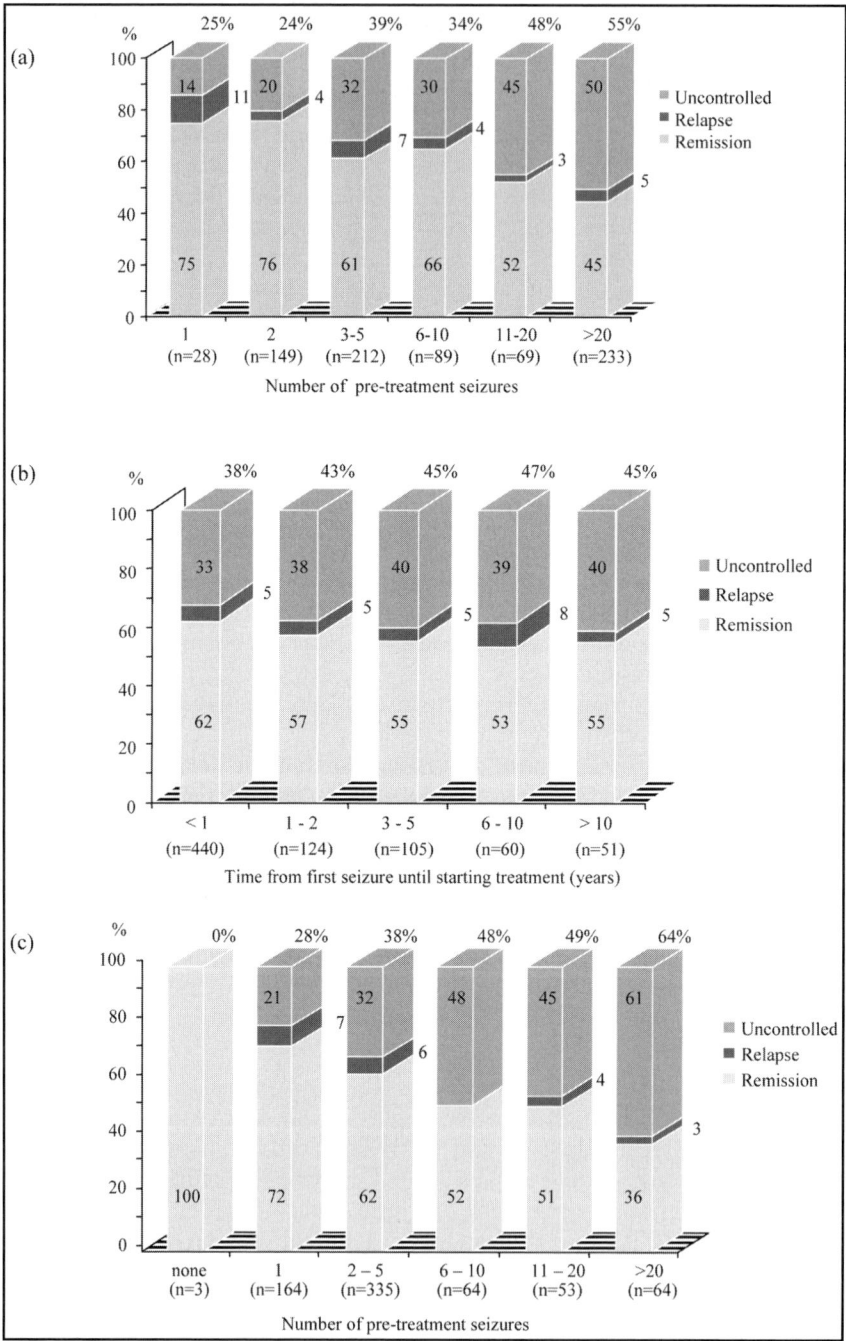

Figure 2. Outcomes (%) by (a) number of pre-treatment seizures (p = 0.024) (b) duration of epilepsy prior to starting treatment (not statistically significant) (c) seizure numbers in the three months before starting treatment (p < 0.0001). Numbers within bars represent percentages. Percentages on top of bars represent patients with refractory epilepsy (uncontrolled and relapsed). Figure taken from Mohanraj & Brodie, 2006.

Table I. Successive responder rates in patients with newly diagnosed epilepsy

	Idiopathic (n = 222)	Symptomatic/cryptogenic (n = 558)	All patients (n = 780)
First drug	58%	47%	50%
Second regimen	13%	12%	12%
Third regimen	3%	3%	3%
Other schedules	0.5%	0.9%	0.8%

Data taken from Mohanraj & Brodie, 2006.

In the 780 patients starting on treatment between July 1982 and May 2001, 245 (31%) never had another seizure after taking their first AED dose, whereas a further 276 (35.4%) never became seizure-free for any 12 month period (*Figure 1*). Median daily doses of carbamazepine, sodium valproate and lamotrigine in the immediate responders were 469 mg, 890 mg and 143 mg, respectively, suggesting substantial pharmacosensitivity in these individuals. Patients with refractory epilepsy were more likely to be male, to have frequent pre-treatment seizures and to have cryptogenic epilepsy.

■ Randomized trials

Many active-controlled, double-blind and pragmatic randomised trials have been undertaken in patients with newly diagnosed epilepsy with the established and newer AEDs (Mohanraj & Brodie, 2003; Kwan & Brodie, 2003; Marson *et al.*, 2007a & b). Comparisons between phenobarbital, primidone, phenytoin, carbamazepine and sodium valproate have shown no difference in efficacy among these drugs, although phenobarbital and primidone in highish doses tended to be less well tolerated (Mattson *et al.*, 1985). Second generation AEDs, such as lamotrigine, gabapentin and oxcarbazepine have demonstrated a tendency toward better tolerability, but again no important differences in efficacy have been reported compared with established AEDs, suggesting that some patients will respond to any appropriate first choice despite differences in their mechanisms of action.

These observations have been augmented by the recently published double-blind, randomised controlled trial comparing controlled-release carbamazepine and levetiracetam in this patient population (Brodie *et al.*, 2007). These drugs have substantial pharmacological differences. Carbamazepine is a traditional narrow spectrum AED that binds to inactivated neuronal Na^+ channels to produce a voltage and frequency-dependent reduction in Na^+ conductance. Levetiracetam has efficacy for some idiopathic generalised epilepsies as well as for partial seizures (Berkovic *et al.*, 2007). It binds to synaptic vesicle 2A protein, thereby interfering with the neuronal release of a range of neurotransmitters. This study was unique in that seizure-free patients could remain on the lowest effective dose of either treatment. The design allowed patients to be followed up until they were seizure-free for a year.

Despite the above pharmacological differences between the comparators, identical outcomes were obtained with both AEDs (Brodie *et al.*, 2007). Interestingly, Kaplan-Meir curves for time to discontinuation due to lack of efficacy or poor tolerability were superimposible using either the per-protocol or intention-to-treat analysis (*Figure 3*). Overall, 56.6% and 58.4% of patients randomized to levetiracetam or controlled-release carbamazepine

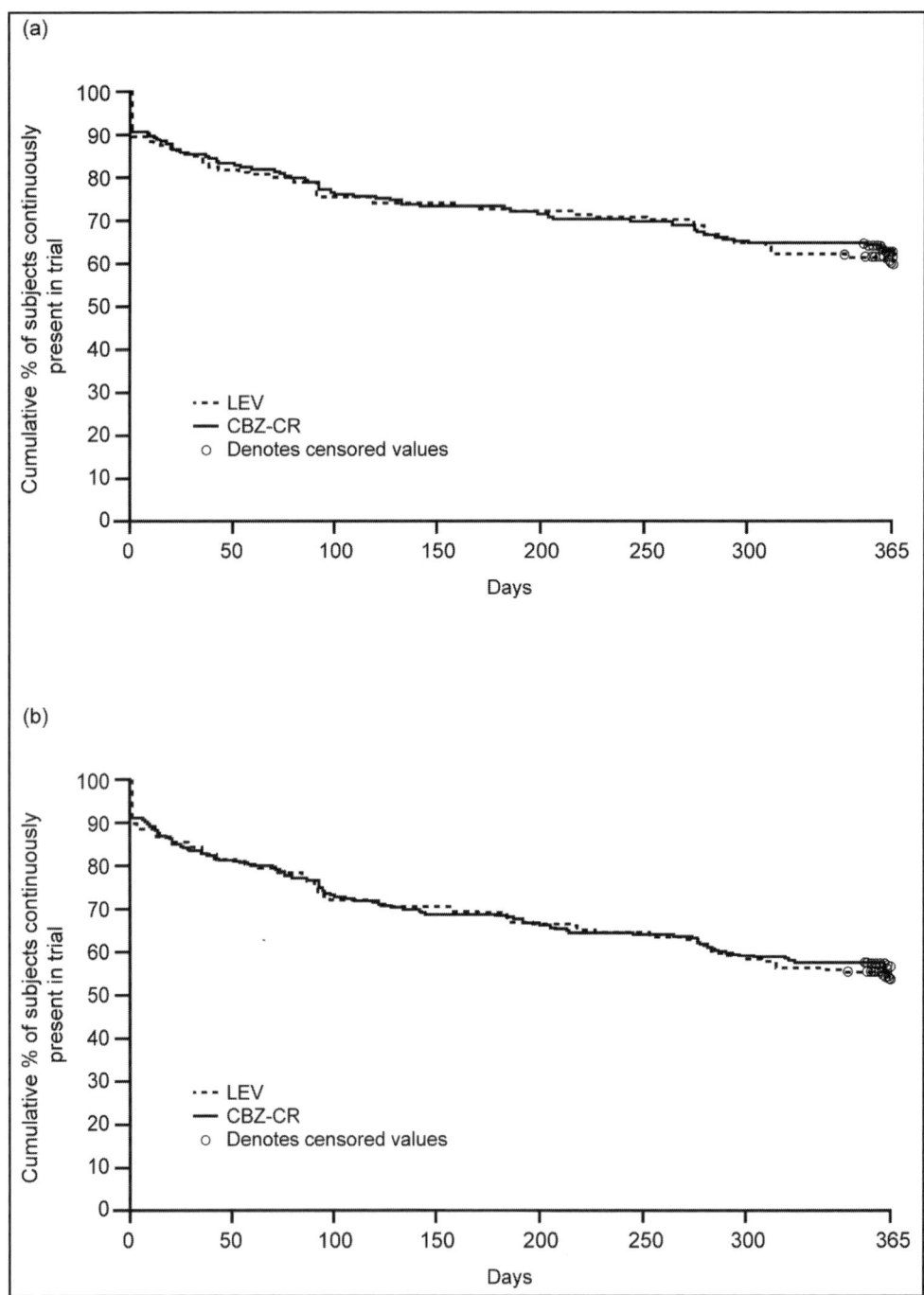

Figure 3. Time to discontinuation due to lack of efficacy or poor tolerability in newly diagnosed patients randomized to levetiracetam (LEV) or controlled-release carbamazepine (CBZ-CR) as their first ever treatment in the (A) per-protocol (LEV, n = 237; CBZ-CR, n = 235) and (B) intention-to-treat, (LEV = 285; CBZ-CR, n = 291) analyses. Figure taken from Brodie et al., 2007.

remained seizure-free for one year using the per-protocol analysis with 89% and 86%, respectively, taking the lowest dose (levetiracetam 500 mg twice daily or carbamazepine 200 mg twice daily). The overall one year seizure free rate in the intention-to-treat population was very similar to the figure obtained from the Glasgow population of newly diagnosed patients (Glasgow database 50%; carbamazepine 53%; levetiracetam 50%). Thus, this trial offered confirmation in a randomized, double-blind setting of previous uncontrolled observations that most people with newly diagnosed epilepsy will respond to their first ever AED at low dosage.

Conclusions

There seems little doubt now that many adolescent and adult patients with the common epilepsies respond readily to any AED at low or moderate dosage, whereas others with apparently similar semiology never achieved seizure freedom from the outset despite treatment with a variety of drugs with different modes of action used singly or in combination. In the Glasgow patient population (n = 780) followed up until the end of 2001, 56.1% remitted on their first AED or second regimen, whereas 35.4% never had a useful period of seizure freedom de novo. The remainder relapsed after a substantial period of perfect control and subsequently developed refractory epilepsy (Mohanraj and Brodie, 2006). Patients with a poorer outcome tended to have a greater seizure density immediately before starting treatment and often had previous or concurrent psychiatric comorbidity, particularly depression, suggesting perhaps a greater underlying degree of brain dysfunction.

The question "Are drug-sensitive and drug-resistant patients the same?" is an important one. If they are not, it should be possible to devise specific therapeutic strategies for individuals who demonstrate refractory epilepsy from the outset rather than persevering with a range of futile drug schedules resulting in an increasing drug burden. Although we now have available more than 20 AEDs with an apparently wide-range of mechanisms of action, all target similar pharmacological endpoints by reducing neuronal excitation and increasing inhibition (Kwan & Brodie, 2007). Thus, one might expect the overall prognosis to improve slowly in the refractory epilepsy population as newer AEDs that work in different ways become more generally available. In support of this suggestion is the emerging evidence that some of the newer broad spectrum drugs may be making inroads into the 30-40% of patients with pharmacoresistant epilepsy (Luciano & Shorvon, 2007; Callaghan et al., 2007). Our ongoing analysis supports this observation with preliminary results being compared to previous published data in Table II. The increase in seizure-free rates with polypharmacy but not monotherapy suggests that newer agents, such as topiramate, levetiracetam and zonisamide, with different mechanisms of action may be having a modest but encouraging positive impact on outcome. These observations provide substantial encouragement for further AED development (Kwan & Brodie, 2007).

Table II. Responder rates in an expanding cohort of patients with newly diagnosed epilepsy

Recruitment	n	Monotherapy	Polypharmacy	Total
1982-1997[1]	470	61%	3.0%	64.0%
1982-2003[2]	780	59%	5.4%	64.6%
1982-2008[3]	1100	61.6%	6.5%	68.1%

Data from [1] Kwan P, Brodie MJ, 2000a; [2] Mohanraj R, Brodie MJ, 2006; [3] Bamagous G, Brodie MJ, in preparation.

Other alternative explanations for the differences between drug-resistant and drug-sensitive patients will be discussed in detail elsewhere in this volume. These include variations in expression of efflux transporter proteins, alterations in ion channels and receptors and genetically determined factors affecting drug response. Lastly, it is possible too that the production of selective brain autoantibodies may result in autoimmune refractory epilepsy in some individuals (Vincent et al., 2006). The unravelling of these intriguing hypotheses will identify new ways to prevent and treat pharmacoresistance and thereby improve the quality of life of many more people with epilepsy (Kwan & Brodie, 2006).

References

Andrade-Valenca LP, Valenca MM, Ribeiro LT, et al. Clinical and neuroimaging features of good and poor seizure control with mesial temporal lobe epilepsy and hippocampal atrophy. *Epilepsia* 2003; 55: 807-14.

Annegers J, Hauser WA, Elverback LR. Remission of seizures and relapse in patients with epilepsy. *Epilepsia* 1979; 20: 729-37.

Berkovic SF, Knowlton RC, Leroy RF, Schiemann J, Falter U on behalf of the Levetiracetam No 1057 Study Group. Placebo-controlled study of levetiracetam in idiopathic generalised epilepsy. *Neurology* 2007; 69: 1751-60.

Brodie MJ, Perucca E, Ryvlin P, Ben-Menachem E, Meenche H-J for the Levetiracetam Monotherapy Study Group. Comparison of levetiracetam and controlled-release carbamazepine in newly diagnosed epilepsy. *Neurology* 2007; 68: 402-8.

Callaghan BC, Anand K, Hesdorffer D, Hauser WA, French JA. Likelihood of seizure remission in adult population with refractory epilepsy. *Ann Neurol* 2007; 62: 382-9.

Cockerell OC, Johnson AL, Sander JWAS, Hart YM, Shorvon SD. Remission of epilepsy: results from the national general practice study of epilepsy. *Lancet* 1995; 346: 140-4.

Collaborative Group for the Study of Epilepsy. Progress of epilepsy in newly referred patients: a multicenter prospective study of the effects of monotherapy on the long-term course of epilepsy. *Epilepsia* 1992; 33: 45-51.

Devinsky O. Patients with refractory seizures. *N Engl J Med* 1999; 340: 1565-70.

Dlugos DJ, Sammel MD, Strom BL, Farrar JT. Response to first drug trial predicts outcome in childhood temporal lobe epilepsy. *Neurology* 2001; 57: 2259-64.

Fosgren L, Beghi E, Oun A, Sillanpää M. The epidemiology of epilepsy in Europe – a systematic review. *Eur J Neurol* 2005; 12: 245-53.

Hititris N, Mohanraj R, Norrie J, Sills GJ, Brodie MJ. Predictors of pharmacoresistant epilepsy. *Epilepsy Res* 2007; 75: 192-6.

Jobe PC. Common pathogenic mechanisms between depression and epilepsy: an experimental perspective. *Epilepsy Behav* 2003; 4: S14-S24.

Kanner AM, Byrne R, Smith MC, Balabanov AJ, Frey M. Does a life-time history of depression predict a worse postsurgical outcome following a left temporal lobectomy? *Ann Neurol* 2006; 60 (suppl 10): S19.

Kobayashi IE, D'Agostino MD, Lopes-Cendes I, Berkovic SF, Andermann E, Andermann F, Cendes F. Hippocampal atrophy and T2-weighted signal changes in familial mesial temporal lobe epilepsy. *Neurology* 2003; 60: 405-9.

Kwan P, Brodie MJ. Early identification of refractory epilepsy. *N Engl J Med* 2000a; 342: 314-9.

Kwan P, Brodie MJ. Epilepsy after the first drug fails: substitution or add-on? *Seizure* 2000b; 9: 464-8.

Kwan P, Brodie MJ. Effectiveness of first antiepileptic drug. *Epilepsia* 2001; 42: 1255-60.

Kwan P, Brodie MJ. Refractory epilepsy: a progressive, intractable but preventable condition? *Seizure* 2002; 11: 77-84.

Kwan P, Brodie MJ. Clinical trials of antiepileptic medications in newly diagnosed patients with epilepsy. *Neurology* 2003; 60 (suppl 4): S2-S12.

Kwan P, Brodie MJ. Refractory epilepsy: mechanisms and solutions. *Expert Rev Neurotherapeutics* 2006; 6: 397-406.

Kwan P, Brodie MJ. Emerging drugs for epilepsy. *Expert Opinion Emerging Drugs* 2007; 12: 407-22.

Leschziner G, Jorgensen AL, Andrew T, *et al*. Clinical factors and ABCB1 polymorphisms in prediction of antiepileptic drug response: a prospective cohort study. *Lancet Neurol* 2006; 5: 668-76.

Luciano AL, Shorvon SD. Results of treatment changes in patients with apparently drug-resistant chronic epilepsy. *Ann Neurol* 2007; 62: 375-81.

Marson AG, Al-Kharusi A, Alwaidh M, *et al*. The SANAD study of effectiveness of carbamazepine, gabapentin, lamotrigine, oxcarbazepine or topiramate for treatment of partial epilepsy: an unblinded randomised controlled trial. Lancet 2007a; 369: 1000-15.

Marson AG, Al-Kharusi A, Alwaidh M, *et al*. The SANAD study of effectiveness of valproate, lamotrigine and topiramate for generalised and unclassifiable epilepsy: an unblinded randomised controlled trial. *Lancet* 2007b; 367: 1016-26.

Mattson RH, Cramer JA, Collins JF, Smith DB, Delgado-Escueta AV, *et al*. Comparison of carbamazepine, phenobarbital, phenytoin and primidone in partial and secondary tonic-clonic seizures. *N Engl J Med* 1985; 313: 145-51.

McKee PJW, Wilson EA, Dawson JA, Larkin JG, Brodie MJ. Managing seizures in the casualty department. *Brit Med J* 1990; 300: 976-9.

Mohanraj R, Brodie MJ. Measuring the efficacy of antiepileptic drugs. *Seizure* 2003; 12: 413-43.

Mohanraj R, Brodie MJ. Pharmacological outcomes in newly diagnosed epilepsy. *Epilepsy Behav* 2005a; 6: 382-7.

Mohanraj R, Brodie MJ. Outcomes in newly diagnosed localisation-related epilepsies. *Seizure* 2005b; 14: 318-23.

Mohanraj R, Brodie MJ. Diagnosing refractory epilepsy: response to sequential treatment schedules. *Eur J Neurol* 2006; 13: 277-82.

Mohanraj R, Brodie MJ. Outcomes of newly diagnosed idiopathic generalised epilepsy syndromes in a non-pediatric setting. *Acta Neurol Scand* 2007; 115: 204-8.

Pugliatti M, Beghi E, Forsgren L, Ekman M, Sobocki P. Estimating the cost of epilepsy in Europe: a review with economic modelling. *Epilepsia* 2007; 48: 2224-33.

Semah F, Picot M-C, Adam C, *et al*. Is the underlying cause of epilepsy a major prognostic factor for recurrence? *Neurology* 1998; 51: 1256-62.

Sillanpää M. Remission of seizures and predictions of intractability in long-term follow-up. *Epilepsia* 1993; 34: 930-6.

Stephen LJ, Kelly K, Mohanraj R, Brodie MJ. Pharmacological outcomes in older people with newly diagnosed epilepsy. *Epilepsy Behav* 2006: 8: 434-7.

Stephen LJ, Kwan P, Brodie MJ. Does the cause of localisation-related epilepsy influence the response to antiepileptic drug treatment? *Epilepsia* 2001; 42: 357-62.

Vincent A, Lang B, Kleopa AK. Autoimmune channelopathies and related neurological disorders. *Neuron* 2006; 52: 123-38.

Refractory versus non-refractory status epilepticus: frequency, differentiating clinical features, and outcome

Aidan Neligan, Simon Shorvon

UCL, Institute of Neurology, London, UK

■ Definitions

First to definitions, for these are necessary to refine the issues addressed in this paper.

Status Epilepticus

Our current definitions derive from the proposals made at the first major meeting devoted to the subject of status epilepticus (SE), the X_{th} Marseille Colloquium, held in 1962 and lead by Henri Gastaut (Gastaut *et al.*, 1967). At the meeting, a new and influential definition of SE was proposed: *a condition characterized by an epileptic seizure which is so frequently repeated or so prolonged as to create a fixed and lasting epileptic condition* and a classification of SE was adopted which paralleled the newly formed International Classification of Seizure Type. The ILAE in its revision of the seizure type classification in 1981, revised the definition (in *an addendum*): *The term "status epilepticus" is used whenever a seizure persists for a sufficient length of time or is repeated frequently enough that recovery between attacks does not occur.*

These definitions of SE, excellent as they are, beg the question how long should a seizure be considered enduring before it is categorized as SE, and this lack of definition of a minimum time period has proved problematic from the point of view of clinical research and epidemiology, and is the subject of continual debate. Gastaut himself suggested that 60 minutes was a reasonable minimum period in which to consider a seizure "enduring" and this became the ILAE standard at the time. The suggested minimum time shortened to 30 minutes (for instance, see Shorvon 1994), then 20 minutes (for instance by Bleck in 1991), to 10 minutes (by Treiman in 1998) and then to 5 minutes by Lowenstein in 1999. The five minute definition was based on the assumption that convulsive seizures lasting longer than 5 minutes seldom were self-terminating (Theodore *et al.*, 1994). Indeed based on their observations of 120 generalised tonic-clonic seizures (GTCSs) in 47 patients, Theodore *et al.* (1994) advocated the use of intravenous antiepileptic drugs if a GTCS persisted longer then 2 minutes. Such a proposition does not to be in accord with common clinical experience where some seizures lasting longer than 5 minutes are self-terminating without therapy. The definitions with 30-60 minute minimum durations are based on physiological criteria and the definitions with 5-10 minute minimum durations have been devised for an essentially operational reason – the highly important goal of encouraging the early application of therapy (a goal which of course we strongly advocate, regardless of the definition of SE adopted).

From the point of view of "refractoriness" however, the adoption of the 5 or 10 minute definition, and the inclusion of short seizures within the rubric of SE, greatly influences estimates of the frequency of SE and also results in a significant decrease in the proportion of refractory cases. These considerations obviously impact on research into, or consideration of, what is refractory SE. These issues were debated at the recent *London Colloquium of Status Epilepticus* (held in April 2007; Shorvon & Trinka 2007) where most, but not all, participants still favoured the 30 minute period (Shorvon et al., 2008; Bleck, 2008).

Refractory status epilepticus

Given the lack of agreement about the definition of SE, it is perhaps not surprising that there is also no accepted definition of refractory SE.

Three factors are commonly used to define "refractoriness" in convulsive SE: the duration of the status, the number of ineffective therapies and the need for anaesthesia. All are arbitrary.

(a) The duration of SE is used by some authors, but this depends when the status episode is deemed to have started and on the time that treatment is started. The initiation of therapy after 5 minutes of continuous seizures will be much more likely to succeed than the initiation of therapy after 60 minutes, a fact well backed up by experimental as well as clinical studies (see for instance Kapur & MacDonald, 1999; Chen & Wasterlain, 2006). Failure of drug treatment after 60 minutes of continuous seizure activity is therefore far more ominous than failure after 5 minutes of continuous seizure activity. Any estimates of the proportion of refractory cases, or description of their characteristics, will be greatly influenced by the bias introduced by considering different time courses.

(b) The number of ineffective therapies which have been tried and failed, is also an inherently unsatisfactory measure – depending on, for instance: dose, choice of drug and method of administration, the hesitancy of therapy; the timing of therapy; and the experience of the treating physician. However, once a patient is deemed "refractory" (i.e. not responding to 2 first line antiepileptic drugs), further non-anaesthetic drug treatment of SE is often ineffective. In the Veterans Affairs Cooperation Study (Treiman et al., 1998) in which a rate of RSE (failure of seizure cessation after 2 ACDs) of 38% for overt convulsive SE and 82% for subtle SE was found, only 2% and 5% respectively responded after the administration of a third ACD.

(c) The time of administration of anaesthesia will depend on local facilities and on the context of the SE. Furthermore, anaesthetic drugs, for instance, achieving the anaesthetic level of burst suppression, will abolish seizure activity in *all* cases; no patient is, in this sense, "refractory" to this therapy, although of course, seizures may return when the anaesthesia is lightened.

Another important point is that the response to antiepileptic therapy is to a very large extent dependent on the underlying aetiology of the status, which is therefore is a very relevant factor when considering refractoriness, but its effect on outcome is largely independent of the seizure activity. Thus, the contribution of seizure activity to the approximately 40% mortality of encephalitis or stroke, for instance, has been estimated to be about 2% (Shorvon, 1994) and the occurrence of SE (and RSE) is essentially a reflection of the severity of the underlying condition. Acute SE due to structural brain disorders (*e.g.* encephalitis or stroke) is particularly likely to have a bad outcome. Conversely, in cases of acute SE in previously non-epileptic patients, where no aetiology is found, the outcome is usually much better, even if the duration of SE is prolonged.

In the literature cited in this paper, refractory SE (RSE) has also been variously defined as the failure to control seizure activity after the administration of 2 anticonvulsants drugs with a minimum duration of seizure activity of 1 hour (for instance Hanley *et al.*, 1998; Maytal *et al.*, 1991) or 2 hours (for instance Strecker *et al.*, 1998; Prasad *et al.*, 2001) or 3 anticonvulsants drugs (for instance: Bleck, 1993; Cascino, 1996; Lowenstein *et al.*, 1998) or failure of 2 or 3 drugs, irrespective of the time elapsed since seizure onset (for instance: America's Working Group on Status Epilepticus, 1993; Lowenstein *et al.*, 1998; Holtkamp *et al.*, 2005). Others have defined refractory SE as an episode of SE resistant to treatment with one first-line antiepileptic drug (benzodiazepines) and one second-line antiepileptic drug (phenytoin, phenobarbital, or valproic acid) (For instance: Mayer *et al.*, 2002; Holtkamp *et al.*, 2005; Rossetti *et al.*, 2005). In a monograph on SE, Shorvon (1994) defined the stage of refractory SE as that in which the patient had failed to respond to benzodiazepine and then to either phenytoin or phenobarbital therapy, and who required anaesthesia. Others have not used the term "refractory" but looked at outcome after the stage of artificial ventilation and anaesthesia (for instance: Koubeissi & Alshekhlee 2007).

In view of the above considerations and the difficulties of definition, we believe that the term "refractory" has little value or meaning and on the whole should be avoided. It makes more sense to consider the severity of SE, not in terms of its refractoriness, but in terms of its outcome, usually measured as mortality, morbidity (intellectual or neurological), or the occurrence of continuing epilepsy.

In this paper in which the primary objective is to define the characteristics of "refractory" and "non-refractory" patients, we propose that four different measures of refractoriness can be used – each of which, in our opinion, has a certain validity but none of which can claim exclusivity:

1. Mortality (especially the 30-day case fatality rate) or morbidity.

2. The need for artificial ventilation.

3. The failure of seizure control within 60 minutes of the onset of continuous seizures.

4. The failure of seizure control despite the use of at least two appropriate antiepileptic drugs (a benzodiazepine and an appropriate IV medication) given appropriately.

In this paper, we will largely confine the discussion to generalised convulsive SE, but in doing so recognise that some forms of non-convulsive status are extremely refractory, although generally with ultimately, a good prognosis and outcome.

Studies of refractory and non-refractory status epilepticus

A recent survey is that of Koubeissi and Alshekhlee (2007), which although has severe methodological limitations, is the biggest published study. A large multi-hospital database was used to ascertain all patients admitted to a sample of hospitals in the United States over a five year period (2000-2005), with a primary diagnosis of "generalised convulsive status epilepticus" (GCSE – ICD – 9,345.3). No other diagnostic criteria were employed. This database, the Nationwide Inpatient Sample, covered about 1,000 hospitals and 5-8 million inpatient stays. The primary outcome was mortality, and the study also provided estimates of the rate of intubation and artificial ventilation – both (as outlined above) measures of refractoriness. In the study, 15,370 cases of GCSE of whom 11,580 were included in the analysis. The overall mortality rate was 3.45%, and it seems clear that many patients with mild seizures were included. Underlying causes were sought, but seem to have been grossly underestimated – the commonest was acute metabolic disturbance (including alcohol intake) found in 2.8% of the cases and ischaemic-hypoxic brain injury in 2.1%. The frequency of SE was highest in young children (21.8% of all cases were less than 10 years of age) and in the elderly (22.3% of all cases were aged 60 years or older). The fatality rate was lowest in young children (1.43% in those under 5 years). The rate was highest in the elderly (7th, 8th and 9th decade), with odds ratio for death of between 10-15 X that in children (1st decade of life). 2,718 (23.47%) of the patients required intubation and ventilation – one measure of "refractoriness". The mortality rate of the ventilated patients was 7.34% – on the face of it surprisingly only 3 times higher than the non-ventilated patients. Patients with cardiovascular disease, with metabolic disorder and those with hypoxic-ischaemic brain injury (which included those in post-anoxic coma in adults after cardiac arrest) were very likely to require ventilation ($p < 0.0001$). The same did not apply to those with tumour, trauma or infection, where there was no significant difference in the numbers requiring and not requiring ventilation.

Other smaller studies have reported mortality and its associations, and most have found higher death rates in refractory SE, particularly in elderly patients (most of whom developed SE due to stroke or hypoxic brain injury), and in those with SE due to an acute brain injury. Claassen and colleagues (2002a) collected 193 patients with refractory epilepsy from 28 published studies. Refractory SE was defined as a failure to respond to 2 antiepileptic drugs. 48% of the episodes were fatal and the patients who died were significantly older (mean 54 years *vs* 42 years in survivors). The mortality rates seem unusually high, and the study has been criticized because the data from the cited source documents do not seem to correspond to the analyses made. Mayer *et al.* (2002) carried out a retrospective survey of 83 episodes of refractory status, defined as failure to respond to benzodiazepine and one IV drug and seizures persisting for more than 60 minutes. The mortality rate was 23% in those with RSE compared to 14% in those with NRSE but the result was not statistically significant. RSE was also associated with prolonged ICU length of stay (7.5 days *vs* 1.0 days, $p < 0.001$) and hospital length of stay (32.5 *vs* 11.0, $p < 0.001$). (Mayer *et al.*, 2002). Rossetti *et al.* found that mortality was 23% in patients with RSE compared to 8% for patients with NRSE ($p = 0.05$). Moreover a return to baseline was more likely in those with NRSE ($p = 0.04$). This study looked at the effect of treatment aggression on prognosis and found that outcome was independent of the anaesthetic agent used or the extent of the EEG burst suppression achieved suggesting that the primary determinant of prognosis is the underlying aetiology. (Rossetti *et al.*, 2005). In a study comparing outcomes in children with NRSE compared to RSE, mortality was significantly higher in RSE (13.3%) compared to NRSE (2.1%) ($p = 0.006$). Children with RSE were more likely to develop a new deficit compared to those with NRSE (71.4% vs 55.1%, p = 0.0001) and more likely to develop subsequent epilepsy (30.6% vs 20.5%, p = 0.004). (Lambrechtsen et al., 2008).

Lowenstein and Alldredge (1993) retrospectively reviewed the clinical course of adult patients treated for generalized SE at the San Francisco General Hospital (SFGH) from 1980 to 1989. 154 patients were included and the four commonest aetiologies were anticonvulsant drug withdrawal (39), alcohol-related (39), drug toxicity (14), and CNS infection (12). Sixty percent of all patients responded to first-line drug treatment (usually phenytoin +/- diazepam). The worst response to therapy was in patients with anoxia, drug toxicity, CNS infection, or other metabolic abnormalities, and the best response was in SE due to tumour, anticonvulsant drug withdrawal, or refractory epilepsy. Of the 22 patients who died, SE was a likely cause of death in only two (i.e., 1.3% of the entire study group). Metabolic abnormalities, stroke, and anoxia were associated with particularly poor outcomes compared with other aetiologies.

One study was conducted with the primary aim of comparing refractory and non-refractory cases was that of Holtkamp and colleagues (2005) (Table I). This was a retrospective study of 83 cases admitted to the neurological intensive care unit (NICU) with de novo SE (convulsive and non-convulsive) ascertained over a ten year period. As only patients admitted to NICU were considered, this was a highly selected cohort. Refractory SE was defined as the failure to respond to benzodiazepines and phenytoin – regardless of time period over which the treatment was administered. In this cohort, the presence of an acute symptomatic CNS lesion was more common in the refractory than non-refractory SE (50% vs 14.9%, p = 0.001). Encephalitis was particularly associated with refractoriness, and low existing antiepileptic drug levels with non-refractoriness. The highly selected nature of the cohort and the relatively small numbers of other aetiologies reduce the power of the study to provide a robust estimate of the prognosis of the other aetiologies. 16.7% of the refractory cases died compared to 8.6% of the non-refractory cases (this difference was not statistically significant). Recurrence of epileptic activity within 24 hours of cessation of SE was more likely in those with refractory SE (45.4%) compared with non-refractory SE (6.5%) (p < 0.001). Prolonged length of stay in the Intensive Care Unit was more likely with refractory SE (median 16.5 days vs 2 days, p < 0.001) and prolonged length of stay in hospital (median 30 days vs 10.5 days, p < 0.01). For those patients with no prior history of seizures, patients with refractory SE were more likely to develop subsequent epilepsy compared with patients with non-refractory SE (87.5% vs 22.2%, p < 0.05).

The most important clinical factor which influences the frequency of occurrence of SE, its "refractoriness" and its outcome is the underlying aetiology. As mentioned above, however, aetiology exerts an influence on the outcome of the SE which is largely independent of the severity of the SE.

Table I. Differences between refractory and non-refractory SE in patients on an NICU

	Non-refractory SE (n = 47)	Refractory SE (n = 36)	p value
CNS disease	23 (48.9%)	32 (88.9%)	p = < 0.001
Acute symptomatic SE	7 (14.9%)	18 (50%)	p = 0.001
Encephalitis	2 (4.3%)	8 (22.2%)	p = 0.018
Low drug levels	13 (27.7%)	0 (0%)	p = < 0.001

For details, see text. (From Holtkamp et al., 2005.)

■ The underlying aetiologies of status epilepticus: frequency, influence on "refractoriness" and outcome

In adults, the majority of cases of SE occur in previously non-epileptic patients. In an analysis of the literature in 1994 (Shorvon 1994), of 1679 patients in 13 hospital series, the SE had no obvious cause in only 19% of cases (11% in children and 13% in the elderly). Febrile SE accounted for 12% of cases, and acute metabolic, toxic and anoxic causes for 14%. Stroke, tumor, trauma, infection, and perinatal causes accounted for between 7-10% each. The underlying cause of SE differs markedly in patients with and without existing epilepsy. In five series of largely adult cases (554 patients), only 41% had a prior history of epilepsy. An acute cause was found in 89% of patients with SE in previously non-epileptic patients, and in only 41% of patients with a previous history of epilepsy. When convulsive SE does occur in patients with a previous history of epilepsy, many cases are due to antiepileptic drug reduction/withdrawal. In these patients, an acute brain insult is much less commonly the precipitating factor.

More recent population-based studies have reported similar findings to those of the older hospital series (6 population-based studies are summarized in *Table II*). In a population-based prospective study of adult patients, from Hessen in Germany, the following aetiologies were recorded: remote stroke 36%, other remote symptomatic 27%, Binswanger disease 17%, acute stroke 14%, tumor 13%, medication induced 11%, metabolic disorders 9%, low antiepileptic drug levels 9%, alcohol 9%, remote trauma 8% and no cause was found in 9%. In a prospective population-based study from Bologna of adults, 41 patients with symptomatic causes were ascertained and the causes were: stroke 41%, systemic metabolic disorders 24%, head injury 10%, alcoholism 7%, tumors 5%, intracranial surgery 2% and other factors in 27% (undefined acute illness in 20%). These findings probably broadly reflect the situation in most Western European adult populations.

In the population-based survey of children with first-ever episodes of SE from London, only 30% of the cohort had a history of prior epilepsy (or neurological abnormality) and the commonest cause of the SE was febrile illness (febrile SE). This accounted for 32% of all cases. 17% had acute symptomatic SE, almost all due to acute metabolic derangement (electrolyte imbalance, hypoglycemia, hypocalcaemia or hypomagnesaemia) or acute CNS infection. Of the 95 children presenting with fever and SE, 12% had bacterial meningitis, emphasizing the importance of this treatable cause in young children (Chin et al., 2006).

Status epilepticus and encephalitis

Encephalitis is an important cause of SE, accounting for about 6-12% of all cases in various series, and is a commoner cause of SE in children then in adults. (Lowenstein et al., 1993). The SE is often refractory. In a review of 22 cases of RSE in children, presumed or agent identified encephalitis was the underlying aetiology in 10 cases. Of these, 4 died, 5 developed seizures and 1 returned to baseline. (Sahin et al., 2001).

The refractory nature of the SE induced by encephalitis and its rather poor outcome has been demonstrated in several hospital-based studies. In a case series of 17 cases of refractory generalised convulsive SE treated with continuous infusion of midazolam, 4 cases were found to be due to viral encephalitis, of whom 1 patient died, 2 patients had moderate to severe encephalopathy and one patient made a full recovery. The mean age was 28. (Yaffe et al., 1993). Holtkamp et al. (2005) found that encephalitis was the cause of refractory

Table II. Six population-based studies of status epilepticus (Table from Shorvon S., 2008)

	Richmond, Virginia, USA	Rochester, Minn, USA	French speaking, Switzerland	Hessen, Germany	Bologna, Italy	London, UK
Year	1989-91	1965-84	1997-98	1997-99	1999-2000	2002-2004
Population (denominator)	202,774	1,090,055	1,735,420	743,285	336,876	605,230
Number of cases	166	199	172	150	44	226 total 176 first-ever episode of SE
Incidence of SE (per 100,000 per year)	41 (raw) 61 (adjusted)	18.3 (adjusted)	9.9 (raw) 10.3 (adjusted)	15.0	13.1	17-23 (adjusted) 12.5-14 (adjusted; first-ever episode of SE)
Female: male ratio of cases	1: 1.2[1]	1: 1.9[2]	1: 1.7[2]	1: 1.9[3]	1: 0.74[2]	1: 1.12
History of prior epilepsy	42%	44%	32.8%	33%	39%	7%[4]
Inclusions/exclusions	Patients one month of age or less were excluded	–	Patients with post anoxic encephalopathy were excluded	Only patients of 18 years of age or over were included	Only patients of 20 years of age or over were included	Only convulsive SE was included; Only children (< 15 yrs of age) were included
Case ascertainment	Prospective hospital record review	Retrospective review using record linkage system	Prospective hospital record review	Prospective hospital record review	Prospective Active surveillance of hospital admissions	Prospective active surveillance through A&E and hospital admissions

[1] Raw data; [2] Adjusted ratio; [3] Adjusted figures, from the regions with the best case ascertainment and least likely to selection bias; [4] Excluding febrile seizures.
Data derived from: DeLorenzo RJ et al., 1996; Hesdorffer et al., 1998; Jallon et al., 1999; Knake et al., 2001; Vignatelli et al., 2003; Chin et al., 2006.

SE in 22% of cases compared with only 4.3% of cases of non-refractory SE ($p < 0.18$). Lin et al. (2008) reviewed all cases of SE related to presumed encephalitis in paediatric intensive care unit over a 4 year period. In this study, RSE was defined as seizures lasting > 2 hours, despite treatment with conventional antiepileptic drugs including initial therapy with a benzodiazepine, followed by therapeutic dosage of both phenytoin and phenobarbital. Out of 46 cases, 20 (43.4%) developed refractory SE with a 30% mortality rate. Of the survivors, all but one developed subsequent epilepsy and/or neurological deficits, and none returned to baseline. For those with non-refractory SE, 4/26 died, 16 developed epilepsy or neurological deficit and only 6 returned to baseline.

Population-based studies tend to show a rather more favorable outcome, with a lower frequency of refractory cases. For instance, in the California Encephalitis Project (CEP) which is an ongoing project aimed at determining the cause of encephalitis, all patients identified with encephalitis were subdivided into 3 categories: Refractory SE, defined as SE requiring anaesthetic coma for management (Group I); Non-refractory SE (Group II); and patients without seizures (Group III). Four percent had refractory SE, 40% non-refractory SE and 56% no seizures. Cases of refractory SE associated with encephalitis tended to be younger (median age = 10) and had a poor outcome with 28% dying within 2 years and 56% neurologically impaired or undergoing rehabilitation (Glaser et al., 2007).

In summary, encephalitis is associated with a high proportion of refractory compared to non-refractory cases, but many patients with encephalitis do not develop SE and the SE is by no means invariably refractory. However, for those who survive both refractory or non-refractory SE caused by encephalitis, there is a substantial risk of developing subsequent epilepsy.

Status epilepticus and stroke

Stroke is a common cause of SE in the elderly particularily in those with no prior history of seizures. In the Richmond study, stroke was the cause of 22% of cases of SE and 85% of all remote symptomatic cases which accounts for a total of almost 50% of adult cases. Adjusted for age, stroke caused 35% of acute cases and 26% of cases were caused by remote symptomatic stroke in patients over 60 (DeLorenzo et al., 1996). In the review of 193 patients with refractory SE, stroke was the underlying cause in 20% (Claassen et al., 2002).

One study has specifically examined the association of SE and stroke. Out of 3,205 patients with first time strokes over an 8 year period, 159 had first time post-stroke seizures. Of these 159, SE was recognised in 31 cases, with SE being the presenting epileptic symptom in 17 cases, in 4 cases stroke began with SE, and in the remaining 17 cases, SE developed after one or more seizures. After follow-up of 47 months, 15 patients had died, 5 cases being directly related to SE. Additional seizures occurred in 8 of the initial SE cases and all 14 patients with SE after one or more seizures. The study concluded that SE in stroke has a poor prognosis but that initial SE as a first epileptic symptom was not predictive of developing subsequent seizures. (Rumbach et al., 2000). A smaller study looked at stroke as a remote symptomatic cause of SE in a cohort of patients with poststroke first time seizures. 180 such cases were identified out of 1,174 patients with stroke. Of these 180, 17 (9%) developed SE. The risk of developing SE was higher in those with higher disability (Rankin scale > 3, odds ratio 4.36). Recurrent SE occurred in 5 cases, all of whom had a first episode of SE within 7 days post-stroke. Early onset SE was associated with a higher risk of recurrence of SE (p = 0.003) and higher mortality (p = 0.04) (Velioglu et al., 2001).

In the population-based study from Germany, Knake et al. (2006) calculated the longer-term mortality rates of those with a first episode of cerebrovascular-related SE compared with those with acute stroke without SE in 166 patients (93 patients with SE, 73 patients with acute stroke without SE). 53/93 SE patients and 35/73 of the acute stroke cases without SE died. Multivariate analysis showed that patients with SE had, after 6 months, twice the risk of death compared with patients with stroke without SE (hazard ratio of 2.12, CI 1.04-4.32, p = 0.0392) (Knake et al., 2006).

In the studies from Switzerland of Rossetti and colleagues (2004, 2006), stroke was the cause of SE in 16% of cases in the population-based sample and had the highest cause-specific mortality (20%), and in the hospital sample of refractory cases, 7 (23%) out of the 31 cases of refractory SE were due to stroke, of whom 3 died.

Holtkamp and colleagues (2005) found that acute stroke accounted for 8.3% (3 patients) of refractory SE and for none of the non-refractory cases. Remote stroke was the cause of 11.1% (4) cases of refractory SE and 14.9% (7) of non-refractory SE. Intracranial haemorrhage was the cause of 5.5% (2) and 4.3% (2) of refractory and non-refractory cases respectively. Sinus venous thrombosis was the cause of 5.5% (2) cases of refractory SE and no cases of non-refractory SE.

Overall stroke (acute or remote symptomatic) is the cause of approximately 20% of cases of SE and carries a generally poor prognosis and high mortality. For those with stroke who develop refractory SE the prognosis is particularly poor and the mortality high. SE as a first epileptic presentation post stroke was found not to be a predictor for the development of subsequent epilepsy.

Alcohol, substance abuse and status epilepticus

Alcohol abuse (intoxication or withdrawal) has been found to be a common cause of SE in both population-based and hospital-based studies, accounting for instance for 25% of cases in SE in the San Francisco Hospital Study (Lowenstein et al., 1993) and 13% of adult cases in the Richmond study (DeLorenzo et al., 1996). Other studies have found smaller proportions (Mayer et al., 2002; Holtkemp et al., 2005; Rossetti et al., 2006).

Ninety per cent (35) of alcohol related cases in the San Francisco had a good outcome compared to 10% (4) of patients who died. (p = 0.001) (Lowenstein et al., 1993). However the total duration of SE was significantly different in the 2 outcome groups (average duration 1.2 hours *versus* 4.1) but the duration was significantly higher for all aetiologies in patients who died. Rossetti et al. found that alcohol was the cause of 6/96 cases of SE with a 50% mortality. (Rossetti et al., 2006). In the study of Holtkamp and colleagues (2005), alcohol abuse was the cause of an equal number (3) of cases of refractory and non-refractory SE.

Drug toxicity or abuse is generally a common cause of SE in hospital-based studies but not in population-based studies, and the rate also varies markedly in different locations. 14% of SE cases in the San Fransisco study were due to drug toxicity (Lowenstein et al., 1993) and only 2% of cases in the Richmond study. (DeLorenzo et al., 1996). Iatrogenic drug-induced SE is also a problem. In a study of medically ill patients who developed SE approximately 1 month after admission, theophylline toxicity was found to be a primary or contributing cause in 25% of patients and was associated with an overall mortality rate of 61% (Delanty et al., 2001).

Refractory SE occurred in 50% of cases of drug toxicity in the San Fransisco study with a mortality rate of 40% (Lowenstein et al., 1993) Drug toxicity was responsible for one case each of refractory and non-refractory SE cases in the study of Holtkamp et al. (2005).

In summary, the reported frequency and prognosis for alcohol-related SE and for SE related to drug-abuse are very variable, but some studies have found significant mortality rates. In iatrogenic drug-induced SE, the mortality is also high but may be influenced by the underlying medical condition.

Anoxia/hypoxia and status epilepticus

Hypoxia, due in adults usually to survival after cardiac arrest, can result in deep coma with myoclonic jerking, and this is assumed by some authorities, but not all, to be a form of "status epilepticus" (see Shorvon 1994). This was the cause of SE in 13% of adult cases in the Richmond study and was associated with a significant mortality. (DeLorenzo et al., 1996). Hypoxia was the cause of 12% of cases of refractory SE in an analysis of 193 cases by Claassen and colleagues (2002).

In a study of 166 postanoxic survivors of cardiac arrest treated with hypothermia, postanoxic SE was present in 24% with a mortality rate of 80% compared to the overall mortality rate of 71% ($p < 0.001$). Post-anoxic SE was associated with a higher mortality regardless of the type of acute cardiac rhythm or hypothermia treatment. (Rossetti A et al., 2007).

In the large study of mortality in convulsive SE by Koubeissi and Alshekhlee (2007), hypoxia-ischaemic brain injury-associated SE was the strongest predictor of mortality with an odds ratio of 9.85 (CI 6.63-14.6). Other studies (Mayer et al., 2002; Rossetti et al., 2004) have shown hypoxia-related SE to have a significant mortality rate and to be the cause of 3 cases of refractory and none of non-refractory SE in the study of Holtkamp and colleagues(2005).

In summary, in cases of myoclonic coma, the SE is almost inevitably refractory, and is associated with a very high mortality rate.

Trauma and status epilepticus

Trauma was the aetiology for 5% of cases in the San Fransisco study with 37% developing refractory SE, all of whom had a good outcome. (Lowenstein et al., 1993). Trauma was responsible for less then 5% of cases in the Richmond study with a 20% mortality (DeLorenzo et al., 1996). Trauma was responsible for 1/31 cases of refractory SE in a study by Rossetti and colleagues (2006), who survived. Post-traumatic brain damage was responsible for 2 cases of NRSE (4.3% of total) and no cases of refractory SE in the study of Holtkamp and colleagues (2005).

In summary, acute trauma is not a common cause of SE and seems largely to result in non-refractory SE with a favourable outcome. How accurate a reflection this is of situations in which patients are anyway artificially ventilated after severe brain trauma and who have significant mortality and morbidity is unclear, and it is possible that ascertainment of such cases was not complete in the large reported series.

Metabolic disorders and status epilepticus

Metabolic disorders accounted for 15% of adult causes in the Richmond study (DeLorenzo et al., 1996) while 4% of cases were due to metabolic disorders in the San Fransisco study, 50% of whom developed refractory SE. In other series, metabolic disorders were the cause of 7% of refractory SE with 0% mortality (Rossetti et al., 2006), 11.5% with a mortality rate of 31% (Towne et al., 1994), 20% (Claassen et al., 2002a), 22% (Mayer et al., 2002) and 26% of RSE cases (8/31) with a mortality rate of 25% (Rossetti et al., 2004). 1 case of RSE was due to encephalopathy in hyperammonaemia in the study by Holtkamp et al. (2005).

However patients with metabolic disorders presenting with GCSE was significantly more likely to require mechanical ventilation (p < 0.0001) with a 3-fold increase in mortality for those requiring mechanical ventilation compared to those who did not (7.43% vs 2.22%, odds ratio 2.79) (Koubeissi et al., 2007).

In summary, acute metabolic disorders are not uncommon causes of SE (10-15%) with a significant mortality rate (20-30%) and an increased risk of mechanical ventilation in acute metabolic disturbance related SE, which is itself an independent risk factor for poorer outcome.

Cerebral tumour and status epilepticus

Tumours were the cause of 7/154 cases in the San Fransisco study causing one case of refractory SE and with a good outcome in all cases (Lowenstein et al., 1993). Tumours were the cause of 5% of cases of SE in the study of Mayer and colleagues (2002), and 4.4% with a mortality rate of 36.4% in the study of Towne et al. (1994). Rossetti et al. (2006) found that tumours were responsible for 14/196 cases of SE in a population-based study with a mortality rate of 20%, and 2/31 cases of refractory SE in a hospital-based study with 0% mortality (Rosseti et al., 2004). In the study of Holtkamp and colleagues (2005), primary brain tumour was responsible for 2 cases of non-refractory SE (4.3% of total) and one case of refractory SE (2.8%) while cerebral metastasis were responsible for 3 cases of non-refractory SE (4.3%) and 2 cases of refractory SE (5.5%).

In summary, primary brain tumours or cerebral tumours are an uncommon cause of SE, perhaps reflecting their subacute or chronic rather than acute nature, and are more likely to be non-refractory than refractory.

Status epilepticus and antiepileptic drug reduction or withdrawal

In the systemic review by Claassen and colleagues (2002) on the treatment of refractory SE, of 193 patients in 28 studies, 34% had a prior history of epilepsy.

A documented nontherapeutic anticonvulsant blood levels at the time of presentation with SE was attributed as the cause of SE in 34% in the Richmond study but associated with a low mortality (4%) (DeLorenzo et al., 1996). Similarly, in the San Francisco Hospital Study, 25% of cases of SE were related to withdrawal of AEDs, with 90% of patients having a good outcome (defined as unchanged from baseline, or mild neurologic deficits that allowed independent living) such that the authors conclude that "[...] patients with a history of epilepsy who develop SE because of anticonvulsant drug withdrawal or breakthrough seizures can be expected to respond well to acute anticonvulsants" (Lowenstein et al., 1993).

Two studies have looked at factors and predictors for the development of refractory. v. non-refractory SE. Holtkamp et al. (2005), in their study of 83 episodes of SE (43% refractory, and 57% non-refractory) found that low levels of AEDs were the primary cause of the SE in 27.7% of the non-refractory cases but none of the refractory cases (p < 0.001) allowing the authors to conclude that "SE caused by insufficient levels of AEDs is usually not refractory". Mayer et al. (2002) found that low AED levels or a recent change in medication was found in 31% of cases, of whom 78% of cases were non-refractory (Mayer et al., 2002). In their study looking at treatment of refractory SE with propofol in 31 cases, 5 cases were found to be due to AED withdrawal, all of whom had a good outcome (Rossetti et al., 2004).

Overall we can conclude that the reduction or withdrawal of antiepileptic drugs is a relatively common cause of SE in patients with a prior history of epilepsy, but that this is very rarely refractory. Furthermore, even when drug reduction or withdrawal does causes refractory SE, there is a low associated mortality.

■ Age and status epilepticus

The nature of SE, its outcome and "refractoriness" differ with age. One important reason for this is the confounding effect of aetiology, and the range of aetiologies of status varies considerably with age.

In children, febrile illness, with or without infection, is a common cause of SE, accounting for 32% of all cases in the North London study by Chin and colleagues (2006). The mortality of febrile SE, in a review of the published literature over the last 15 years found that febrile SE has a low mortality (14 out of 876 patients with febrile SE; 1.6%) and this has fallen significantly from the early 1970s probably due to early and aggressive treatment of SE (Chungath and Shorvon 2008). In a follow-up of 613 children diagnosed with epilepsy over 8 years, 58 (9.5%) had one or more episodes of SE (usually febrile SE). A previous episode of SE was strongly predicitive of subsequent episodes (18/56 [32.1%] vs 40/557 [7.2%]; p < 0.0001). The first episode of SE occurred at a median age of 2.5 years after diagnosis and younger age was an independent risk factor for developing SE (Berg et al., 2004). In the Dutch study of epilepsy in childhood, a total of 494 children with newly diagnosed epilepsy were followed up prospectively for 5 years. SE occurred in 47 (9.5%) and SE was the first seizure in 32 (78%). Termission remission or mortality was not significantly worse in children with SE (Stroinlk et al., 2007).

Analysis of a cohort of 193 children with SE (mean age 5 years) causes were classified as idiopathic in 46, febrile in 46, acute symptomatic in 45 and progressive neurologic in 11. All 7 deaths occurred in the progressive neurologic group and of the 186 survivors, new neurologic deficits were found in 17 (9.1%). Fifteen of the 17 sequelae occurred in children with acute or progressive neurologic deficits while only 2 cases occurred in the 137 children with other causes (idiopathic or febrile). Thirty-two per cent of children had a prior history of unprovoked seizures and of the 125 surviving children with no previous history of seizures, 30% subsequently had a further unprovoked seizure (Maytal et al., 1989).

In an retrospective study of SE in 154 children from a single institution, 60 (39%) had refractory status defined as seizures lasting more than 60 minutes and unresponsive to benzodiazepines and at least one IV antiepileptic drug. Refractory SE was more likely to occur (with a significance level of P = < 0.001), in patients with: a family history of seizures, higher seizure frequency, higher number of maintenance AEDs, non-convulsive SE and focal or electrographic seizures on initial EEG. Predictors for poor outcome in both groups were long seizure duration (p < 0.001), acute symptomatic aetiology (p = 0.04) which included causes like acute metabolic disorders (32.5%), encephalitis (25%), acute brain trauma (12.5%), stroke (12.5%), hypoxia-ischaemic encephalopathy (10%) and AED noncompliance (9%), non-convulsive SE (p = 0.001) and age at admission < 5 years at admission (p = 0.05). The number of children who returned to baseline was significantly less in those with RSE (66.6% vs 82.9%; p = 0.05) and they had a higher risk of developing a new deficit (71.4% vs 55.1%; p = 0.0001) or subsequent epilepsy (30.6% vs 16%; p = 0.004) (Lambrechtsen et al., 2008).

For children who develop refractory SE, prognosis is poor with high mortality and morbidity as evidenced in a study of 22 children with refractory SE (Sahin et al., 2001). The mortality rate of 32% (7/22) and 53% of survivors (8/15) developed subsequent seizures. Prognosis was related to aetiology with the worst prognosis in the acute symptomatic group where out of 8 children, 3 died and 5 developed a neurological deficit or seizures with none returning to baseline. (all cases presumed or confirmed encephalitis). Other causes associated with a poor outcome were CNS lymphoproliferative disease, brainstem neoplasm, Alpers disease, MCAD disease and previous haemorrhage. On the other hand, those with a previous diagnosis of epilepsy with breakthrough seizures had a much more favourable prognosis.

Sub-analysis by age found that the youngest (< 3 years: 3 died, 1 new deficit, 0 return to baseline) had the worst prognosis compared to older groups (3-10 years: 3 died, 6 new deficit, 3 RTB; > 10 years: 1 died, 1 new deficit, 4 RTB) and these findings are similar to those of others (Maytal et al., 1989; Lambrechtsen et al., 2008).

The prognosis of SE in the adult population is poorer as judged by mortality in the Richmond study where the adult mortality rate was 14% compared to 3% in the paediatric population. The difference is more apparently in the over 60s with a mortality rate of 38% (DeLorenzo et al., 1996). The main reason is largely the increased frequency in adults of systematic metabolic disorders, stroke, and progressive symptomatic disorders such as tumour and dementia. In an analysis of prognosis of SE in 96 cases, Rossetti et al. found that in those aged = 65 the mortality rate was 29% compared to an overall mortality rate of 15.6% and accounted for 60% of all deaths. On multivariate analysis to predict death, age = 65 had a odd ratio of 5.41 (p = 0.02) (Rossetti et al., 2006).

Towne et al. found that mortality rates increase with increasing age [Age (yr) 16-30: Mortality (%): 12.5; 30-60: 15.2; 60-: 32.3] (Towne et al., 1994). In an analysis of predictors of functional disability and mortality after SE in 74 patients, Claassen et al. (2002b) found that on multiple logistic regression analysis that increased age was predictive of death (Odds Ratio 1.1, p = 0.02). Koubeissi and Alshekhlee (2007) found that mortality rates for Generalised Convulsive Status Epilepticus increased with age, with the lowest rate (0.67%) for those aged $\leqslant$ 10 years and increasing steadily with age to mortality rates of 6.78% for those aged 61-70, 8.13% for those aged 71-80 and 10.15% for those aged > 80.

In summary, the refractoriness of the SE and its prognosis and mortality rate vary with age, but this variation is largely a reflection of the differing underlying aetiologies at different ages. There is a generally worse outcome for younger children than older children, and in those with an acute symptomatic cause. For those children who develop refractory SE, prognosis is poor with high mortality and morbidity and high rates of subsequent epilepsy. In adults, increasing age is associated with a poorer prognosis with increased risk of functional morbidity and mortality and therefore more likely to be associated with refractory SE. Prognosis for those aged > 80 years with SE is especially poor.

▪ The duration of status epilepticus and its relation to outcome

Since the landmark studies of Aicardi and colleagues (1970), it has been recognised that the longer the seizure continues, the more difficult it is to control and the worse the outcome. This has been confirmed in numerous experimental studies, for instance related to acute changes in GABAergic receptor function, excessive NMDA receptor mediated transmission, mitochondrial changes and receptor trafficking (Kapur & MacDonald, 1997; Chen & Wasterlain, 2006; Shorvon & Trinka, 2007). The recognition of this point has lead to earlier and more aggressive treatment (and indeed is the main reason for the shortening of the minimum time period necessary to define SE). One example is the study of Towne and colleagues (1994) who found that a seizure duration of > 1 hour was associated with a mortality rate of 32% compared with a mortality rate of 2.7% for seizure duration < 1 hour. In the San Fransisco study, a correlation for poorer outcome and the duration of seizures was observed in all 4 major aetiological groups (good outcome: n = 115: duration: 2.4 hrs; poor outcome: n = 34: duration 18.2 hrs; p = 0.0001) but only achieved statistical significance in 2 groups (alcohol-related and CNS infection) (Lowenstein et al., 1993).

In summary, the longer the seizure persists (typically > 1 hour), the more likely is the seizure to be unresponsive to antiepileptic drug therapy, the higher is the mortality and the worse is the prognosis in survivors.

▪ Conclusion

From this review, the following general conclusions can be drawn:

1. The published definitions of "refractoriness" are unsatisfactory and essentially arbitrary (discussed above). In our view, the concept of "refractory" status should be avoided. The severity of the condition can be reflected better by consideration of its outcome.

2. What is clear is that the most important variable which influences "refractoriness" (and outcome) is the underlying aetiology.

3. Acute structural brain disorders resulting in SE in previously non-epileptic patients are particularly likely to be refractory.

4. In acute SE, in previously non-epileptic patients, without obvious cause, the SE is less likely to be refractory, and the prognosis is much better.

5. In patients with previous epilepsy, a common cause of SE is injudicious drug reduction/withdrawal. Such cases are less likely to be refractory, and have a good ultimate outcome.

6. The duration of the SE is also a factor influencing "refractoriness" and outcome. This is confirmed in experimental and clinical studies, and reflects the rapid physiological changes that occur as seizure activity progresses. Because of this, it is important to apply urgent early therapy in all cases of convulsive SE.

7. Age is also a factor influencing refractoriness and outcome, but this is largely due to the confounding influence of underlying aetiology, which varies with age.

Acknowledgments

SDS is supported by an MRC co-operative group grant. Neither author has any conflict of interests to declare.

References

Aicardi J, Chevrie JJ. Convulsive status epilepticus in infants and children. *Epilepsia* 1970; 11: 187.

Berg AT, Shinnar S, Testa FM et al. Status Epilepticus after the initial diagnosis of epilepsy in children. *Neurology* 2004; 63: 1027-34.

Bleck TP. Convulsive disorders: status epilepticus. *Clin Neuropharmacol* 1991; 14: 191-8.

Bleck TP. Transatlantic similarities and differences in the management of status epilepticus. *Epilepsia* 2008: 49 (in press).

Cascino GD. Generalized convulsive status epilepticus. *Mayo Clin Proc* 1996; 71: 787-92.

Chen JWY, Wasterlain CG. Status epilepticus: pathophysiology and management in adults. *Lancet Neurol* 2006; 5: 246-56.

Chin RF, Neville BG, Peckham C, Bedford H, Wade A, Scott RC. Incidence, cause, and short-term outcome of convulsive status epilepticus in childhood: prospective population-based study. *Lancet* 2006; 368: 222-9.

Chungath M and Shorvon SD. The outcome of febrile seizures. *Nature Clinical Practice Neurology* 2008 (in press).

Claassen J, Hirsch LJ, Emerson RG, Mayer SA. Treatment of Refractory Status Epilepticus with Phenobarbital, Propofol, or Midazolam: A Systemic Review. *Epilepsia* 2002a; 43: 146-53.

Claassen J, Lokin JK, Fitzsimmons BFM, Mendelsohn BA, Mayer SA. Predictors of functional disability and mortality after status epilepticus. *Neurology* 2002b; 58: 139-42.

Claassen J, Hirsch LJ, Mayer SA. Treatment of status epilepticus: a survey of neurologists. *J Neurol Sci* 2003; 211: 37-41.

Coeytaux A, Jallon P, Galobardes B et al. Incidence of status epilepticus in French-speaking Switzerland: (EPISTAR). *Neurology* 2000; 55: 693-7.

Commission on Classification and Terminology of the International League against Epilepsy. Proposal for revised clinical and electroencephalographic classification of epileptic seizures. From the Commission on Classification and Terminology of the International League Against Epilepsy. *Epilepsia* 1981; 22: 489-501.

Delanty N, French JA, Labar DR, Pedley TA, Rowan AJ. Status epilepticus arising de novo in hospitalized patients: an analysis of 41 patients. *Seizure* 2001; 10: 116-9.

DeLorenzo RJ, Hauser WA, Towne AR, Boggs JG, Pellock JM, Penberthy L, Garnett L, Fortner CA, Ko D. A prospective, population-based epidemiologic study of status epilepticus in Richmond, Virginia. *Neurology* 1996; 46: 1029-35.

Gastaut H, Roger J, Loh H ed. *Les états de mal épileptiques*. Paris: Masson, 1967.

Glaser CA, Gilliam S, Honarmand S, Tureen JH, Lowenstein DH, Anderson LJ et al. Refractory Status Epilepticus in Suspected Encephalitis. *Neurocrit Care* 2007 Dec 21.

Hanley DF, Kross JF. Use of midazolam in the treatment of refractory status epilepticus. *Clin Ther* 1998; 20: 1093-105.

Hesdorffer DC, Logroscino G, Cascino G, Annegers JF, Hauser WA. Incidence of status epilepticus in Rochester, Minnesota, 1965-1984. *Neurology* 1998; 50: 735-41.

Holtkamp M, Mashur F, Harms L, Einhaupl KM, Meierkord H, Buckheim K. The management of refractory generalised convulsive and complex partial status epilepticus in three European countries: a survey among epileptologists and critical care neurologists. *J Neurol Neurosurg Psychiatry* 2003; 74: 1095-9.

Holtkamp M, Othman J, Buchheim K, Meierkord H. Predictors and prognosis of refractory status epilepticus treated in a neurological intensive care unit. *J Neurol Neurosurg Psychiatry* 2005; 76: 534-9.

Kapur J, Macdonald RL. Rapid seizure-induced reduction of benzodiazepine and Zn2+ sensitivity of hippocampal dentate granule cell GABA A receptors. *J Neurosci* 1997; 17: 7532-40.

Knake S, Rochon J, Fleischer S *et al.* Status epilepticus after stroke is associated with increased long-term case fatality. *Epilepsia* 2006; 47: 2020-6.

Knake S, Rosenov F, Vescovi M, *et al.* Incidence of status epilepticus in adults in Germany: a prospective, population-based study. *Epilepsia* 2001; 42: 714-8.

Koubeissi M, Alshekhlee A. In-hospital mortality of generalized convulsive status epilepticus: A large US sample. *Neurology* 2007; 69: 886-93.

Lambrechßen FA, Buchhalter JA. Aborted and refractory status epilepticus in children: A comparative analysis. *Epilepsia* 2008; 49: 615-25.

Lin JJ, Lin KL, Wang HS, Hsia SH, Wu CT. Analysis of status epilepticus related presumed encephalitis in children. *Eur J Paediatr Neurol* 2008; 12: 32-7.

Lowenstein DH, Alldredge BK. Status epilepticus at an urban public hospital in the 1980s. *Neurology* 1993; 43: 483-8.

Lowenstein DH, Alldredge BK. Status Epilepticus. *N Engl J Med.* 1998; 338: 970-96.

Lowenstein DH, Bleck T, Macdonald RL. It's Time to Revise the Definition of Status Epilepticus. *Epilepsia* 1999; 40: 120-22.

Mayer SA, Claassen J, Lokin J, Mendelsohn F, Dennis LJ, Fitzsimmons BF. Refractory Status Epilepticus: frequency, risk factors, and impact on outcome. *Arch Neurol* 2002; 59: 205-10.

Maytal J, Shinnar S, Moshé SL, Alvarez LA. Low morbidity and mortality of status epilepticus in children. *Paediatrics* 1989; 83: 323-31.

Prasad A, Worrall BB, Bertram EH, Bleck TP. Propofol and midazolam in the treatment of refractory status epilepticus. *Epilepsia* 2001; 42: 380-6.

Rossetti AO, Reichhart MD, Schaller MD, Despland PA, Bogousslavsky J. Propofol Treatment of Refractory Status Epilepticus: A Study of 31 Episodes. *Epilepsia* 2004; 45: 757-63.

Rossetti AO, Logroscino G, Bromfield EB. Refractory Status Epilepticus: Effect of Treatment Aggressiveness on Prognosis. *Arch Neurol* 2005; 62: 1698-702.

Rossetti AO, Hurwitz S, Logroscino G, Bromfield EB. Prognosis of status epilepticus: role of aetiology, age, and consciousness impairment at presentation. *J Neurol Neurosurg Psychiatry* 2006; 77: 611-5.

Rossetti AO, Logroscino G, Liaudet L *et al.* Status Epilepticus: An independent outcome predictor after cerebral anoxia. *Neurology* 2007; 69: 255-60.

Rumbach L, Sablot D, Berger E, Tatu L, Vullier F, Moulin T. Status epilepticus in stroke: Report on a hospital-based stroke cohort. *Neurology* 2000; 54: 350-4.

Sahin M, Menache C, Holmes GL, Riviello JR. Outcome of Severe Refractory Status Epilepticus in Children. *Epilepsia* 2001; 42: 1461-7.

Sahin M, Menache CC, Holmes GL, Rivello JR. Prolonged treatment for acute symptomatic refractory status epilepticus: Outcome in children. *Neurology* 2003; 61: 398-401.

Shinnar S, Berg AT, Moshe SL, Shinnar R. How long do new-onset seizures in children last? *Ann Neurol* 2001; 49: 659-64.

Shorvon S. *Status Epilepticus: its clinical features and treatment in children and adults.* Cambridge, UK: Cambridge University Press, 1994.

Shorvon S. The management of status epilepticus. *J Neurol Neurosurg Psychiatry* 2001; 70 (suppl 2): 1122-7.

Shorvon SD and Trinka E. The Proceedings of the First London Colloquium on Status Epilepticus. *Epilepsia* 2007; 48 (suppl 8): 1-109.

Shorvon SD. Epidemiology: Status Epilepticus. In: Schwartzkroin P ed. *Encyclopedia of basic science of epilepsy*. Elsevier: New York. 2008a (in press).

Shorvon S, Baulac M, Cross H, Trinka E, Walker M. The drug treatment of status epilepticus in Europe – consensus document from a workshop at the 1_{st} London Colloquium on Status Epilepticus. *Epilepsia* 2008; 49 (in press).

Strecker MM, Kramer TH, Raps, EC, O'Meeghan R, Dulaney E, Skaar DJ. Treatment of refractory status epilepticus with profolol. *Epilepsia* 1998; 39: 18-26.

Stroink H, Geerts AT, van Donselaar CA *et al*. Status epilepticus in children with epilepsy: Dutch study of epilepsy in childhood. *Epilepsia* 2007; 48: 1708-15.

Theodore W, Porter R, Albert P *et al*. The secondarily generalized tonic-clonic seizure: a videotape analysis. *Neurology* 1994; 44: 1403-7.

Towne AR, Pellock JM, Ko D, Delorenzo RJ. Determinants of Mortality in Status Epilepticus. *Epilepsia* 1994; 35: 27-34.

Treatment of convulsive status epilepticus. Recommendations of the Epilepsy Foundation of America's Working Group on Status Epilepticus. *JAMA* 1993; 270: 854-9.

Treiman DM, Meyers PD, Walton NY, *et al*. A comparison of four treatments for generalized convulsive status epilepticus: Veterans Affairs Status Epilepticus Cooperative Study Group. *N Engl J Med* 1998; 339: 792-8.

Velioglu SK, Özmenoglu M, Cavit B, Alioglu Z. Status Epilpeticus After Stroke. *Stroke* 2001; 32: 1169-72.

Vignatelli L, Tonan C, D'Alessandro R. Incidence and short-term prognosis of status epilepticus in adults in Bologna, Italy. *Epilepsia* 2003; 44: 964-8.

Yaffe K, Lowenstein DH. Prognostic factors of pentobarbital therapy for refractory generalized status epilepticus. *Neurology* 1993; 43: 895-900.

Current knowledge on basic mechanisms of drug resistance

Wolfgang Löscher

Department of Pharmacology, Toxicology, and Pharmacy, University of Veterinary Medicine Hannover, and Center for Systems Neuroscience, Hannover, Germany

---

Pharmacoresistance is the major problem in epilepsy therapy. This is defined as the persistence of seizures despite treatment with a range of antiepileptic drugs (AEDs) with different mechanisms of action used singly or in combination at maximum tolerated doses. Consequently, there is a pressing need to develop more effective treatments and strategies. For this goal, we need to understand the mechanisms underlying drug resistance. A number of plausible hypotheses have been proposed *(Figure 1)*, including:

(1) acquired alterations to the structure and/or functionality of target ion channels and neurotransmitter receptors *(target hypothesis)*;

(2) inadequate penetration of AEDs across the blood-brain barrier *(transporter hypothesis)*;

(3) an inherent resistance governed by genetic variants of proteins involved in the pharmacokinetics and pharmacodynamics of AED action *(gene variant hypothesis)*; and

(4) structural brain alterations and/or network changes (*e.g.*, hippocampal sclerosis) *(network hypothesis)*.

These hypotheses are almost exclusively been based on observations in surgically resected brain specimens from patients with drug resistant temporal lobe epilepsy (TLE) and data from animal models of TLE (Löscher & Potschka, 2005a,b; Schmidt & Löscher, 2005; Remy & Beck, 2006; Szoeke *et al.*, 2006). These four hypotheses, which are both plausible and based on a reasonable body of evidence, will be discussed in the following.

■ The target hypothesis

To exhibit antiepileptic activity, a drug must act on one or more target molecules in the brain. These targets include voltage-dependent ion channels, neurotransmitter receptors, and transporters or metabolic enzymes involved in the release, uptake and metabolism of neurotransmitters (Rogwaski & Löscher, 2004). The target hypothesis is primarily based on studies with carbamazepine on voltage-gated sodium channels in hippocampal neurons.

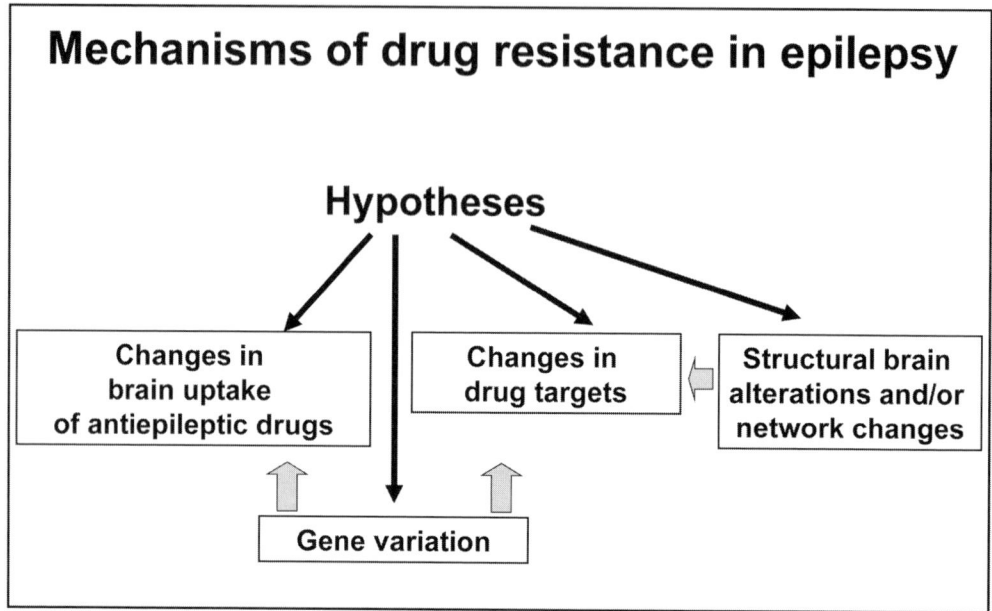

Figure 1. The four hypotheses of pharmacoresistance discussed in this review. The brain alterations underlying these hypotheses are not exclusive but may occur together in the same patient, thus explaining that patients with pharmacoresistant epilepsy are resistant to many, if not all AEDs, irrespective of differences in mechanism of action.

Voltage-gated Na^+ channels are ubiquitously expressed in excitable cells and appear to be targets for multiple first-line AEDs, including carbamazepine, phenytoin and lamotrigine. To my knowledge, Wytse Wadman's group was the first to report a loss of carbamazepine's modulatory effects on sodium channels in hippocampal neurons of patients with intractable epilepsy (Vreugdenhil et al., 1998). The latter group found that the modulation of sodium current inactivation by carbamazepine in hippocampal CA1 neurons from patients with TLE and mesial temporal sclerosis was only half of that encountered in neocortical neurons from the same patients, and only half of that encountered in CA1 neurons from patients without mesial temporal sclerosis (Vreugdenhil et al., 1998). Similar observations were obtained in the kindling model of TLE in that the carbamazepine-response of sodium channels of CA1 neurons isolated from the epileptic focus of fully kindled rats was only half of that in control rats (Vreugdenhil & Wadman, 1999).

More recently, Heinz Beck's group substantiated and extended these data by showing that the use-dependent block of voltage-dependent Na^+ channels of dentate granule cells by carbamazepine is completely lost in patients with carbamazepine-resistant TLE in comparison to patients clinically responsive to this AED (Remy et al., 2003a). In addition to the loss of use-dependent inhibition of Na^+ channels by carbamazepine, the fast recovery from inactivation of the fast Na^+ current was carbamazepine-insensitive in pharmacoresistant patients, whereas recovery was markedly slowed in cells from carbamazepine-responsive patients (Remy et al., 2003a). Consistent with these data from patients with intractable TLE, Remy et al. (2003a) also showed that use-dependent block of Na^+ channels by carbamazepine in dentate granule cells is absent in the pilocarpine rat model of TLE. Based on these data, the authors suggested that a loss of Na^+ channel drug sensitivity may explain the development of drug-resistant epilepsy. In a subsequent study in the rat pilocarpine model in TLE, Remy et al. (2003b) demonstrated that the effects of phenytoin on fast recovery from inactivation of Na$^+$ channels of hippocampal granule neurons were significantly reduced, though not as pronounced as observed with carbamazepine, substantiating the concept that reduced pharmacosensitivity of Na$^+$ channels may contribute to the development of drug resistance. In contrast to carbamazepine and phenytoin, lamotrigine slowed the time course of recovery from fast inactivation both in epileptic and control rats without significant inter-group difference (Remy et al., 2003b). In the pilocarpine model, a loss of sensitivity of sodium channels to carbamazepine and phenytoin was also found in hippocampal CA1 neurons, although the loss of AED-sensitivity was less pronounced in CA1 neurons than in dentate granule neurons (Schaub et al., 2007). Thus, the results of Beck and colleagues suggested that target mechanisms of drug resistance are cell type and AED specific.

Which mechanisms can account for altered sensitivity of Na$^+$ channels in CA1 or dentate granule cells in epileptic tissue? One possibility is that the subunit composition of these channels is altered, resulting in channels with lower AED sensitivity (Remy & Beck, 2006). Several changes in Na$^+$ subunit expression have been observed in both human and experimental epilepsy (Remy and Beck, 2006). For instance, in the pilocarpine model of TLE, the accessory β1 and β2 subunits were down-regulated, which was suggested to play a role in the altered pharmacosensitivity of Na$^+$ channels (Ellerkmann et al., 2003). This view is supported by a study of Lucas et al. (2005) showing that a mutation in the β1 subunit of the voltage-gated sodium channel results in a dramatic loss of channel sensitivity to phenytoin.

A critical question in studying target alterations in epilepsy is the relation of changes on the cellular level to AED sensitivity *in vivo*. While such a correlation has been observed in patients with TLE (Remy et al., 2003a; Jandova et al., 2006), such a correlative analysis has not yet been performed for the pilocarpine model of TLE, which has been used in most studies of Beck's group. We used the kindling model of TLE to study whether AED responders and nonresponders differ in pharmacological sensitivity of voltage-dependent sodium channels (Jeub et al., 2002). Responders and nonresponders were selected by repeated testing with phenytoin *in vivo*, followed by evaluation of phenytoin's *in vitro* effects on voltage-gated Na$^+$ channels of hippocampal CA1 neurons. The *in vivo* resistance to phenytoin was not associated with altered tonic block of Na$^+$ channels by phenytoin, but recovery from Na$^+$ channel inactivation and use-dependent blocking effects were not analyzed in this study (Jeub et al., 2002).

Apart from voltage-dependent Na$^+$ channels, other drug targets, such as GABA-mediated inhibition, may be altered in patients with intractable epilepsy. Using the rat pilocarpine model of TLE, Brooks-Kayal et al. (1998) demonstrated that expression of GABA$_A$ receptor subunit mRNAs is substantially altered in hippocampal dentate granule cells of pilocarpine-treated rats *vs* controls. These changes in GABA$_A$ receptor subunit expression correlated with profound alterations in receptor function and pharmacology (Brooks-Kayal et al., 1998; Coulter 2000; Coulter, 2001). In normal granule cells, GABA$_A$ receptors of dentate granule cells are insensitive to zinc which is released from mossy fibers and functions as a negative allosteric modulator of GABA$_A$ receptors. This zinc insensitivity of normal GABA$_A$ receptors is a result of high levels of expression of the α1 subunit in these cells (Coulter, 2000). In epileptic rats, expression of the α1 and β1 subunits decreases and expression of α4 and δ subunits increases, leading to an assembly of GABA$_A$ receptors that are strikingly zinc sensitive. In addition to the enhanced zinc sensitivity, GABA$_A$

receptors from the epileptic hippocampus loose their sensitivity to augmentation by the benzodiapine type site I modulator zolpidem (Cohen et al., 2003). Coulter (2000, 2001) has proposed that this temporal and spatial juxtaposition of these pathophysiological alterations may compromise normal "gatekeeper" function of the dentate gyrus through dynamic zinc-induced failure of inhibition, predisposing the hippocampal circuit to generate seizures. Of course, assuming that similar alterations in $GABA_A$ receptor function and pharmacology also take place in the epileptogenic human hippocampus, this could lead to reduced efficacy of AEDs acting *via* GABA-mediated inhibition.

We have recently used a rat model of TLE that allows selecting AED responsive and resistant rats for studying whether AED nonresponders differ from responders in expression and pharmacological sensitivity of $GABA_A$ receptors (Volk et al., 2006; Bethmann et al., 2008). In this model, spontaneous recurrent seizures develop after a status epilepticus induced by prolonged electrical stimulation of the basolateral amygdala. Prolonged daily administration of phenobarbital at maximum tolerable doses in epileptic rats of this model results in two subgroups, *i.e.*, a responder subgroup with control of seizures and a nonresponder subgroup without any significant reduction in seizure frequency. The resistance to phenobarbital extends to other AEDs, including phenytoin, thus resembling the multidrug type of AED resistance in patients with intractable TLE. This model thus offers unique approaches to the biological basis of refractoriness, particularly because pathological alterations in AED resistant such rats can be directly compared with those of rats that respond to AEDs. With respect to $GABA_A$ receptors, phenobarbital resistant rats strikingly differed from responsive rats in autoradiographic imaging of diazepam-sensitive and diazepam-insensitive $GABA_A$ receptor binding in the dentate gyrus with a significant shift to enhanced diazepam-insensitive binding in nonresponders (Volk et al., 2006). These diazepam-insensitive receptors likely contain the $\alpha 4$ and δ-subunit, which correspond to a major population mediating tonic inhibition in the dentate gyrus. To directly address this possibility, expression of various $GABA_A$ receptor subunits was determined in AED responders and nonresponders (Bethmann et al., 2008). In nonresponders, decreased expression of various subunits, including $\alpha 1$, $\beta 2/3$ and $\gamma 2$, was observed in CA1, CA2, CA3, and dentate gyrus, whereas much less widespread alterations were determined in responders. Furthermore, upregulation of the $\alpha 4$-subunit was observed in CA1 pyramidal cells of nonresponders. Phenobarbital's anticonvulsant effect is thought to be primarily related to enhancement of GABA-mediated inhibitory synaptic transmission *via* modulation of $GABA_A$ receptors (Rogawski and Löscher, 2004). Although the effects of barbiturates on the $GABA_A$ receptor depend largely on the β-subunit, their agonist activity is substantially influenced by the α-subunit subtype. The marked decreases in β- and α-subunits observed in phenobarbital-nonresponders are likely to reduce the effect of phenobarbital on $GABA_A$ receptors and thus could be involved in the lack of anticonvulsant efficacy of phenobarbital in these animals. These data substantiate the hypothesis that alterations in $GABA_A$ receptor subtypes may be involved in resistance to AEDs. Profound alterations in $GABA_A$ receptor subtype expression have also been reported in patients with AED-resistant TLE (Loup et al., 2000).

Further evidence that changes in $GABA_A$ receptors such as occurring during epileptogenesis can lead to drug resistance comes from a series of studies of Bob Macdonald's and Claude Wasterlain's groups using the pilocarpine model (Kapur & Macdonald, 1997; Mazarati et al., 1998; Macdonald & Kapur, 1999; Jones et al., 2002). The latter groups demonstrated that during a pilocarpine-induced status epilepticus there is a substantial reduction of potency for termination of seizures by AEDs that enhance $GABA_A$-mediated inhibition, such as benzodiazepines and phenobarbital. This progressive development of pharmacoresistance during a sustained status epilepticus is paralleled by alterations in the functional properties of dentate granule cell $GABA_A$ receptors. The authors concluded that rapid modulation of $GABA_A$ receptors during status epilepticus may result in pharmacoresistance to AEDs that enhance $GABA_A$ receptor-mediated inhibition (Jones et al., 2003). More recently, Goodkin et al. (2005) and Naylor et al. (2005) showed that internalization of $GABA_A$ receptors, i.e., trafficking of these receptors from the synaptic membrane to submembranous compartments, causes a decrease in the number of functional postsynaptic $GABA_A$ receptors that is likely to explain the pharmacoresistance to GABAmimetic AEDs in status epilepticus.

Apart from alterations in $GABA_A$ receptor subunit expression and receptor trafficking, a third potential mechanism to explain loss of pharmacological sensitivity of these receptors is a shift from adult inhibitory to neonatal excitatory $GABA_A$ receptors, recapitulating ontogenesis (Ben-Ari and Homes, 2005). Such a shift in GABAergic response polarity from hyperpolarizing to depolarizing has been described in human epileptic neurons recorded in the subiculum of hippocampal slices obtained from resections in patients suffering from mesial TLE (Cohen et al., 2002). This shift is thought to be a result of increased intraneuronal Cl^- levels, caused by increased neuronal expression of NKCC1, an inwardly directed Na^+ K^+ $2Cl^-$ cotransporter that facilitates the accumulation of intracellular Cl^-, and downregulation of KCC2, an outwardly directed K^+ Cl^- cotransporter (Köhling, 2002; Ben-Ari & Holmes, 2005; Rivera et al., 2005; Palma et al., 2006). Upregulation of NKCC1 and downregulation of KCC2 in the hippocampus have been described both in patients with TLE and the kindling model of TLE (Okabe et al., 2002; Rivera et al., 2002; Okabe et al., 2003; Palma et al., 2006; Huberfeld et al., 2007). We currently plan to examine whether the brain expression of these chloride transporters differs in phenobarbital responsive and resistant epileptic rats.

As a proof-of-principle for the target hypothesis, it will be important to demonstrate that AED-resistant subgroups of patients differ from AED-responsive subgroups in their AED-target sensitivity. Such a proof-of-principle is difficult to obtain in patients, because, in contrast to patients with intractable epilepsy, patients responding to AEDs in general do not undergo surgical treatment for their epilepsy. Although Remy et al. (2003a) obtained surgical "reference" specimens from two patients who responded well to treatment with carbamazepine for comparison with 10 patients with carbamazepine-resistant TLE, differences in age, gender, history of epilepsy and AED treatment and various other variables may form a bias for such a comparison. As illustrated by our recent studies, animal models of TLE allowing to select age-matched AED responders and nonresponders may be useful to further evaluate the target hypothesis. Although the target hypothesis is a novel and biologically plausible theory to explain drug resistance, the fact that most patients resistant to AED treatment are resistant to a broad range of AEDs with different mechanisms of action suggest that other, less specific mechanisms contribute to drug resistance. The most prominent hypothesis in this respect, the transporter hypothesis, which was first explored in chemotherapy-resistant cancer, currently attracts growing interest as a putative mechanism to explain drug resistance in epilepsy by reduced penetration of AEDs into the brain.

■ The multidrug transporter hypothesis

The importance of (multi)drug efflux transporters such as P-glycoprotein (P-gp) in disease processes and treatment has become increasingly evident in recent years (Leonard et al., 2003; Lee & Bendayan, 2004; Löscher & Potschka, 2005a,b). Drug efflux transporters have a major impact on the pharmacological behavior of most clinically used drugs, critically affecting drug absorption, disposition, and elimination in the body (Schinkel & Jonker, 2003). Furthermore, such transporters are involved in the emergence of "multidrug resistance" (MDR) which plays an important role in the failure of treatments of tumors, infectious diseases and several brain disorders, including epilepsy (Leonard et al., 2003; Lee & Bendayan, 2004; Löscher & Potschka, 2005a,b). P-gp, the encoded product of the human *multidrug-resistance-1* (*MDR1*; *ABCB1*) gene, is of particular clinical relevance in that this transporter has a broad substrate specificity (which led to the term "multidrug transporter"), including a variety of structurally divergent drugs in clinical use today (Fromm, 2004). Furthermore, P-gp is expressed by tissues with excretory function (small intestine, liver and kidney) and at blood-tissue barriers (blood-brain barrier [BBB], blood-testis barrier and placenta), thus limiting drug entry into the body after oral administration, promoting drug elimination into bile and urine, and limiting drug penetration into sensitive tissues such as the brain (Fromm, 2004).

In the BBB, multidrug transporters such as P-gp, members of the multidrug resistance protein (MRP) family and breast cancer related protein (BCRP) are located in brain capillary endothelial cells that form the BBB and combine to reduce the brain penetration of many drugs (Sun et al., 2003; Begley, 2004; Hermann et al., 2006). This phenomenon of multidrug resistance is a major hurdle when it comes to the delivery of therapeutics to the brain, including brain cancer chemotherapy. Therefore, the development of strategies for bypassing the influence of these drug efflux transporters, for the design of effective drugs that are not substrates, and for the development of inhibitors for the transporters has become a high imperative for the pharmaceutical industry (Begley, 2004).

Tishler et al. (1995) were the first to report that brain expression of *MDR1*, which encodes P-gp in humans, is markedly increased in the majority of patients with medically intractable partial (mostly temporal lobe) epilepsy. *MDR1* mRNA levels were determined in brain specimens removed from patients during resective surgery for intractable epilepsy and were compared with normal brain control specimens obtained from patients undergoing removal of arteriovenous malformations. In line with enhanced *MDR1* expression in epileptogenic brain tissue, immunohistochemistry for P-gp showed increased staining in capillary endothelium and astrocytes. Tishler et al. (1995) proposed that P-gp may play a clinically significant role by limiting access of AEDs to the brain parenchyma, so that increased P-gp expression may contribute to the refractoriness of seizures in patients with treatment-resistant epilepsy.

Following the report by Tishler et al. in 1995, the finding of *MDR1*/P-gp overexpression in epileptogenic brain tissue of patients with drug-refractory epilepsy was confirmed by several other groups (cf. Kwan & Brodie, 2005; Löscher & Potschka, 2005a,b; Schmidt & Löscher, 2005). Furthermore, it was shown that, in addition to P-gp, several MRPs, but not BCRP, are overexpressed in brain capillary endothelial cells and/or astrocytes of pharmacoresistant patients (cf. Kwan & Brodie, 2005; Löscher & Potschka, 2005b; Schmidt & Löscher, 2005). In some of these studies, the overexpression of drug efflux transporters in astrocytes appeared most marked around blood vessels. In view of data indicating that the endothelial barrier function of the BBB is transiently disrupted during seizures (cf. Oby & Janigro, 2006), overexpression of multidrug transporters in astroglial end-feet covering the blood vessels may represent a "second barrier" under these conditions (Abbott et al., 2002; Sisodiya et al., 2002). Sisodiya et al. (2002) proposed that overexpressed multidrug transporters lower the extracellular concentration of AEDs in the vicinity of the epileptogenic pathology and thereby render the epilepsy caused by these pathologies resistant to AED treatment.

An open question is whether the overexpression of P-gp and MRPs in epileptogenic brain tissue of patients with intractable epilepsy is intrinsic (constitutive) or acquired, *i.e.*, a consequence of epilepsy, of uncontrolled seizures, of chronic treatment with AEDs, or of combinations of these factors. Because treatment-resistant patients have the same extent of neurotoxic side effects under AED treatment as patients who are controlled by AEDs, the overexpression of drug transporters in treatment-resistant patients is most likely restricted to the epileptic focus or circuit. This is substantiated by a previous study of Sisodiya *et al.* (2002) in which overexpression of P-gp and MRP1 was found in epileptogenic tissue but not in adjacent normal tissue of the same patients.

In animal models of TLE, such as the kindling and kainate models, a transient overexpression of P-gp was found in brain capillary endothelial cells, astroglia and neurons following seizures (*cf.* Löscher & Potschka, 2005b; Schmidt & Löscher, 2005), indicating that seizures themselves can induce overexpression of drug transporters. This could explain the observation that one of the major predictors of pharmacoresistance is high seizure frequency (or density) prior to initiation of treatment (Regesta & Tanganelli, 1999). However, constitutive rather than induced or acquired overexpression of multidrug transporters has been reported in patients with malformations of cortical development (Sisodiya *et al.*, 1999). In addition to intrinsic or acquired overexpression of multidrug transporters in the BBB of patients with epilepsy, polymorphisms in transporter genes may play a role in pharmacoresistance (see below). Furthermore, alterations in expression and functionality of multidrug transporters in patients with intractable epilepsy need not necessarily be restricted to the brain, but could also occur in other tissues, such as the small intestine, where P-gp is thought to form a barrier against entrance of drugs from the intestinal lumen into the bloodstream, thereby limiting their oral bioavailability (Fromm, 2004). In this respect, it is interesting to note that Lazarowski *et al.* (2007) have reported persistent subtherapeutic plasma levels of AEDs (including phenytoin and phenobarbital) despite aggressive and continuous AED administration in patients with refractory epilepsy associated with overexpression of *MDR1*.

In view of the emerging evidence that multidrug transporters are overexpressed in epileptogenic brain tissue, particularly in capillary endothelial cells and astrocytes contributing to BBB permeability, it is of major clinical interest to evaluate whether AEDs are substrates for these transporters. Only then, overexpression of P-gp or MRPs could critically contribute to pharmacoresistance in epilepsy. The first indication that AEDs are substrates for P-gp came from experiments of Tishler *et al.* (1995) who found that intracellular phenytoin levels in a *MDR1*-expressing neuroectodermal cell line were only one fourth that in *MDR1*-negative cells, suggesting that P-gp significantly contributes to the transport of phenytoin out of the cell. Phenytoin transport by P-gp was also demonstrated in a kidney epithelial cell line transfected with the rodent *mdr1a* cDNA, which could be blocked by the P-gp inhibitor PSC833 (Schinkel *et al.*, 1996).

More recently, Rizzi *et al.* (2002) demonstrated that *mdr1a/b* knockout mice, which lack P-gp, exhibit a significant, 50% increase in phenytoin levels in the hippocampus compared to wildtype mice. *Mdr1* knockout mice were also used to demonstrate P-gp transport of carbamazepine (Rizzi *et al.*, 2002) and topiramate (Sills *et al.*, 2002). By using a rat microdialysis model with microdialysis probes in both brain hemispheres and local (cerebral) inhibition of multidrug transporters in one hemisphere, we have previously demonstrated that several major AEDs are substrates for either P-gp or MRPs or both (Löscher & Potschka, 2005b). Overall, current data from these different experimental approaches described above indicate that at least eight major AEDs (phenytoin, phenobarbital, carbamazepine, oxcarbazepine, lamotrigine, gabapentin, felbamate, topiramate) are substrates for P-gp and some of them (phenytoin, carbamazepine, valproate) seem also to be transported by MRPs at the BBB (Löscher & Potschka, 2005b).

However, more recent data from our group demonstrated species differences in the transport of AEDs by P-gp in that significant transport could be demonstrated with rodent but not human P-gp in an *in vitro* transport assay (Baltes et al., 2007). In this respect, it is important to consider that most AEDs are highly lipophilic, which could conceal asymmetrical transport in *in vitro* transport assays that are commonly used for identifying P-gp substrates. This prompted us to modify such assay in a way that allows evaluating active transport independently of the passive permeability component, demonstrating transport of several major AEDs, including phenytoin, phenobarbital, and lamotrigine, by human P-gp (Luna Tortos et al., 2007). Using an *in vitro* BBB model with human capillary endothelial cells from either normal brain or drug-resistant epileptic brain, Cucullo et al. (2007) recently reported a dramatically reduced permeability of phenytoin across the *in vitro* BBB formed from endothelial cells of patients with refractory epilepsy, which could be partially counteracted by the selective Pgp inhibitor tariquidar, substantiating transport of AEDs by human P-gp.

In view of the overexpressed efflux transporters found in epileptogenic brain tissue of patients with pharmacoresistant epilepsy and animal models of epilepsy, another important question is whether this overexpression lowers brain uptake of AEDs. By using the kainate model of TLE in mice, Rizzi et al. (2002) demonstrated that the significant increase in *mdr1* mRNA expression measured by RT-PCR in the hippocampus after kainate-induced seizures was associated with a 30% decrease in the brain/plasma ratio of phenytoin, thus substantiating that P-gp alterations significantly affect concentrations of AEDs in the brain. A decrease in phenytoin concentrations of similar magnitude was also determined in the hippocampus of amygdala-kindled rats (Potschka & Löscher, 2002). More recently, van Vliet et al. (2007) reported decreased brain levels of phenytoin that were restricted to brain regions with increased expression of P-gp in epileptic rats, which could be counteracted by inhibiting P-gp. In patients with oxcarbazepine (OXC)-resistant epilepsy, the brain tissue expression of *ABCB1* mRNA was found to be inversely correlated with brain levels of 10-OHCBZ (10,11-dihydro-10-hydroxy-5H-dibenzo(b,f)azepine-5-carboxamide), the active metabolite of OXC, indicating that Pgp may play a role in the pharmacoresistance to OXC by causing insufficient concentrations of its active metabolite at neuronal targets (Marchi et al., 2005).

A further important step in the evaluation of the multidrug transporter hypothesis of drug resistant epilepsy was the demonstration that rats that do not respond to AEDs exhibit significantly higher expression levels of P-gp in brain capillary endothelial cells of the BBB than AED-responsive rats (Potschka et al., 2004b; Volk & Löscher, 2005). This was demonstrated for two different rat models of TLE, phenytoin-resistant kindled rats and phenobarbital-resistant rats with spontaneous recurrent seizures (Potschka et al., 2004b; Volk & Löscher, 2005).

With respect to the ultimate proof of a hypothesis of drug resistance, *i.e.*, demonstration that inhibition or avoidance of the resistance-mediating mechanism counteracts drug resistance in epilepsy, some indirect, correlative evidence came from experiments with diverse

AEDs in pharmacoresistant kindled rats, selected by repeated testing with phenytoin (Löscher, 2002). As described above, these phenytoin-resistant rats have an increased expression of P-gp in focal epileptogenic brain tissue. All AEDs that were substrates for P-gp showed absent or low anticonvulsant efficacy in phenytoin nonresponders (Löscher, 2002; Löscher and Potschka, 2002). Levetiracetam, which seems not to be a substrate for rat P-gp (Potschka et al., 2004a), was as efficacious in phenytoin responders as in nonresponders (Löscher, 2002). For direct proof of principle, it has to be examined whether P-gp inhibitors counteract multidrug resistance as previously shown for brain cancer (Fellner et al., 2002). For this purpose, we used epileptic rats that were either responsive or resistant to phenobarbital (Brandt et al., 2006). In resistant animals, co-administration of the selective P-gp inhibitor, tariquidar, together with phenobarbital reversed resistance, leading to seizure control in animals that were resistant to phenobarbital alone (Brandt et al., 2006). That such a strategy may be functioning in patients with epilepsy is suggested by a report by Summers et al. (2004) on a patient with intractable epilepsy in whom the P-gp inhibitor verapamil was added to the AED regimen. This addition was associated with improved overall seizure control and subjective quality of life (Summers et al., 2004). A similar clinical improvement after verapamil was reported by Iannetti et al. (2005). However, these observations should be interpreted with caution because of their uncontrolled nature, and because verapamil has additional properties beyond inhibition of P-gp. The practical importance of the multidrug transporter hypothesis in the treatment of epilepsy needs to be further proven, using more selective P-gp inhibitors such as tariquidar or elacridar.

■ The gene variant hypothesis

Drug treatment of epilepsy is characterized by unpredictability in efficacy, adverse drug reactions and optimal doses in individual patients, which, at least in part, is thought to be a consequence of genetic variation. It is becoming increasingly clear that genetic polymorphisms play a role in variability of both AED pharmacokinetics and pharmacodynamics (Ferraro & Buono, 2005; Depondt, 2006; Szoeke et al., 2006; Tate & Sisodiya, 2007). Single nucleotide polymorphisms (SNPs), variations at a single site in the DNA, are the most frequent form of sequence variations in the human genome and may affect the efficacy, tolerability and duration of action of AEDs. With respect to drug resistance, both drug targets and drug transporters may be affected by genetic variation, forming the gene variant hypothesis. In terms of AED targets, so far the most interesting data have been accrued for voltage dependent Na^+-channels (Depondt, 2006). In studies on genetic variation in SCN1A, the gene encoding for the alpha-subunit of the voltage-gated neuronal sodium channel, associations of functional SNPs with clinical response to phenytoin, carbamazepine, lamotrigine and oxcarbazepine were reported (Tate et al., 2005; Depondt, 2006).

With respect to drug transporters, various candidate gene studies have evaluated whether polymorphisms in MDR1 (ABCB1), the gene encoding P-gp, are associated with AED response in patients with epilepsy (Ferraro & Buono, 2005; Depondt, 2006; Szoeke et al., 2006; Tate & Sisodiya, 2007). A common SNP (C3435T) identified within exon 26 of the MDR1 gene has been reported to be associated with a differential expression and function of P-gp (Hoffmeyer et al., 2000). Siddiqui et al. (2003) were the first to report that patients with multidrug-resistant epilepsy were significantly more likely to be homozygous for the C allele than the T allele, which, however, was not confirmed by several subsequent studies (Szoeke et al., 2006; Tate & Sisodiya, 2007). One major reason for inconsistent data on this polymorphism may be that several of the association genetics studies involved AEDs, such as valproate or carbamazepine, that do not seem to be substrates of human P-gp. Two recent studies on patients undergoing monotherapy with AEDs (phenytoin or phenobarbital) that are transported by human P-gp showed that pharmacoresistance was much more frequent in patients with the CC genotype of the *MDR1* C3435T polymorphism (Ebid et al., 2007; Basic et al., 2008). Furthermore, the study by Basic et al. (2008) indicated that the CC genotype is associated with lower CSF levels of phenobarbital than the CT or TT genotype. However, causality has not been proven in any of these studies, but all reported findings remain associations. Future ongoing studies with specific Pgp inhibitors may be able to extend the evidence from association to causation.

■ The network hypothesis

Hippocampal sclerosis is a common finding in patients with pharmacoresistant TLE, so that it is often suggested that hippocampal sclerosis plays a causal role in the mechanisms underlying AED resistance (Schmidt & Löscher, 2005). In the hippocampal formation, the dentate gyrus normally functions as a high-resistance gate or filter, preventing the propagation of synchronized activity from the entorhinal cortex into the seizure-prone hippocampus (Nadler, 2003). In patients with TLE and in animal models of TLE, this filter or "gatekeeper" attribute of the dentate gyrus is compromised in that dentate granule cells form an interconnected synaptic network associated with loss of GABAergic hilar interneurons (Nadler, 2003). Indeed, loss of neurons in the hilus of the dentate gyrus, which is closely associated with development of granule cell disinhibition and hyperexcitability, has been proposed to be the common pathological denominator and primary network defect underlying development of a hippocampal seizure focus (Sloviter, 1994; Sloviter, 1999; Nadler, 2003). To directly address whether morphological alterations in the hippocampus are causally related to AED resistance, we recently compared hippocampal damage in epileptic rats that either responded or did not respond to phenobarbital (Volk et al., 2006; Bethmann et al., 2008). A significant loss of neurons in the CA1, CA3c/CA4 and dentate hilus was found in most (> 90%) of nonresponders, whereas most (> 90%) of responders did not differ in this respect from non-epileptic controls, resulting in a highly significant difference between pharmacoresistant and responsive epileptic rats. Based on these observations, it appears that the functional alterations in the dentate gyrus developing as a response to hilar cell loss are critically involved in the mechanisms underlying the refractoriness of seizures to AED treatment. As indicated in *Figure 1*, such structural and functional network changes will also affect AED targets, as demonstrated by the concomitant alterations in hippocampal morphology and $GABA_A$ receptor expression in pharmacoresistant rats of our model of TLE (Volk et al., 2006; Bethmann et al., 2008) and in patients with AED resistant TLE (Loup et al., 2000).

■ Conclusions

Although AEDs are very useful in blocking seizures, many patients do not respond adequately to these agents. In order to enhance our understanding about the mechanisms of pharmacoresistance in epilepsy and thereby develop new strategies for more efficacious treatments, studies on brain tissue from drug-resistant patients and suitable experimental models of intractable epilepsy are mandatory. There is increasing evidence from studies on epileptic brain tissue that AED target alterations and overexpression of multidrug transporters may be important mechanisms of pharmacoresistance, and both mechanisms of refractoriness may coexist in the same epileptogenic brain tissue. Target and transporter alterations in patients with epilepsy may be a consequence of the disease, the treatment, genetic factors or combinations of these possibilities. In addition to target and transporter alterations, the long-term, progressive changes in neural networks during development and progression of epilepsy may lead to reduced pharmacosensitivity. However, none of these hypotheses is really verified as yet, but much of the evidence is correlative in nature. Furthermore, there are certainly other mechanisms contributing to pharmacoresistance that have to be dealt with when thinking about effective therapeutic agents for hitherto intractable types of epilepsy. Thus, development of novel pharmacologic strategies for improved treatment of drug-refractory epilepsy will be a complex venture.

References

Abbott NJ, Khan EU, Rollinson CMS, et al. Drug resistance in epilepsy: the role of the blood-brain barrier. In: Ling V (ed). *Mechanisms of drug resistance in epilepsy. Lessons from oncology*. Chichester: Wiley, 38-46.

Baltes S, Gastens AM, Fedrowitz M, Potschka H, Kaever V, Löscher W. Differences in the transport of the antiepileptic drugs phenytoin, levetiracetam and carbamazepine by human and mouse P-glycoprotein. *Neuropharmacology* 2007; 52: 333-46.

Basic S, Hajnsek S, Bozina N, et al. The influence of C3435T polymorphism of ABCB1 gene on penetration of phenobarbital across blood-brain barrier in patients with generalized epilepsy. *Seizure Eur J Epilepsy* 2008; Mar 6.

Begley DJ. ABC transporters and the blood-brain barrier. *Curr Pharm Des* 2004; 10: 1295-312.

Ben Ari Y, Holmes GL. The multiple facets of gamma-aminobutyric acid dysfunction in epilepsy. *Curr Opin Neurol* 2005; 18: 141-5.

Bethmann K, Fritschy JM, Brandt C, Löscher W. Antiepileptic drug resistant rats differ from drug responsive rats in GABAA-receptor subunit expression in a model of temporal lobe epilepsy. *Neurobiol Dis* 2008; 31: 169-87.

Brandt C, Bethmann K, Gastens AM, Löscher W. The multidrug transporter hypothesis of drug resistance in epilepsy: proof-of-principle in a rat model of temporal lobe epilepsy. *Neurobiol Dis* 2006; 24: 202-11.

Brooks-Kayal AR, Shumate MD, Jin H, Rikhter TY, Coulter DA. Selective changes in single cell $GABA_A$ receptor subunit expression and function in temporal lobe epilepsy. *Nature Medicine* 1998; 4: 1166-72.

Cohen AS, Lin DD, Quirk GL, Coulter DA. Dentate granule cell GABA(A) receptors in epileptic hippocampus: enhanced synaptic efficacy and altered pharmacology. *Eur J Neurosci* 2003; 17: 1607-16.

Cohen I, Navarro V, Clemenceau S, Baulac M, Miles R. On the origin of interictal activity in human temporal lobe epilepsy in vitro. *Science* 2002; 298: 1418-21.

Coulter DA. Mossy fiber zinc and temporal lobe epilepsy: pathological association with altered "epileptic" gamma-aminobutyric acid A receptors in dentate granule cells. *Epilepsia* 2000; 41 (suppl 6): S96-S99.

Coulter DA. Epilepsy-associated plasticity in gamma-aminobutyric acid receptor expression, function, and inhibitory synaptic properties. *Int Rev Neurobiol* 2001; 45: 237-52.

Cucullo L, Hossain M, Rapp E, Manders T, Marchi N, Janigro D. Development of a humanized in vitro blood-brain barrier model to screen for brain penetration of antiepileptic drugs. *Epilepsia* 2007; 48: 505-16.

Depondt C. The potential of pharmacogenetics in the treatment of epilepsy. *Eur J Paediatr Neurol* 2006; 10: 57-65.

Ebid AH, Ahmed MM, Mohammed SA. Therapeutic drug monitoring and clinical outcomes in epileptic Egyptian patients: a gene polymorphism perspective study. *Ther Drug Monit* 2007; 29: 305-12.

Ellerkmann RK, Remy S, Chen J, et al. Molecular and functional changes in voltage-dependent Na(+) channels following pilocarpine-induced status epilepticus in rat dentate granule cells. *Neuroscience* 2003; 119: 323-33.

Fellner S, Bauer B, Miller DS, et al. Transport of paclitaxel (Taxol) across the blood-brain barrier in vitro and in vivo. *J Clin Invest* 2002; 110: 1309-18.

Ferraro TN, Buono RJ. The relationship between the pharmacology of antiepileptic drugs and human gene variation: an overview. *Epilepsy Behav* 2005; 7: 18-36.

Fromm MF. Importance of P-glycoprotein at blood-tissue barriers. *Trends Pharmacol Sci* 2004; 25: 423-9.

Goodkin HP, Yeh JL, Kapur J. Status epilepticus increases the intracellular accumulation of GABAA receptors. *J Neurosci* 2005; 25: 5511-20.

Hermann DM, Kilic E, Spudich A, Kramer SD, Wunderli-Allenspach H, Bassetti CL. Role of drug efflux carriers in the healthy and diseased brain. *Ann Neurol* 2006; 60: 489-98.

Hoffmeyer S, Burk O, von Richter O, et al. Functional polymorphisms of the human multidrug-resistance gene: multiple sequence variations and correlation of one allele with P-glycoprotein expression and activity in vivo. *Proc Natl Acad Sci USA* 2000; 97: 3473-8.

Huberfeld G, Wittner L, Clemenceau S, et al. Perturbed chloride homeostasis and GABAergic signaling in human temporal lobe epilepsy. *J Neurosci* 2007; 27: 9866-73.

Iannetti P, Spalice A, Parisi P. Calcium-channel blocker verapamil administration in prolonged and refractory status epilepticus. *Epilepsia* 2005; 46: 967-9.

Jandova K, Pasler D, Antonio LL, et al. Carbamazepine-resistance in the epileptic dentate gyrus of human hippocampal slices. *Brain* 2006; 129: 3290-306.

Jeub M, Beck H, Siep E, et al. Effect of phenytoin on sodium and calcium currents in hippocampal CA1 neurons of phenytoin-resistant kindled rats. *Neuropharmacology* 2002; 42: 107-16.

Jones DM, Esmaeil N, Maren S, Macdonald RL. Characterization of pharmacoresistance to benzodiazepines in the rat Li-pilocarpine model of status epilepticus. *Epilepsy Res* 2002; 50: 301-12.

Kapur J, Macdonald RL. Rapid seizure-induced reduction of benzodiazepine and Zn2+ sensitivity of hippocampal dentate granule cell GABAA receptors. *J Neurosci* 1997; 17: 7532-40.

Köhling R. Neuroscience. GABA becomes exciting. *Science* 2002; 298: 1350-1.

Kwan P, Brodie MJ. Potential role of drug transporters in the pathogenesis of medically intractable epilepsy. *Epilepsia* 2005; 46: 224-35.

Lazarowski A, Czornyj L, Lubienieki F, Girardi E, Vazquez S, D'Giano C. ABC transporters during epilepsy and mechanisms underlying multidrug resistance in refractory epilepsy. *Epilepsia* 2007; 48 (suppl 5): 140-9.

Lee G, Bendayan R. Functional expression and localization of P-glycoprotein in the central nervous system: relevance to the pathogenesis and treatment of neurological disorders. *Pharm Res* 2004; 21: 1313-30.

Leonard GD, Fojo T, Bates SE. The role of ABC transporters in clinical practice. *Oncologist* 2003; 8: 411-24.

Loup F, Wieser HG, Yonekawa Y, Aguzzi A, Fritschy JM. Selective alterations in GABAA receptor subtypes in human temporal lobe epilepsy. *J Neurosci* 2000; 20: 5401-19.

Löscher W, Potschka H. Role of multidrug transporters in pharmacoresistance to antiepileptic drugs. *J Pharmacol Exp Ther* 2002; 301: 7-14.

Löscher W. Animal models of drug-resistant epilepsy. *Novartis Found Symp* 2002; 243: 149-59; discussion: 159-66.

Löscher W, Potschka H. Drug resistance in brain diseases and the role of drug efflux transporters. *Nature Rev Neurosci* 2005a; 6: 591-602.

Löscher W, Potschka H. Role of drug efflux transporters in the brain for drug disposition and treatment of brain diseases. *Prog Neurobiol* 2005b; 76: 22-76.

Lucas PT, Meadows LS, Nicholls J, Ragsdale DS. An epilepsy mutation in the beta1 subunit of the voltage-gated sodium channel results in reduced channel sensitivity to phenytoin. *Epilepsy Res* 2005; 64: 77-84.

Luna Tortos C, Fedrowitz M, Löscher W. Several major antiepileptic drugs are substrates for human P-glycoprotein. *Epilepsia* 2007; 48 (suppl 6): 365.

Macdonald RL, Kapur J. Acute cellular alterations in the hippocampus after status epilepticus. *Epilepsia* 1999; 40: S9-S20.

Marchi N, Guiso G, Rizzi M, *et al*. A pilot study on brain-to-plasma partition of 10,11-dyhydro-10-hydroxy-5H-dibenzo(b,f)azepine-5-carboxamide and MDR1 brain expression in epilepsy patients not responding to oxcarbazepine. *Epilepsia* 2005; 46: 1613-9.

Mazarati AM, Baldwin RA, Sankar R, Wasterlain CG. Time-dependent decrease in the effectiveness of antiepileptic drugs during the course of self-sustaining status epilepticus. *Brain Res* 1998; 814: 179-85.

Nadler JV. The recurrent mossy fiber pathway of the epileptic brain. *Neurochem Res* 2003; 28: 1649-58.

Naylor DE, Liu H, Wasterlain CG. Trafficking of GABA(A) receptors, loss of inhibition, and a mechanism for pharmacoresistance in status epilepticus. *J Neurosci* 2005; 25: 7724-33.

Oby E, Janigro D. The blood-brain barrier and epilepsy. *Epilepsia* 2006; 47: 1761-74.

Okabe A, Ohno K, Toyoda H, Yokokura M, Sato K, Fukuda A. Amygdala kindling induces upregulation of mRNA for NKCC1, a Na(+), K(+)-2Cl(-) cotransporter, in the rat piriform cortex. *Neurosci Res* 2002; 44: 225-9.

Okabe A, Yokokura M, Toyoda H, *et al*. Changes in chloride homeostasis-regulating gene expressions in the rat hippocampus following amygdala kindling. *Brain Res* 2003; 990: 221-6.

Palma E, Amici M, Sobrero F, *et al*. Anomalous levels of Cl- transporters in the hippocampal subiculum from temporal lobe epilepsy patients make GABA excitatory. *Proc Natl Acad Sci USA* 2006; 103: 8465-8.

Potschka H, Löscher W. A comparison of extracellular levels of phenytoin in amygdala and hippocampus of kindled and non-kindled rats. *Neuroreport* 2002; 13: 167-71.

Potschka H, Baltes S, Löscher W. Inhibition of multidrug transporters by verapamil or probenecid does not alter blood-brain barrier penetration of levetiracetam in rats. *Epilepsy Res* 2004a; 58: 85-91.

Potschka H, Volk HA, Löscher W. Pharmacoresistance and expression of multidrug transporter P-glycoprotein in kindled rats. *Neuroreport* 2004b; 19: 1657-61.

Regesta G, Tanganelli P. Clinical aspects and biological bases of drug-resistant epilepsies. *Epilepsy Res* 1999; 34: 109-22.

Remy S, Gabriel S, Urban BW, *et al*. A novel mechanism underlying drug resistance in chronic epilepsy. *Ann Neurol* 2003; 53: 469-79.

Remy S, Urban BW, Elger CE, Beck H. Anticonvulsant pharmacology of voltage-gated Na+ channels in hippocampal neurons of control and chronically epileptic rats. *Eur J Neurosci* 2003; 17: 2648-58.

Remy S, Beck H. Molecular and cellular mechanisms of pharmacoresistance in epilepsy. *Brain* 2006; 129: 18-35.

Rivera C, Li H, Thomas-Crusells J, et al. BDNF-induced TrkB activation down-regulates the K+-Cl-cotransporter KCC2 and impairs neuronal Cl- extrusion. *J Cell Biol* 2002; 159: 747-52.

Rivera C, Voipio J, Kaila K. Two developmental switches in GABAergic signalling: the K+-Cl-cotransporter KCC2 and carbonic anhydrase CAVII. *J Physiol* 2005; 562: 27-36.

Rizzi M, Caccia S, Guiso G, et al. Limbic seizures induce P-glycoprotein in rodent brain: functional implications for pharmacoresistance. *J Neurosci* 2002; 22: 5833-9.

Rogawski MA, Löscher W. The neurobiology of antiepileptic drugs. *Nat Rev Neurosci* 2004; 5: 553-64.

Schaub C, Uebachs M, Beck H. Diminished response of CA1 neurons to antiepileptic drugs in chronic epilepsy. *Epilepsia* 2007; 48: 1339-50.

Schinkel AH, Wagenaar E, Mol CA, van Deemter L. P-glycoprotein in the blood-brain barrier of mice influences the brain penetration and pharmacological activity of many drugs. *J Clin Invest* 1996; 97: 2517-24.

Schinkel AH, Jonker JW. Mammalian drug efflux transporters of the ATP binding cassette (ABC) family: an overview. *Adv Drug Deliv Rev* 2003; 55: 3-29.

Schmidt D, Löscher W. Drug resistance in epilepsy: putative neurobiologic and clinical mechanisms. *Epilepsia* 2005; 46: 858-77.

Siddiqui A, Kerb R, Weale ME, et al. Association of multidrug resistance in epilepsy with a polymorphism in the drug-transporter gene ABCB1. *N Engl J Med* 2003; 348: 1442-8.

Sills GJ, Kwan P, Butler E, de Lange EC, van den Berg DJ, Brodie MJ. P-glycoprotein-mediated efflux of antiepileptic drugs: preliminary studies in mdr1a knockout mice. *Epilepsy Behav* 2002; 3: 427-32.

Sisodiya SM, Heffernan J, Squier MV. Over-expression of P-glycoprotein in malformations of cortical development. *Neuroreport* 1999; 10: 3437-41.

Sisodiya SM, Lin W-R, Harding BN, Squier MV, Keir G, Thom M. Drug resistance in epilepsy: expression of drug resistance proteins in common causes of refractory epilepsy. *Brain* 2002; 125: 22-31.

Sloviter RS. The functional organization of the hippocampal dentate gyrus and its relevance to the pathogenesis of temporal lobe epilepsy. *Ann Neurol* 1994; 35: 640-54.

Sloviter RS. Status epilepticus-induced neuronal injury and network reorganization. *Epilepsia* 1999; 40: S34-S39.

Summers MA, Moore JL, McAuley JW. Use of verapamil as a potential P-glycoprotein inhibitor in a patient with refractory epilepsy. *Ann Pharmacother* 2004; 38: 1631-4.

Sun H, Dai H, Shaik N, Elmquist WF. Drug efflux transporters in the CNS. *Adv Drug Deliv Rev* 2003; 55: 83-105.

Szoeke CE, Newton M, Wood JM, et al. Update on pharmacogenetics in epilepsy: a brief review. *Lancet Neurol* 2006; 5: 189-96.

Tate SK, Depondt C, Sisodiya SM, et al. Genetic predictors of the maximum doses patients receive during clinical use of the anti-epileptic drugs carbamazepine and phenytoin. *Proc Natl Acad Sci USA* 2005; 102: 5507-12.

Tate SK, Sisodiya SM. Multidrug resistance in epilepsy: a pharmacogenomic update. *Expert Opin Pharmacother* 2007; 8: 1441-9.

Tishler DM, Weinberg KT, Hinton DR, Barbaro N, Annett GM, Raffel C. MDR1 gene expression in brain of patients with medically intractable epilepsy. *Epilepsia* 1995; 36: 1-6.

van Vliet EA, van Schaik R, Edelbroek PM, et al. Region-specific overexpression of P-glycoprotein at the blood-brain barrier affects brain uptake of phenytoin in epileptic rats. *J Pharmacol Exp Ther* 2007; 322: 141-7.

Volk HA, Löscher W. Multidrug resistance in epilepsy: rats with drug-resistant seizures exhibit enhanced brain expression of P-glycoprotein compared with rats with drug-responsive seizures. *Brain* 2005; 128: 1358-68.

Volk HA, Arabadzisz D, Fritschy JM, Brandt C, Bethman K, Löscher W. Antiepileptic drug resistant rats differ from drug responsive rats in hippocampal neurodegeneration and GABAA-receptor ligand-binding in a model of temporal lobe epilepsy. *Neurobiol Dis* 2006; 21: 633-46.

Vreugdenhil M, Vanveelen CWM, Vanrijen PC, Dasilva FHL, Wadman WJ. Effect of valproic acid on sodium currents in cortical neurons from patients with pharmaco-resistant temporal lobe epilepsy. *Epilepsy Res* 1998; 32: 309-20.

Vreugdenhil M, Wadman WJ. Modulation of sodium currents in rat CA1 neurons by carbamazepine and valproate after kindling epileptogenesis. *Epilepsia* 1999; 40: 1512-22.

What should the characteristics be of a pertinent model to identify new treatments for drug resistant epilepsy?

Edward H. Bertram

Department of Neurology, University of Virginia, Charlottesville, Virginia, USA

In this chapter we will discuss the process of finding new drugs for epilepsy, specifically drugs that will succeed against drug resistant epilepsy. Although the definition of drug resistant epilepsy has been discussed extensively in another chapter, there is a major aspect of this condition that is often not discussed or completely recognized. Although the term implies or is often interpreted to mean that the patient with drug resistant epilepsy does not respond to the currently available drugs, the reality is that most patients do respond to the drugs with a reduced seizure frequency, but the response is incomplete with occasional break through seizures. How many of the patients with drug resistant epilepsy are truly resistant (no effect of the drug) or are incompletely responsive (significant reduction but seizures do continue) is not known. Further, there are many patients who do respond quite well, but the drugs that do suppress the seizures completely have such significant toxicity, either systemic or neurologic, that the medication must be stopped. These are important issues to consider, because it could be that less toxic drugs with similar mechanisms could solve the resistance problem. With the ultimate goal, as is often stated, of no seizures and no side effects, we need to consider the potential mechanisms of drug resistance (or, perhaps more correctly, incomplete drug efficacy) and make use of models that possess these mechanisms and allow us to predict more accurately the effect of treatments on seizures as well as neurological function in people with epilepsy.

There are many possible but as yet unproved reasons for drugs to fail to control seizures completely, and in designing or selecting better models, these potential mechanisms of resistance must be taken into consideration. The issue of systemic toxicity (*e.g.*, allergic reactions, liver toxicity) can be predicted and avoided up to a point in preclinical testing and by particular structural characteristics in the design of the molecule, but many of the reactions are ultimately unique to individual patients. In this chapter we will not discuss this potential cause of drug failure. Another common cause of drug failure not secondary to efficacy is neurologic toxicity (*e.g.*, ataxia, psychiatric symptoms). Because psychiatric and cognitive functions are higher cortical function issues, they may be hard to predict in animal screens, but, as we will discuss later, designing or selecting drugs that are more specific for epileptic circuits while avoiding the "normal" circuits may help avoid this group of problems. Two potential reasons for the drugs to fail to suppress seizures on purely mechanistic as opposed to toxicologic reasons are that the drugs are directed at the wrong target or that the drug is directed at the correct target, but just can't get to it (Table I). It is these two potential causes of incomplete drug response (which we will refer to hereafter as drug resistance) that we will focus on in choosing ideal or at least improved, models.

The ideal model for therapy discovery for drug resistant epilepsy will be one that can perfectly predict ultimate clinical efficacy in patients with all forms of refractory epilepsy, as well as identify major toxicities. Inasmuch as drug resistant epilepsy consists of a number of syndromes with likely diverse pathophysiologies at different developmental or degenerative stages, the likelihood the goal can be achieved with a single model is not high. The problem is further exacerbated by the lack of good models for the many syndromes. Because of this issue we will describe in generalities the problems faced in identifying new therapies for intractable epilepsy and then discuss how some of the existing models might provide the means for identifying better drugs.

The primary issue for epilepsy pharmacotherapy is not that we need more drugs but that we need drugs that are better than what we now have. To be effective a therapy has to target a key mechanism involved with the seizure and reach the area of the brain that will have the desired effect. In view of the diversity of the epilepsies it is not known whether there is a component that is common to all seizure types, but ideally, in order to find that one drug with broad efficacy, identifying a single mechanism that is the key to seizure suppression in multiple epilepsy syndromes would be ideal. However, pursuing a "universal target" that could treat all types of epilepsy may result in a target that is common to many normal functions as well, resulting in greater degrees of toxicity. For the purposes of this article we will focus on partial epilepsy as it is the most common group of epilepsies that are drug resistant.

■ Relevant Epilepsy Physiology

As we consider pertinent models for therapy discovery, we should first consider the physiology of the partial seizure and the stages of an epileptic seizure that could be targeted. There are at least three: seizure initiation (transition from interictal to ictal), seizure buildup (the early phase of activity that occurs within the initiating circuit) and seizure spread (the process of recruiting additional regions and circuits) (Figure 1). The importance of breaking seizures down into these phases is that each is likely associated with different mechanisms that may involve different potential molecular targets for drug interaction. The ideal model should incorporate all three of those stages and each of these

Table I. Possible contributors to drug resistance

Lowered affinity of target for drug
Reduced efficacy of drug at receptor
Limited access of drug to target
Targetting wrong molecule
Distribution of drug to non critical circuits (toxicity over efficacy)
Primary effect wrong neuron type (e.g. interneurons)
Primary effect wrong part of the circuit (e.g. thalamus vs cortex)

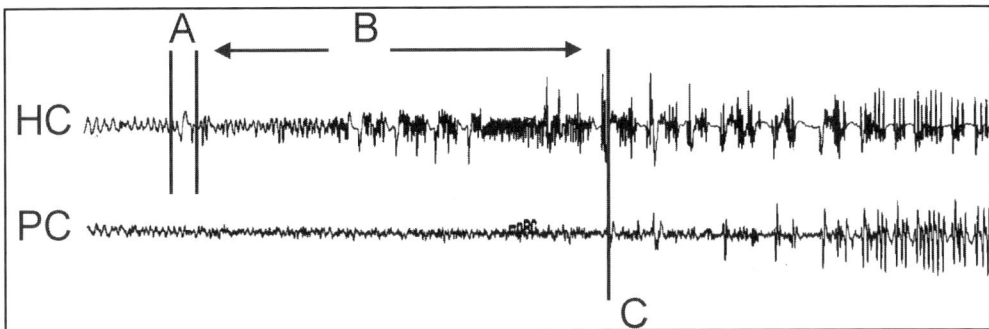

Figure 1. Stages of seizure evolution. The three stages of seizure evolution in a seizure recorded from the hippocampus (HC) and piriform cortex (PC) in a rat with limbic epilepsy. A: narrow window of seizure initiation in the HC, in which the seizure transitions from interictal to ictal; B: seizure buildup, in which the seizure activity continues and intensifies; C: seizure spread, when the seizure in the initial circuits begins to recruit additional areas.

stages should have mechanisms similar to human epilepsy. Although many of the currently used acutely induced models have the second and third phases (buildup and spread), few, especially the models for partial epilepsy, have the spontaneous initiation stage, and it is this stage which may be the most appropriate to target, although prevention of buildup or spread could also be clinically useful by the prevention of clinically significant seizures. In addition to the stages of seizures that should be considered in identifying models for epilepsy, one needs to consider the circuits in which the seizures arise, as there is a potential that a single drug can have very different effects depending on where in the seizure circuit it has the greatest effect. Thus having models that have intact seizure circuits may also be a key element in the ideal model, combined with all three seizure stages.

■ What should the targets be? Where should drugs work?

Answering these questions should be a major focus of drug discovery, and one that new models should help us answer. At the moment we don't have an answer to what the molecular targets should be in general, and where on the neurons the compounds should be working. We also don't have an answer to the question about where in the brain in general the drugs should be going. Although there has been much discussion about the first question regarding which molecules should be targeted, there is little agreement about the places on the neurons we should be targeting. Should they be post-synaptic receptors, voltage gated channels (depolarizing channel antagonists *vs* hyperpolarizing channel agonists), neuromodulators, axon initial segments, presynaptic excitatory or inhibitory terminals, somatic *versus* dendritic receptors and channels? Inhibitory or excitatory neurons? Projection systems or local circuits?

One of the problems that we face is that at the moment we really don't know where the drugs are acting, either a particular molecular target (we have some idea about a few: sodium channels, GABA receptors) or on which population of neurons (Kwan & Brodie, 2007; Rogawski, 2006; Sankar & Holmes, 2004; Sills, 2006). For this reason it is possible that the right mechanism of action could affect the wrong neuronal populations or regions of the brain. For example, using a proinhibitory agent could inhibit the interneurons more than it does the excitatory projection neurons, with a resultant overall disinhibition and worsened seizures. There may not be much we can do to target specific neuronal populations and regions at the moment, as little is known about how drugs enter and traffic in the brain, but as we consider choosing potential molecular targets for drug development it may be important to select those potential targets which are more specific for particular neuronal populations such as hippocampal pyramidal cells. This type of approach requires a much greater understanding of the local physiology and regional network interactions than we currently have. For this reason, focusing more on the epilepsy specific changes in receptors and channels may be the more rewarding approach for the moment.

Choosing the best molecular targets for drugs has become more complicated because there is rapidly expanding evidence for pathological expression of different isoforms of receptors and channels (Aronica et al., 2001; Brooks-Kayal, et al., 2001; Mangan & Lothman, 1996) These aberrantly expressed drug targets have a very different pharmacologic profile than the normally expressed channels. These altered expressions and the associated changes in physiology and pharmacology have been extensively studied and documented for voltage gated sodium channels and GABA receptors especially in rat models of chronic limbic epilepsy (Mangan & Bertram, 1997; Ketelaars et al., 2001; Shumate et al., 1998). Many of the currently used AEDs are less effective on these epilepsy associated channel isoforms (Mtchedlishvili et al., 2001; Remy et al., 2002; Vreugdenhil & Wadman, 1999). Although it is not clear whether these changes are contributing to drug resistance, it is certainly a plausible explanation for the failure of some drugs to control the seizures of epilepsy. For this reason using normal brain systems to identify drugs may fail to identify molecules that would be much more effective if directed at the "epileptic" channels. As we consider pertinent models we therefore need to consider these changes, and choose models that incorporate them so that epilepsy specific molecules might be identified. However, if we wish to identify the single epilepsy cure-all, determining a mechanism or target that crosses epilepsy types might depend on identifying a mechanism and target that is common to a particular stage for all seizures (perhaps the spread phase).

▪ Where should the drugs go?

We turn now to the the earlier question, where should the drugs go. Another way of asking that question is how well do we target particular regions of the brain that might be key components of the seizure circuitry? The currently employed models (such as maximal electroshock, subcutaneous pentylene tetrazole and kindling) have the buildup and spread phases (phase 2 and 3), but, with the possible exception of kindling, the circuits in which these seizure phases occur are not well defined and may be different from the circuits that support those seizure stages in the human epilepsies. Few of the usually employed screening models have endogenously spontaneous seizures, and those that do (genetic spike and wave seizure models) may not be as relevant to the more intractable forms of human epilepsy. Thus one feature that future models should incorporate is spontaneous onset, as seizure onset may involve a group of mechanisms that are unique to that seizure phase and can only be identified by the models that have spontaneous onsets. In addition because of issues of region specific physiology and pharmacology, as well as the issue of drug access (or lack thereof) it would also be appropriate that the model use the same circuits for seizure initiation and buildup as in human epilepsy.

A pertinent model should be able to identify molecules that will be effective at one of the seizure stages involved with seizure initiation and spread and thus incorporate a mechanism or the mechanisms that are key at that particular stage. But which mechanism? To identify which mechanism to target we should first consider the potential mechanisms underlying seizure initiation, build up and spread, which is, for the moment, largely speculation. For the purposes of discussion, let's focus on one type of epilepsy (limbic) for which we have at least some data about the potential alterations. As noted earlier, these changes include alternate expression of sodium channel isoforms as well as different GABA receptor subtypes (Aronica et al., 2001; Brooks-Kayal et al., 2001; Mangan & Lothman, 1996) (there are other changes as well) that result in increased excitability of the affected neurons. However, these changes by themselves do not cause the animal or person to seize continuously. These changes may increase the predisposition to seize, as the individual only has a seizure every now and again. There must therefore be other mechanisms that are in a regular ebb and flow, that, when enough factors converge on a population of neurons that are predisposed to seize, they will push the predisposed neurons over into a seizure. Such a scenario would imply that there would be greater probability that a seizure would occur at certain times than at others, that the seizures would follow an endogenously controlled ebb and flow of neurotransmitters and neuromodulators. Thus knowing the key combination of neuromodulators that will push the brain over into a seizure can provide another group of potential molecular targets for epilepsy drug development.

What evidence do we have that neuromodulators might play a role in at least some types of seizures? There are several lines of evidence, although none are direct. Among the induced seizure models, agonists for the central acetylcholine receptor, a major neuromodulator in the central nervous system, are a common and effective means of inducing seizures (Cavalheiro et al., 1991). There is clear evidence that neuroactive steroids play a significant role in neuronal excitability and some forms of human epilepsy (e.g., catamenial seizures tied to particular phases of the menstrual cycle) (Herzog & Fowler, 2008; Scharfman & MacLusky, 2006; Smith et al., 2007). Among the epilepsies, limbic seizures clearly follow a diurnal pattern, both in man and in animals, with seizures twice as likely to occur during the day than at night (Quigg et al., 1998). Other seizure types may occur more commonly at night or exclusively at night (Scheffer et al., 1995). There is one report of a patient with two separate seizure foci, one parietal and one mesial temporal. The former focus was associated with seizures that occurred exclusively at night, whereas the mesial temporal seizures were most commonly seen during the day (Quigg & Straume, 2000). All of these observations suggest strongly that there are endogenous, fluctuating influences on the occurrence of seizures. The observations also suggest that influencing the ups and downs of these neuromodulators may be a new approach to epilepsy. The acute models of induced seizures used in the current drug discovery process are less likey to uncover the role of some of these neuromodulators, so that models with spontaneous seizures may be of potential great utility for identifying new approaches to epilepsy pharmacotherapy.

As we consider the problem of drug resistant epilepsy and the process of drug discovery, perhaps the biggest challenge we face is the absence of established epilepsy specific targets. Although some attempts have been made to place some logic into the discovery process, many of the drugs that have come into clinical practice have been cold hits that had no clearly defined mechanisms (De Smedt et al., 2007; Sills, 2006; Yang et al., 2007). Although some have at least some ill-defined mechanism of action or target that was discovered after approval, it remains unclear whether those named mechanisms are truly the means of seizure control. It is this lack of defined targets which truly impedes the development of new therapies. Perhaps it is in this area that the new models could provide the greatest benefit. As noted earlier, there are specific stages that a seizure evolves through and it is likely that each stage has a unique pharmacology. It is also quite likely that a mechanism of action that will be effective at one stage will be completely ineffective at another. The molecule that might prevent seizure initiation could be completely ineffective at preventing seizure buildup. As we try to put some logic into the drug discovery process we should consider using models that have all of the typical seizure stages so that we can determine which targets are involved with which stages.

■ What should we model?

Although many of the acute models currently employed in the discovery process have the buildup and spread, few have a well defined endogenous initiation, so it is likely that those acutely induced models will not identify molecules that could prevent seizure initiation (Meldrum, 1997). Of the animal models with "spontaneous" seizures many are a form of genetic spike wave seizures or are stimulated by environmental stimuli (*e.g.* audiogenic seizures), and these seizure types are not a major focus of new drug discovery. Few use the effect on EEG as a measure of drug efficacy. The post status epilepticus limbic epilepsy models do have spontaneous seizures and have EEGs that are similar to the ictal EEGs in human limbic epilepsy (Ben-Ari *et al.*, 1980; Bertram & Cornett, 1994; Cavalheiro *et al.*, 1991; Goffin *et al.*, 2007). Although we are a long way from demonstrating that these models could identify compounds that would be highly effective, one could develop a fervent belief that such models could lead us to a therapeutic promised land after years in the desert. But how?

Before we describe how we might use one of the chronic epilepsy models to identify new therapies, we should review the features of human epilepsy that should be modeled (*Table II*). First, the seizures arise should spontaneously. It's a key feature that is missing in the models that we now use to identify potential AEDs, and there are likely a number of, at the moment unidentified, mechanisms that push the brain over into a seizure. The transition from the interictal state to a seizure likely has a number of unique mechanisms that may provide one of the best potential targets for seizure prevention. It is possible that blocking the mechanisms of seizure initiation will have little effect on the latter two stages of a seizure and thus drugs targeting those mechanisms might not be effective in the acute seizure models. As in human epilepsy the chronic limbic epilepsy rodent models have spontaneous seizures.

Another aspect of majority of the human focal epilepsies is that there is an associated pathology. This pathology has a number of potential implications for pharmacotherapy, as noted earlier, including alterations in the expressed isoforms of a particular molecular drug target associated with a presumed change in the pharmacology of that target. There are other changes that may limit or alter the distribution of the drugs to key parts of the brain. The ideal model should, therefore, contain those changes so that there would be

Table II. Features of human drug resistant epilepsy to model

Altered channels and receptors
Spontaneous seizure onset
Pathology
Seizures in same circuits
Intact seizure circuits
Seizure physiology
Endogenous mechanisms of seizure onset

good parallels between the model and the real condition, because, in theory, success of a molecule in such a model should be highly predictive of clinical success, at least in terms of seizure suppression.

The chronic limbic epilepsy models have a number of these changes. They have patterns of neuronal loss that are quite similar to the patterns that are seen in human limbic epilepsy (variable, in multiple limbic structures) (Ben-Ari et al., 1980, Bertram & Scott, 2000; Cavalheiro et al., 1991) changes in receptors and channels (Aronica et al. 2001; Brooks-Kayal et al., 2001; Mathern et al., 1997), expression of drug resistant proteins (Löscher, 2007; Sisodiya, 2003), and spontaneous seizures that, at least on EEG, are similar to the spontaneous seizures recorded from limbic structures in humans (Bertram & Cornett, 1994). For these reasons these models would appear to have the ideal combination for drug identification Whether the changes in the expression of the receptors have the same changes in pharmacosensitivity for all receptors and channels as might occur in people remains to be determined, but using models that have alterations in receptor expression that are similar to humans may well be the path to uncovering drugs that are more specific to the molecules that help generate seizures. One clear issue with this approach that may diminish its value is whether these key changes are universal to the many varieties of human focal epilepsy. Unfortunately for the moment we will have to satisfy ourselves with this one group of models as it is the only one that has many of the features of this one type of drug resistant human epilepsy and hope that the new drugs that are discovered to be effective in these models will be effective not only for human limbic epilepsy but also for other forms of focal epilepsy. An additional potential limiting factor with these models, as we will discuss later, is that they are highly labor intensive so that they are not well suited to mass screening of hundreds of compounds in a year. However, they could have a very specific niche in identifying targets or in making a final decision to move to clinical trial.

■ Using chronic epilepsy models

Although there are a number of reports using the chronic limbic epilepsy models to study antiepileptic drugs (Bethmann et al., 2007; Nissinen & Pitkanen, 2007; van Vliet et al., 2007 van Vliet et al., 2008), the reports also make it clear this approach to drug testing is very labor intensive and technologically sophisticated and may not be suited to mass, blind screening programs. How then can these models best be used? What data do we need that will indicate that these models are models for drug resistant epilepsy? The goal is to determine whether these models can identify drugs that do a better job in resistant epilepsy (and ideally we want better drugs, not just more drugs). As a first step we need to know how well the current drugs work, and they should show a similar level of efficacy that we see in human drug resistant epilepsy: a partial, but incomplete effect (these models should be incompletely drug responsive, not completely drug resistant just as in the human counterpart) (Stables et al., 2003).

Assuming that the rodent models of chronic limbic epilepsy show incomplete responses, the question then becomes how do we use these models in the drug discovery process? In the traditional screening procedure using acutely induced seizures, the typical practice is to give the drug, wait a defined period of time (usually within 30 minutes) and induce the seizure (White, 2003). Matching drug dosing (and, therefore, drug levels) to the onset (induction) of the seizure is a straightforward issue. In models with spontaneous (and usually irregularly spontaneous) seizures, matching potentially therapeutic levels to seizure onset is often an issue of chance. Some rats may have many (20 or more) seizures in a day whereas others may seize as infrequently as once a week or less. For this reason the traditional means of dosing the animals in screening protocols (single dose just before the seizure) is difficult if not impossible, as the seizures are difficult to predict and match with potentially therapeutic drug levels. The problem of matching seizures to therapeutic levels is further compounded by the usually very short half lives of most drugs in rodents (several hours is typical) (Löscher, 2007) For this reason, multiple dosing becomes essential, often multiple doses in a day. The amount of drug necessary is often high enough (100 mg or more per day) that implantable reservoirs can't supply sufficient amounts over multiple days. Because most of the drugs are poorly soluble in water, organic solvents are necessary, and their compatibility with pumps is quite variable. One potential solution to these many obstacles is to use animals with high seizure frequencies so that the chances of the animal's having a seizure while the drug is at a therapeutic level is high.

In addition to the problems with dosing is the problem of documenting seizures and the effect that drugs have on them. Rats are unable to report their own seizures or the seizures of their neighbors, so that a monitoring system to document not only the seizures by EEG but also their severity (convulsive or nonconvulsive). There are a number of approaches to recording prolonged video EEGs in rodents with epilepsy, so the technique is well established (Bertram, 2006). The real, and limiting issue is the effort that is necessary to operate such a system, especially in the setting of measuring the effects of drugs. To maintain and keep a single system operational while obtaining and analyzing the data from 10 to 15 rats undergoing continuous EEG and video recording while analyzing the data takes the full time attention of a single skilled technician. For this reason alone, using these models cannot be considered as a component of an initial mass drug screen. Although these limbic epilepsy models have great potential to identify new compounds of new mechanisms, their use and the associated issues must be carefully considered and planned so that these models can be used at appropriate points in the drug discovery process (*Table III*).

It is clear that the limbic epilepsy models are far from the ideal in which we could screen potential drugs quickly and cheaply, and the results in these theoretically easy screens would be more broadly predictive for success in multiple seizure types. The limbic epilepsy models do have many of the key features of epilepsy (pathology and spontaneity of seizures) but they are expensive to create and labor and technology intensive in use. Still, these post status epilepticus models may have a place in the lengthy therapy discovery process. They will almost certainly not play a significant role in the initial screening of the thousands of potential drugs that are created each year, but they may play a role in identifying potential new targets for drug development as well as in deciding which among a limited

Table III. Problems with chronic epilepsy models as screening tools

Irregular seizures
Unpredictable seizures
Short drug half lives
Large amounts of drug required
Expensive
Low throughput
Technically complex
Labor intensive

number of compounds of similar mechanisms of action will be selected for clinical development. Before we take a compound or related compounds to these limbic epilepsy models, we should know what is/are the compound's potential mechanism(s) of action and does that one compound get into the brain? For these issues *in vitro* screens for receptor affinity and action to determine a mechanism of drug action together with the several acute *in vivo* seizure models (*e.g.* maximal electroshock or kindling) to determine if these compounds could get into the brain would likely reduce the number of candidate compounds to be tested in these more realistic although more complex limbic epilepsy models significantly. Is it possible that we would miss some compounds by this approach (no demonstrated mechanism of action or failure to suppress an acutely induced seizure) that would likely do well clinically? Almost certainly, but we have to have a means of narrowing the compounds to a manageable number before screening them in one of the chronic models. There are almost certainly compounds in the past that would have done as well or better than those currently in use that never went to clinical trial, and there will no doubt be other potentially great AEDs that go unrecognized regardless of the screening tool used. We just hope that there are enough good ones that get identified so that the failure to recognize others ultimately has little effect on finding better drugs than we now have. Defining a mechanism of drug action that is effective in this group of models should eventually lead to "best in class" drugs for that target that achieve the goal of "no seizures, no side effects".

How should information from these models of real epilepsy be used? Ideally the test will be used to predict clinical success. However, for the moment, successful results in these models should be viewed with some degree of cautious optimism as it regards potential efficacy in people. At the moment there is no evidence that these models are more accurate at predicting clinical efficacy in people than the acute seizure models in current use. It is an act of faith to believe that these new epilepsy models will be more predictive, although there are lots of theoretical reasons why they should be. The hypothesized tight efficacy parallels between epileptic man and beast exist because of the many similarities between the two: the models have spontaneous seizures and many of the pathological changes found in patients with limbic epilepsy, and the pathological changes suggest that the pathological alterations cause similar changes in pharmacological profiles. However, until this group of limbic epilepsy models is truly clinically validated, it will only be speculation. By validation of a model we mean that the results obtained in the model closely parallel those in humans. Until at least one drug that shows efficacy in these models predicts similar efficacy in clinical trials, the added benefit of these models is justifiably open to question. It is also unlikely (but this point is also open to criticism) that a drug that fails in the model would be sent to clinical trials, so parallels with negative results in the animals will not often be made in the clinic. Until these models are validated they should be viewed simply as another tool in the process of identifying new and, ideally, more efficacious AEDs.

Although identifying the most efficacious (and truly better) AEDs is the real goal of using these models, we are a long way from that goal. In the meantime there is still a very good use for these models: the identification of mechanisms to target. Until now there has never been an organized approach to deciding which of a number of potential mechanisms should be targeted, and certainly not in a model of epilepsy. Although drugs with a defined neuronal mechanism have been tested, none have been compared in an epilepsy model. One of the missing pieces in epilepsy drug development is a well defined target or targets to develop drugs for. These models could provide that set of targets. The other benefit to using these models is that there are parts of the brain that are involved in seizure generation and spread and parts that are not (Bertram, 1997; Bertram et al., 1998) Although the distribution of drugs within the brain will likely vary significantly from drug to drug, some may preferentially go to the epileptogenic zones and be highly effective. Because the pathology is similar to human pathology, the distribution of the drugs may well be different than what we see in normal brain. So by using drugs of a defined mechanism of action in an *in vivo* system that has "human" pathology, we may improve the chances of discovering drugs of outstanding potential, at least for limbic epilepsy. It is in the potential to discover classes of compounds that these models may have their best initial usefulness.

In summary, the need for models that have real epilepsy with strong human parallels to assist in the drug discovery process is clear. There are so many changes in the brain in epilepsy that it is not reasonable to think that "normal" brains can be used to discover better drugs. Although models of true epilepsy with appropriate changes exist, their use for broad screening is limited by a number of technical challenges that make them expensive and slow to use. However for discovering "best" targets and as a late stage screen to determine potential efficacy or best in class drugs before a clinical trial, these models may provide a new and important path to better therapies that will reduce the burden of drug resistance in epilepsy. However, these potentials remain largely theoretical until the model is properly validated in a clinical trial with a new compound. Ultimately, however, to move the field forward significantly, which is what we all want, we need a number of models of different human epilepsy types, because each syndrome may respond better to different drugs. Having multiple models may also lead us to the real goal: finding the one drug that will treat all forms of epilepsy.

Acknowledgments

This work was supported in part by grant NS 25605 and NS 49617 from the National Institute of Neurological Disorders and Stroke of the National Institutes of Health.

References

Aronica E, Yankaya B, Troost D, van Vliet EA, Lopes da Silva FH, Gorter JA. Induction of neonatal sodium channel II and III alpha-isoform mRNAs in neurons and microglia after status epilepticus in the rat hippocampus. *Europ Jour Neurosci* 2001; 13: 1261-6.

Ben-Ari Y, Tremblay E, Ottersen OP. Injections of kainic acid into the amygdaloid complex of therat: an electrographic, clinical and histological study in relation to the pathology of epilepsy. *Neurosci* 1980; 5: 515-28.

Bertram EH. Monitoring for seizures in rodents. In: *Models of Seizures and Epilepsy,* Chapter 46. A Pitkänen, PA Schwartzkroin & SL Moshé (eds). Amsterdam: Elsevier, 2006: 569-82.

Bertram EH. The functional anatomy of spontaneous seizures in a rat model of chronic limbic epilepsy. *Epilepsia*, 1997; 38: 95-105.

Bertram EH, Cornett J. The evolution of a rat model of chronic limbic epilepsy. *Brain Res* 1994; 661: 157-62.

Bertram EH, Scott C. Pathological substrate for limbic epilepsy: is the medial dorsal thalamic nucleus the unifying abnormality. *Epilepsia* 2000; 41 (suppl 6): S3-S9.

Bertram EH, Zhang DX, Mangan P, Fountain N, Rempe D. Functional anatomy of limbic epilepsy: a proposal for central synchronization of a diffusely hyperexcitable network. *Epilepsy Res*. 1998; 32: 194-205.

Bethmann K, Brandt C, Löscher W. Resistance to phenobarbital extends to phenytoin in a rat model of temporal lobe epilepsy. *Epilepsia* 2007; 48: 816-26.

Brooks-Kayal AR, Shumate MD, Jin H, Rikhter TY, Kelly ME, Coulter DA. gamma-Aminobutyric acid(A) receptor subunit expression predicts functional changes in hippocampal dentate granule cells during postnatal development. *J Neurochem* 2001; 77: 1266-78.

Cavalheiro EA, Leite JP, Bortolotto ZA, Turski WA, Ikonomidou C, Turski L: Long-term effects of pilocarpine in rats: structural damage of the brain triggers kindling and spontaneous recurrent seizures. *Epilepsia* 1991; 32: 778-82.

De Smedt T. Raedt R. Vonck K. Boon P. Levetiracetam: the profile of a novel anticonvulsant drug-part I: preclinical data. *CNS Drug Reviews* 2007; 13: 43-56.

Goffin K. Nissinen J. Van Laere K. Pitkanen A. Cyclicity of spontaneous recurrent seizures in pilocarpine model of temporal lobe epilepsy in rat. *Experiment Neurol* 2007; 205: 501-5.

Herzog AG. Fowler KM. NIH Progesterone Trial Study Group. Sensitivity and specificity of the association between catamenial seizure patterns and ovulation. *Neurology* 2008; 70: 486-7.

Ketelaars SO, Gorter JA, van Vliet EA, Lopes da Silva FH, Wadman WJ. Sodium currents in isolated rat CA1 pyramidal and dentate granule neurones in the post-status epilepticus model of epilepsy. *Neurosci* 2001; 105: 109-20.

Kwan P, Brodie MJ. Emerging drugs for epilepsy. *Expert Opinion on Emerging Drugs* 2007; 12: 407-22.

Löscher W. The pharmacokinetics of antiepileptic drugs in rats: consequences for maintaining effective drug levels during prolonged drug administration in rat models of epilepsy. *Epilepsia* 2007; 48: 1245-58.

Löscher W. Drug transporters in the epileptic brain. *Epilepsia* 2007; 48 (suppl 1): 8-13.

Mangan P, Bertram E. Shortened-duration $GABA_A$ receptor mediated synaptic potentials underlie enhanced CA1 excitability in a chronic model of temporal lobe epilepsy. *Neurosci* 1997; 80: 1101-11.

Mangan PS, Lothman EW. Profound disturbances of pre- and post synaptic $GABA_B$ receptor-mediated processes in region CA1 in a chronic model of temporal lobe epilepsy. *J Neurophysiol* 1996; 76: 1282-96.

Mathern GW, Pretorius JK, Leite JP, *et al*. Differential changes in hippocampal AMPA and NMDA mRNA levels and subunit immunoreactivity in human temporal lobe epilepsy and a rodent model of chronic limbic epilepsy. *Epilepsy Res* 1998; 32: 154-71.

Meldrum BS. Identification and preclinical testing of novel antiepileptic compounds. *Epilepsia* 1997; 38 (suppl 9): S7-15.

Mtchedlishvili Z, Bertram EH, Kapur J. Diminished allopregnanolone enhancement of $GABA_A$ receptor currents in a rat model of chronic temporal lobe epilepsy. *Journ Physiol* 2001; 537: 453-65.

Nissinen J, Pitkanen A. Effect of antiepileptic drugs on spontaneous seizures in epileptic rats. *Epilepsy Res* 2007; 73: 181-91.

Quigg M, Straume M, Menaker M, Bertram EH. Temporal Distribution of Partial Seizures: Comparison of an Animal Model with Human Partial Epilepsy. *Ann Neurol* 1998; 43: 748-55.

Quigg M, Straume M. Dual epileptic foci in a single patient express distinct temporal patterns dependent on limbic versus nonlimbic brain location. *Ann Neurol* 2000; 48: 117-20.

Remy S, Chen J, Gabriel S, *et al*. A novel mechanism underlying pharmaco-resistance in chronic epilepsy: reduced pharmacosensitivity of voltage-dependent sodium channels. *Epilepsia* 2002: 43 (suppl 7): 4.

Rogawski MA. Diverse mechanisms of antiepileptic drugs in the development pipeline. *Epilepsy Res* 2006; 69: 273-94.

Sankar R. Holmes GL. Mechanisms of action for the commonly used antiepileptic drugs: relevance to antiepileptic drug-associated neurobehavioral adverse effects. *Jour Child Neurol* 2004; 19 (suppl 1): S6-14.

Scharfman HE, MacLusky NJ. The influence of gonadal hormones on neuronal excitability, seizures, and epilepsy in the female. *Epilepsia* 2006; 47: 1423-40.

Scheffer IE, Jones L, Pozzebon M, Howell RA, Saling MM, Berkovic SF. Autosomal dominant rolandic epilepsy and speech dyspraxia: a new syndrome with anticipation. *Ann Neurol* 1995; 38: 633-42.

Shumate MD, Lin DD, Gibbs JW, Holloway KL, Coulter DA. GABA-A receptor function in epileptic human dentate granule cells: comparison to epileptic and control rat. *Epilepsy Res* 1998; 32: 114-28.

Sills GJ. The mechanisms of action of gabapentin and pregabalin. *Curr Opin Pharmacol.* 2006; 6: 108-13.

Sisodiya SM. Mechanisms of antiepileptic drug resistance. *Curr Opin Neurol* 2003; 16: 197-201.

Smith SS, Shen H, Gong QH, Zhou X. Neurosteroid regulation of GABA(A) receptors: Focus on the alpha4 and delta subunits. *Pharmacol Therapeut* 2007; 116: 58-76.

Stables JP, White HS, Dudek FE, *et al.* Models for identifying treatments for pharmacoresistance in and prevention of epilepsy. NINDS Workshop Report. *Epilepsia* 2003; 44: 1472-8.

van Vliet EA, van Schaik R, Edelbroek PM, *et al.* Inhibition of the multidrug transporter P-glycoprotein improves seizure control in phenytoin-treated chronic epileptic rats. *Epilepsia* 2006; 47: 672-80.

van Vliet EA, van Schaik R, Edelbroek PM, Wadman WJ, Lopes da Silva FH, Gorter JA. Development of tolerance to levetiracetam in rats with chronic epilepsy. *Epilepsia* 2008; 49: 1151-9.

Vreugendenhil M, Wadman WJ. Modulation of sodium currents in rat CA1 neurons by carbamazepine and valproate after kindling epileptogenesis. *Epilepsia* 1999; 40: 1512-22.

White HS. Preclinical development of antiepileptic drugs: past, present, and future directions. *Epilepsia* 2003; 44 (suppl 7): 2-8.

Yang XF, Weisenfeld A. Rothman SM. Prolonged exposure to levetiracetam reveals a presynaptic effect on neurotransmission. *Epilepsia* 2007; 48: 1861-9.

Pertinent approaches for genetic identification of resistance to AEDs

Sanjay Sisodiya

Department of Clinical and Experimental Epilepsy, UCL Institute of Neurology, National Hospital for Neurology and Neurosurgery, London, UK

Drug resistance in epilepsy is a thorny problem from many perspectives, as illustrated by several other chapters in this collection. We certainly do not know, in most cases, what causes it – but at a more fundamental level, we have trouble defining it, or even knowing if it is a unitary state. Thoughtful commentaries from experienced researchers have contributed to many of these debates: definitions matter, and in genomic studies, phenotype remains king. The focus of this chapter is to consider what contribution genetics might have to the understanding, treatment, and prevention of drug resistance in epilepsy. Where issues such as definition are integral to considerations of genetics, these will also be considered. At this time, there is no proven common genetic basis to drug resistance in epilepsy, but we are now in a position to undertake comprehensive studies – provided we can define the problem – that might at least allow us to define the extent and identity of any common genetic contribution, or alternatively to exclude common variation of given effect size. In either case, this should permit some understanding of what is left to do, and how it might be achieved. The purpose of genetic study of drug resistance must be to identify (new) underlying mechanisms, to thence generate treatments or prevention, because successful prediction of the state of drug resistance alone is an insufficient achievement, as we do not currently have effective treatments other than antiepileptic drugs to offer most patients with drug-resistant epilepsy.

Most genetic studies in epilepsy have been "traditional" linkage studies in kindreds with particular syndromes, leading sometimes to the discovery of causative pathological mutations in a gene. In contrast, there have been comparatively few direct genetic studies of response – or resistance – to antiepileptic drugs or other treatment (surgery).

Recent studies of drug resistance have largely, but not uniquely, focused on two hypotheses, the transport and the target hypotheses. It is generally considered that these need not be mutually exclusive, and that whatever the reality behind drug resistance, however defined, the phenomenon is likely to be multifactorial. Nevertheless, even within the most recent history of the study of drug resistance, a start needed to be made somewhere. Both these hypotheses were reasonable starting points, because, even if one considers only a genetic perspective, preliminary evidence across human disease had already indicated more than five years ago that genes influencing drug response tended to encode drug targets, drug metabolisers and drug transporters, all key components of the interaction between drug and organism (Goldstein et al., 2003).

■ Target issues

With regard to the target hypothesis (Remy & Beck, 2006), our quantitative trait association study demonstrated that common variation in SCN1A was associated with the maximum dose used in clinical practice both of carbamazepine, and as a functional replication in a partially-overlapping cohort, of phenytoin (Tate et al., 2005). The associated variant in SCN1A was not initially known to be functional, but was picked as a tagging polymorphism, i.e. a polymorphism that reflected the state of a number of other polymorphisms, and thus allowed greater cost efficiency in the association study. The variant accounted for only a small percentage of the total variation in the chosen carbamazepine or phenytoin dosage phenotype. Extensive further molecular genetics and in vitro modelling work have demonstrated that the associated variant is very likely itself to be functional, as it appears to govern the splicing of alternative exons in SCN1A (Tate et al., 2005; Heinzen et al., 2007). Of note, this alternative splicing event also influences the regulation of SCN1A gene expression by NOVA2 (Heinzen et al., 2007). It remains to be shown whether the alternative encoded protein isoforms themselves have different biophysical properties and different responses to antiepileptic drugs, and whether this ties in with other evidence in support of the target hypothesis, much of which is drug- and cell population-specific and otherwise difficult to access (Schaub et al., 2007; Jandová et al., 2006). It should also be noted that the original association has not been independently replicated (Zimprich et al., 2008). Nevertheless, this tentative first pharmacodynamic pharmacogenetic variant in epilepsy provides some support for a genetic approach to drug resistance in human epilepsy, and to the target hypothesis in particular.

It does need to be borne in mind that the original phenotype (Tate et al., 2005) was a complex composite phenotype, and was not purely one of drug resistance. It also remains important to establish a theoretical framework for studying the pharmacogenetic basis of the target hypothesis. We need to be clear what we will accept as criteria for proof. We need to know how to test the hypothesis in vivo in man. We need to establish how commonly target variation may be responsible for pharmacoresistance. We need to understand how target variation might explain non-response to multiple antiepileptic drugs in individual patients. We need to understand broadly whether there is a genetic basis for the target hypothesis, and whether this genetic basis is constitutive – or purely inherited – or may be acquired. Even though there is much to do, the importance of the approach again lies not particularly in the possibility of prediction of drug dosage in individual patients (which is likely to be influenced by other factors as well), but in the identification of targets, pathways and mechanisms leading to novel approaches to treatment.

"Target" might be more broadly interpreted. A "pharmacogenetic" study of seizure response after temporal lobectomy as treatment for drug-resistant temporal lobe epilepsy reported an association between a variant in the prion protein gene PRNP and mesial temporal lobe epilepsy and outcome after surgical treatment in 100 consecutive patients (Walz et al., 2003). We were unable to find the reported variant in a Western European population of 121 patients with drug-resistant temporal lobe epilepsy with hippocampal sclerosis (Cavalleri et al., 2005).

■ Metabolism issues

Pharmacokinetic genetic variation in epilepsy is of course long-established. Allelic variants in the gene encoding CYP2C9 are well known to influence the rate of metabolism of phenytoin (Tate et al., 2005; Aynacioglu et al., 1999). CYP2C19 has a small contribution to phenytoin metabolism in general; alleles in the gene encoding CYP2C19 with distributions more restricted to specific populations have been suggested to contribute to phenytoin pharmacokinetics (Hung et al., 2004). Most of these variants with quantitative effects on metabolism are rare. In routine clinical practice, most such variants are easily accommodated, by alteration in drug dosage. This is the likely explanation for the absence of routine testing of CYP2C9 allelic status prior to prescription of phenytoin, and serves as a useful reminder that identified pharmacogenetic variants may not always be of direct clinical utility.

■ Transport issues

The transport hypothesis has received perhaps more attention, and certainly generated more controversy. Overall, we are at the point now that some, even those who until recently were strong supporters, believe there is little or no real evidence in support of a role in humans for the best studied multidrug transporter, P-glycoprotein (Löscher & Sills, 2007; Anderson & Shen, 2007), whilst others hold the opposite position. Pharmacogenetic studies have focused on *ABCB1*, the gene encoding P-glycoprotein. Our own initial pharmacogenetic study was a candidate SNP study, and adopted a particular definition of drug resistance (and responsiveness) (Siddiqui et al., 2003). There have been at least twelve separate association studies since (Ebid et al., 2007; Kwan et al., 2007; Leschziner et al., 2007; Ozgon et al., 2008; Shahwan et al., 2007; Kim et al., 2006a; Kim et al., 2006b; Seo et al., 2006; Hung et al., 2005; Sills et al., 2005; Tan et al., 2004; Zimprich et al., 2004). Only one has been structured as an exact replication, on the basis of definitions alone (Tan et al., 2004) – and, as is well-known, this larger replication effort did not support the original finding. Some have suggested that *ABCB1* variation may affect antiepileptic drug dose requirements (Ebid et al., 2007; Simon et al., 2007), whilst others submit that there is a relationship between some measure of *ABCB1* expression and antiepileptic drug levels in human brain (Marchi et al., 2005), but cause and effect have not been conclusively linked. Whilst there are subtleties to consider (Kimchi-Sarfaty et al., 2007; Sisodiya & Goldstein, 2007; Wang et al., 2005), there is no consensus on any possible role for genetic variation in *ABCB1* and drug resistance in epilepsy.

Other transporter, or putative transporter, proteins have been postulated to have a role in drug resistance in epilepsy, for example, RLIP76 (Awasthi et al., 2005); pharmacogenetic studies considering the encoding gene as a candidate gene variation within which might associate with clinical phenotypes of drug resistance have not shown any such association (Soranzo et al., 2007; Leschziner et al., 2007b). A lack of genetic association does not, however, exclude a role in drug resistance for the encoded protein.

Future prospects: lessons from achievements to date in studies of other diseases

A survey of real achievements across genetics and genomics is beyond the scope of this chapter, but a brief assessment shows that such achievements are possible – it is not a hopeless task.

The outstanding example of success in pharmacogenetics must be for warfarin. People vary widely in their daily requirements for warfarin for anticoagulation. The therapeutic index for this drug is so narrow, and the consequences of both inadequate and excessive anticoagulation so potentially catastrophic, that pharmacogenetic investigation was of undoubted importance. Vitamin K epoxide reductase has been known since 1974 as the target of warfarin (Zimmerman & Matschiner, 1974), but its molecular constitution and encoding gene(s) remained elusive. Warfarin resistance was subsequently mapped to rat chromosome 1 and vitamin K-dependent protein deficiencies were mapped to the syntenic region of human chromosome 16 – using traditional genetic techniques. In 2004, contemporaneous genetic studies in humans with combined vitamin K-dependent clotting factor deficiency or warfarin resistance and in other animal species resulted in the identification of *VKORC1*, vitamin K epoxide reductase complex subunit 1, as the target of warfarin (Rost et al., 2004; Li et al., 2004). This result might have remained of small print relevance. Within a year, however, a population genetic association study of (only) 147 patients requiring warfarin anticoagulation demonstrated that common variation in *VKORC1* strongly influenced daily dosage requirements (D'Andrea et al., 2005), with rapid confirmation and extension of an effect of common variation in *VKORC1* (Rieder et al., 2005). One key polymorphism identified (rs9923231) lies within the *VKORC1* promoter and appears to be the major pharmacodynamic pharmacogenetic determinant. That polymorphic variants in the gene encoding the chief metabolizing enzyme of warfarin, *CYP2C9*, influenced daily dose was already known (Voora et al., 2005). These findings support the assertion that genes encoding drug target(s) and drug metabolizing enzyme(s) are prime candidates for pharmacogenetic study – in general, and if these proteins and their genes are known (Goldstein et al., 2003).

The stage was then set for rapid translation to clinical application. Variation in clinical demographic factors account for some 20% of dose differences; *CYP2C9* variation accounts for another 20%; *VKORC1* variation accounts for some 14%: together perhaps 60% of dose variation can be predicted. This is a significant achievement for a drug with a narrow therapeutic index. The FDA has approved the use of genetic testing for warfarin dosage (http://www.fdanews.com/newsletter/article?articleId=98705&issueId = 10747). In the succeeding three years since the discovery of *VKORC1*, clinical pharmacogenetic guidelines for warfarin usage, including pharmacogenetic variants and patient age, sex and weight have been devised, but formal recommendation for their implementation in warfarin-naïve patients awaits prospective trials (Flockhart et al., 2008).

Without a doubt, the key value of this pharmacogenetic discovery is in the improved understanding it allows – clinical application follows from such understanding. For example, preliminary studies suggest that co-medication with warfarin and low-dose Vitamin K (80-100 micrograms/day) greatly improves the stability of anticoagulation and the actual time spent within the therapeutic window (Sconce et al., 2006). The potential of pharmacogenetics – in this case, a candidate gene study of drug response – has been realized, and its power demonstrated, with several postulated principles being upheld. Perhaps most interestingly from the perspective of epilepsy, in warfarin pharmacogenetics we have the best example of pathway genetics generating clinically-important results.

There are now several examples of such pharmacogenetic findings (see review by Eichelbaum et al., 2006), including of course an important study in epilepsy showing a very powerful association between the *HLA-B*1502* allele and Stevens-Johnson syndrome caused by carbamazepine exposure in Han Chinese (Chung et al., 2004). This was a candidate SNP and allele study of 44 patients, and is now considered sufficiently established for an FDA advisory for genotyping prior to carbamazepine usage in patients of South Asian origin (http://www.fda.gov/cder/drug/InfoSheets/HCP/carbamazepineHCP.htm).

Clearly in circumscribed areas of human disease treatment there has been remarkable progress. Yet, the majority of drugs prescribed in humans do not have replicated, convincing pharmacogenetic associations, if indeed any studies have been undertaken. What can be learnt from existing successes for application to other drugs and diseases? Why have those studies that have succeeded done so? The following framework might be extrapolated from successful disease susceptibility association studies:

The drug appears to have a relatively clean mechanism of action, target, metabolism or transport.

The drug has a narrow therapeutic index, often with serious adverse reactions resulting from inappropriate usage or dosing.

A clear clinical phenotype is thus definable and identifiable in regular clinical practice.

The target or mechanism of drug action may be at least partly known, or Mendelian diseases have been identified which result from mutations in genes thus identified as the drug target-encoding gene, both facilitating a candidate gene approach.

The combination of effect size and minor allele frequencies have permitted comparatively small studies to identify putatively causal associations – the common disease (or common phenotype) – common variant hypothesis in these cases at least has been supported.

Chance findings have been assiduously pursued: rare kindreds with Mendelian traits, traditional linkage genetics and cytogenetics have permitted candidate regions or genes to be identified and narrowed down.

Technological aspects, though often sophisticated, have, in general, not been the key to these discoveries. Bioinformatics and other disciplines have been employed where necessary and applicable.

In the past, studies have mainly been of candidate genes – genes selected because they encode proteins which are drug targets, drug transporters or drug metabolisers, or proteins within pathways defined by these elements. In fact, many previous pharmacogenetic studies have been candidate SNP studies, where one or a few chosen polymorphisms have been studied, without necessarily any regard to haplotype structure or coverage of variation in the entire gene. Such studies were often the only ones feasible. Where biological motivation is very strong for a given polymorphism or gene, this approach remains, barely, justifiable.

However, we no longer need to limit ourselves to selection and study of candidate polymorphisms or candidate genes. The concepts, technology, biological and funding resources are now available to undertake an examination of the effect on phenotypes of interest of specified common variation across the entire genome. Most authorities consider that there are of the order of 10-15 million single nucleotide polymorphisms in the human genome. Current genome-wide genotyping technology enables examination of 500,000 SNPs in a given individual. Higher density chips are available, and becoming more widely used. Association studies for drug response, based on the common disease-common variant (CD/CV) model, are thus now possible at the whole genome level, and when considering drug phenotypes, should be called pharmacogenomic rather than pharmacogenetic studies.

There are no published genome-wide pharmacogenomic association studies in epilepsy. There is, on the other hand, a rich literature already for genome-wide association studies for disease susceptibility (reviewed in Altshuler & Daly, 2007; Bowcock, 2007; Gibson & Goldstein, 2007). An empirical view has emerged that for disease susceptibility studies at least, cohorts of at least 2,000 cases are likely to be able to identify disease-associated variants (http://www.wtccc.org.uk/). We do not know what parameters might apply to GWAS of drug response, though it is worth bearing in mind that significant and important associations have been revealed in candidate gene studies of as few as 44 patients for Stevens-Johnson syndrome with carbamazepine (Chung et al., 2004) and 147 patients for warfarin dosing (D'Andrea et al., 2005).

The key component of any proposed study design framework is the phenotype. The challenge is to identify a bioclinical phenotype that is robust, meaningful and analysable. With regard to drug resistance in epilepsy, the key will be the definition and modelling of drug resistance. The least certain aspect is cohort size, and it is to be hoped that far smaller cohorts may enable clinically-important drug responses to be understood at a genetic level – only empirical evidence will determine this. If further efforts to examine drug resistance in epilepsy at a candidate gene level are made, then models used for gene selection will need to be explicitly considered. Antiepileptic drug pharmacogenetics is not equivalent to the genetics of drug resistance: the sets of genes implicated in each case are not identical and may not necessarily be overlapping. Such considerations are unnecessary for GWAS: pharmacogenomic studies offer a major advantage despite their several drawbacks – there is no need to postulate candidate genes *a priori*.

There are no published genome-wide studies of drug resistance in epilepsy. There are, however, several ongoing genome-wide association studies of various aspects or phenotypes of epilepsy. These efforts include EPICURE (www.epicureproject.eu), funded by the European Union, the Epilepsy Phenome-Genome Project (www.epgp.org), funded by the NIH and the EPIGEN consortium (www.epilepsygenetics.eu), partially funded by the Wellcome Trust. In each case, multicentre collaborations have been established, with shared phenotyping protocols, genotyping platforms and association strategies. The possibility exists for large metacollaborative initiatives to examine drug resistance – if a common definition can be agreed. Genomic studies may contribute to understanding of the apparent benefits of postulated interventions for drug-resistant epilepsy, such as repetitive transcranial magnetic stimulation (Cantello et al., 2007; Fregni et al., 2006).

Finally, on the current horizon is individual-subject whole genome sequencing for large cohorts of patients. In this setting, it will not be necessary to type a set of surrogate markers representing the entirety of common variation(s), but instead it will be possible to directly type all variation, including rare variants that might contribute to empirical confirmation of the CD/RV model. This will generate truly immense possibilities across human diseases, not least for epilepsy (for a series of opinions on the impact of accessible whole genome sequencing, see http://www.nature.com/ng/qoty/index.html) At this time, whole *gene* (not genome) resequencing in large cohorts for mutation discovery is proving just feasible, and is yielding important results in other fields, such as diabetes (Edghill *et al.*, 2008), and is underway in epilepsy (The Human Channelopathy Project, http://www.bcm.edu/fromthe-lab/vol03/is8/04oct_b.htm). Data from this study may allow testing of aspects of the common disease-rare variant model, including the phenomenon of drug resistance.

■ Caveats

Genomics is likely to prove a powerful tool. But it will not be the solution to all our problems in epilepsy. For example, there may be relevant genetic variation that population genetic association studies cannot identify because it is not common across patients (*i.e.* common disease/rare variant), or because it is not unitary (multigenic trait, perhaps with different combinations of common variants in different patients, all leading to the same phenotypic outcome), or because any common variant is not currently tagged (*i.e.* singleton untaggable polymorphism). It may also be that a single polymorphism is not of major enough effect size, or that it is population-specific, or that it is genetically complex, or that there is epigenetic modification. We may identify an associated common variant but then not be able to determine the causal variant – an unlikely but not impossible scenario. It is also possible that there is no relevant genetic variation in or around the controlling gene of interest – so then genetics cannot offer us a clue to the phenotype of interest. Phenocopies will present another confounding factor. It may prove necessary to iteratively refine phenotypes using genotyping and phenotypic information.

■ Conclusions

Drug resistance in epilepsy is an important clinical problem. A genomic approach may allow better understanding of its basis, with a view to novel therapeutic approaches. There is no guarantee that a genomic approach will achieve this aim. A well-constructed study – or international, multicentre initiative – may, however, at least allow us the chance to understand the boundaries constraining any genomic influence, thus permitting us to understand the size of the problem that remains beyond genomics. We must also remember the ethical, social and moral aspects of genetic and genomic research (Shostak & Ottman, 2006).

Acknowledgments

The author's work is supported by grants from the UK MRC and Wellcome Trust.

References

Altshuler D, Daly M. Guilt beyond a reasonable doubt. *Nat Genet* 2007; 39 (7): 813-5.

Anderson GD, Shen DD. Where is the evidence that p-glycoprotein limits brain uptake of antiepileptic drug and contributes to drug resistance in epilepsy? *Epilepsia* 2007; 48 (12): 2372-4.

Awasthi S, Hallene KL, Fazio V, *et al*. RLIP76, a non-ABC transporter, and drug resistance in epilepsy. *BMC Neurosci* 2005; 27 (6): 61.

Aynacioglu AS, Brockmöller J, Bauer S, *et al*. Frequency of cytochrome P450 CYP2C9 variants in a Turkish population and functional relevance for phenytoin. *Br J Clin Pharmacol* 1999; 48 (3): 409-15.

Bowcock AM. Genomics: guilt by association. *Nature* 2007 7; 447 (7145): 645-6.

Cantello R, Rossi S, Varrasi C, *et al.* Slow repetitive TMS for drug-resistant epilepsy: clinical and EEG findings of a placebo-controlled trial. *Epilepsia* 2007; 48 (2): 366-74.

Cavalleri GL, Lynch JM, Depondt C, *et al.* Failure to replicate previously reported genetic associations with sporadic temporal lobe epilepsy: where to from here? *Brain* 2005; 128 (Pt 8): 1832-40.

Chung WH, Hung SI, Hong HS, *et al.* Medical genetics: a marker for Stevens-Johnson syndrome. *Nature* 2004 1; 428 (6982): 486.

D'Andrea G, D'Ambrosio RL, Di Perna P, *et al.* A polymorphism in the VKORC1 gene is associated with an interindividual variability in the dose-anticoagulant effect of warfarin. *Blood* 2005 15; 105 (2): 645-9.

Ebid AH, Ahmed MM, Mohammed SA. Therapeutic drug monitoring and clinical outcomes in epileptic Egyptian patients: a gene polymorphism perspective study. *Ther Drug Monit* 2007; 29 (3): 305-12.

Edghill EL, Flanagan SE, Patch AM, *et al.* Insulin Mutation Screening in 1,044 Patients with Diabetes: Mutations in the INS gene are a Common Cause of Neonatal Diabetes but a Rare Cause of Diabetes Diagnosed in Childhood or Adulthood. *Diabetes* 2008; 11.

Eichelbaum M, Ingelman-Sundberg M, Evans WE. Pharmacogenomics and individualized drug therapy. *Annu Rev Med* 2006; 57: 119-37.

Flockhart DA, O'Kane D, Williams MS, *et al.* ACMG Working Group on Pharmacogenetic Testing of CYP2C9, VKORC1 Alleles for Warfarin Use. Pharmacogenetic testing of CYP2C9 and VKORC1 alleles for warfarin. *Genet Med* 2008; 10 (2): 139-50.

Fregni F, Otachi PT, Do Valle A, *et al.* A randomized clinical trial of repetitive transcranial magnetic stimulation in patients with refractory epilepsy. *Ann Neurol* 2006; 60 (4): 447-55.

Gibson G, Goldstein DB. Human genetics: the hidden text of genome-wide associations. *Curr Biol* 2007 6; 17 (21): R929-32.

Goldstein DB, Tate SK, Sisodiya SM. Pharmacogenetics goes genomic. *Nat Rev Genet* 2003; 4: 937-47.

Heinzen EL, Yoon W, Tate SK, *et al.* Nova2 interacts with a cis-acting polymorphism to influence the proportions of drug responsive splice variants of SCN1A. *Am J Hum Genet* 2007; 80 (5): 876-83.

Hung CC, Lin CJ, Chen CC, Chang CJ, Liou HH. Dosage recommendation of phenytoin for patients with epilepsy with different CYP2C9/CYP2C19 polymorphisms. *Ther Drug Monit* 2004; 26 (5): 534-40.

Hung CC, Tai JJ, Lin CJ, Lee MJ, Liou HH. Complex haplotypic effects of the ABCB1 gene on epilepsy treatment response. *Pharmacogenomics* 2005; 6 (4): 411-7.

Jandová K, Päsler D, Antonio LL, *et al.* Carbamazepine-resistance in the epileptic dentate gyrus of human hippocampal slices. *Brain* 2006; 129 (Pt 12): 3290-306.

Kim YO, Kim MK, Woo YJ, *et al.* Single nucleotide polymorphisms in the multidrug resistance 1 gene in Korean epileptics. *Seizure* 2006a; 15 (1): 67-72.

Kim DW, Kim M, Lee SK, Kang R, Lee SY. Lack of association between C3435T nucleotide MDR1 genetic polymorphism and multidrug-resistant epilepsy. *Seizure* 2006b; 15 (5): 344-7.

Kimchi-Sarfaty C, Oh JM, Kim IW, *et al.* A "silent" polymorphism in the MDR1 gene changes substrate specificity. *Science* 2007 Jan 26; 315 (5811): 525-8; Erratum in: *Science* 2007 30; 318 (5855): 1382-3.

Kwan P, Baum L, Wong V, *et al.* Association between ABCB1 C3435T polymorphism and drug-resistant epilepsy in Han Chinese. *Epilepsy Behav* 2007; 11 (1): 112-7.

Leschziner GD, Andrew T, Leach JP, *et al.* Common ABCB1 polymorphisms are not associated with multidrug resistance in epilepsy using a gene-wide tagging approach. *Pharmacogenet Genomics* 2007a; 17 (3): 217-20.

Leschziner GD, Jorgensen AL, Andrew T, et al. The association between polymorphisms in RLIP76 and drug response in epilepsy. *Pharmacogenomics* 2007b; 8 (12): 1715-22.

Li T, Chang CY, Jin DY, Lin PJ, Khvorova A, Stafford DW. Identification of the gene for vitamin K epoxide reductase. *Nature* 2004 5; 427 (6974): 541-4.

Löscher W, Sills GJ. Drug resistance in epilepsy: why is a simple explanation not enough? *Epilepsia* 2007; 48 (12): 2370-2.

Marchi N, Guiso G, Rizzi M, et al. A pilot study on brain-to-plasma partition of 10,11-dyhydro-10-hydroxy-5H-dibenzo (b,f)azepine-5-carboxamide and MDR1 brain expression in epilepsy patients not responding to oxcarbazepine. *Epilepsia* 2005; 46 (10): 1613-9.

Ozgon GO, Bebek N, Gul G, Cine N. Association of MDR1 (C3435T) polymorphism and resistance to carbamazepine in epileptic patients from Turkey. *Eur Neurol* 2008; 59 (1-2): 67-70.

Remy S, Beck H. Molecular and cellular mechanisms of pharmacoresistance in epilepsy. *Brain* 2006; 129 (Pt 1): 18-35.

Rieder MJ, Reiner AP, Gage BF, et al. Effect of VKORC1 haplotypes on transcriptional regulation and warfarin dose. *N Engl J Med* 2005; 352: 2285-93.

Rost S, Fregin A, Ivaskevicius V, et al. Mutations in VKORC1 cause warfarin resistance and multiple coagulation factor deficiency type 2. *Nature* 2004 5; 427 (6974): 537-41.

Schaub C, Uebachs M, Beck H. Diminished response of CA1 neurons to antiepileptic drugs in chronic epilepsy. *Epilepsia* 2007; 48 (7): 1339-50.

Sconce E, Avery P, Wynne H, Kamali F. Vitamin K supplementation can improve stability of anticoagulation for patients with unexplained variability in response to warfarin. *Blood* 2006; 109: 2419-23.

Seo T, Ishitsu T, Ueda N, et al. ABCB1 polymorphisms influence the response to antiepileptic drugs in Japanese epilepsy patients. *Pharmacogenomics* 2006; 7 (4): 551-61.

Shahwan A, Murphy K, Doherty C, et al. The controversial association of ABCB1 polymorphisms in refractory epilepsy: an analysis of multiple SNPs in an Irish population. *Epilepsy Res* 2007; 73 (2): 192-8.

Shostak S, Ottman R. Ethical, legal, and social dimensions of epilepsy genetics. *Epilepsia* 2006 Oct; 47 (10): 1595-602.

Siddiqui A, Kerb R, Weale M, et al. Multidrug resistance in epilepsy is associated with a polymorphism in ABCB1. *N Engl J Med* 2003; 348: 1442-48.

Sills GJ, Mohanraj R, Butler E, et al. Lack of association between the C3435T polymorphism in the human multidrug resistance (MDR1) gene and response to antiepileptic drug treatment. *Epilepsia* 2005; 46 (5): 643-7.

Simon C, Stieger B, Kullak-Ublick GA, et al. Intestinal expression of cytochrome P450 enzymes and ABC transporters and carbamazepine and phenytoin disposition. *Acta Neurol Scand* 2007; 115 (4): 232-42.

Sisodiya SM, Goldstein DB. Drug resistance in epilepsy: more twists in the tale. *Epilepsia* 2007; 48 (12): 2369-70.

Soranzo N, Kelly L, Martinian L, et al. Lack of support for a role for RLIP76 (RALBP1) in response to treatment or predisposition to epilepsy. *Epilepsia* 2007; 48 (4): 674-83.

Tan NC, Heron SE, Scheffer IE, et al. Failure to confirm association of a polymorphism in ABCB1 with multidrug-resistant epilepsy. *Neurology* 2004 28; 63 (6): 1090-2.

Tate SK, Depondt C, Sisodiya SM, et al. Genetic predictors of clinical use of the anti-epileptic drugs phenytoin and carbamazepine. *Proc Natl Acad Sci USA* 2005; 102: 5507-12.

Voora D, Eby C, Linder MW, et al. Prospective dosing of warfarin based on cytochrome P-450 2C9 genotype. *Thromb Haemost* 2005; 93: 700-5.

Walz R, Castro RM, Velasco TR, et al. Surgical outcome in mesial temporal sclerosis correlates with prion protein gene variant. *Neurology* 2003 11; 61 (9): 1204-10.

Wang D, Johnson AD, Papp AC, Kroetz DL, Sadée W. Multidrug resistance polypeptide 1 (MDR1, ABCB1) variant 3435C>T affects mRNA stability. *Pharmacogenet Genomics* 2005; 15 (10): 693-704.

Zimmerman A, Matschiner JT. Biochemical basis of hereditary resistance to warfarin in the rat. *Biochem Pharmacol* 1974; 23: 1033-40.

Zimprich F, Sunder-Plassmann R, Stogmann E, *et al.* Association of an ABCB1 gene haplotype with pharmacoresistance in temporal lobe epilepsy. *Neurology* 2004 28; 63 (6): 1087-9.

Zimprich F, Stogmann E, Bonelli S, *et al.* A functional polymorphism in the SCN1A gene is not associated with carbamazepine dosages in Austrian patients with epilepsy. *Epilepsia* 2008; 49 (6): 1108-9.

Molecular targets of antiepileptic drugs

Graeme J. Sills

Division of Neurological Science, School of Clinical Sciences, University of Liverpool, UK

The issue of drug resistance in epilepsy has received considerable attention in recent years, and the search for mechanisms that might explain why around 30% of patients fail to respond to current medications continues apace. A number of plausible hypotheses have been proposed, including inadequate penetration of antiepileptic drugs across the blood-brain barrier; acquired alterations to the structure and/or functionality of ion channels and neurotransmitter receptors that represent the principal targets of antiepileptic drugs; and an inherent resistance, governed by genetic variants of proteins involved in the pharmacokinetics and pharmacodynamics of antiepileptic drug action (Schmidt & Löscher, 2005). What is commonly forgotten, however, is that drug resistance is, by definition, a function of the availability of drugs, the mechanisms by which those drugs work, and the appropriateness of those mechanisms for the disease process. One could argue that the term "drug resistance" has commonly been employed to hide our lack of basic understanding of the pathophysiology of epilepsy and the pharmacology of drugs used in its treatment. That understanding has improved immeasurably in the past 20 years. At the same time, an unprecedented number of new antiepileptic drugs have reached the marketplace.

The serendipitous discovery of the anticonvulsant properties of phenobarbital in 1912 marked the foundation of the modern pharmacotherapy of epilepsy. The subsequent 70 years saw the introduction of phenytoin, ethosuximide, carbamazepine, sodium valproate and a range of benzodiazepines. Collectively, these agents have come to be regarded as the "established" antiepileptic drugs (Brodie & Dichter, 1996). A concerted period of drug development for epilepsy throughout the 1980s and 1990s has resulted in eleven new agents being licensed as add-on treatment for difficult-to-control adult epilepsy with some becoming available as monotherapy for newly diagnosed patients. These have become known as the "new" or "modern" antiepileptic drugs (Schachter, 2007).

Whether by either accident or design, the drug treatment of epilepsy has traditionally relied upon the control of symptoms, *i.e.* suppression of seizures. Recurrent seizure activity is the manifestation of an intermittent and excessive hyperexcitability of the nervous system and, while the pharmacological minutiae of currently marketed antiepileptic drugs remain to be completely unravelled, these agents essentially redress the balance between neuronal excitation and inhibition. At the cellular level, three major mechanisms of action are recognised; modulation of voltage-gated ion channels, enhancement of (γ-aminobutyric acid (GABA) mediated inhibitory neurotransmission, and attenuation of glutamate mediated excitatory neurotransmission (Kwan et al., 2001; Rogawski & Löscher, 2004). The principal pharmacological targets of currently available antiepileptic drugs are highlighted in Table I.

Current antiepileptic drug targets

Voltage-gated ion channels

Ion channels regulate the flow of positively and negatively charged ions across neuronal cell membranes and ultimately control the intrinsic excitability of the nervous system (Barchi, 1998). Voltage-gated sodium channels are responsible for depolarisation of the nerve cell membrane and conduction of action potentials across the surface of neuronal cells. At nerve terminals, voltage-gated calcium channels are recruited by sodium channel dependent depolarisation, leading to calcium entry, neurotransmitter release and chemical signalling across the synapse. Sodium channels are expressed throughout the neuronal cell membrane, on dendrites, soma, axons, and nerve terminals, with no current evidence to suggest differential distribution on the basis of channel sub-type (see below, however). In contrast, calcium channels are distributed, on a cellular and anatomical basis, according to physiologically-defined sub-types (Hofmann et al., 1994). The high-voltage-activated (HVA) calcium channels, denoted N-, P/Q-, and R-type, are typically found on pre-synaptic nerve terminals and believed to regulate neurotransmitter release. The L-type channel is also a member of the HVA family but expressed on the soma and dendrites of post-synaptic cells where it is involved in the processing of synaptic inputs. The low-voltage-activated (LVA) calcium channel (T-type) is also post-synaptic but predominantly localised to thalamocortical relay neurones where it has been postulated to underpin the rhythmic 3 Hz spike-wave discharges that are characteristic of absence seizures (Coulter et al., 1989a).

Inhibitory neurotransmission

GABA is the predominant inhibitory neurotransmitter in the mammalian central nervous system and is released at up to 40% of all synapses in the brain (Olsen & Avoli, 1997). GABA is synthesised from glutamate by the action of the enzyme glutamic acid decarboxylase. Following release from GABAergic nerve terminals, it acts on the post-synaptic ionotropic $GABA_A$ receptor which responds to GABA binding by increasing chloride ion conductance, resulting in fast neuronal hyperpolarisation or inhibition (Rabow et al., 1995). In contrast, the G-protein-coupled $GABA_B$ receptor mediates slow hyperpolarisation of the post-synaptic membrane and is also found pre-synaptically where it acts as an auto-receptor, with activation limiting further GABA release (Bowery, 2006). GABA is removed from the synaptic cleft into localised nerve terminals and glial cells by a family of transport proteins, denoted GAT-1, GAT-2, GAT-3, and BGT-1. Thereafter, GABA is either recycled to the readily releasable neurotransmitter pool or inactivated by the mitochondrial enzyme GABA-transaminase.

Table I. Summary of molecular targets of current antiepileptic drugs (+++ = principal target, ++ = probable target, + = possible target)

	Voltage-gated Na⁺ channels	HVA Ca²⁺ channels	LVA Ca²⁺ channels	GABA$_A$ receptors	GABA turnover	Glutamate receptors	Synaptic vesicle protein 2A	Carbonic anhydrase
Phenobarbital		+		+++		+		
Phenytoin	+++							
Ethosuximide			+++					
Carbamazepine	+++							
Sodium valproate	++		++		++			
Benzodiazepines				+++				
Vigabatrin					+++			
Lamotrigine	+++	++						
Gabapentin	+	++			+			
Felbamate	++	++		++		++		
Topiramate	++	++		++		++		+
Tiagabine					+++			
Oxcarbazepine	+++	+						
Levetiracetam		++		+			+++	
Pregabalin		++						
Zonisamide	+++		++					+
Rufinamide	+++							

Excitatory neurotransmission

Glutamate is the principal excitatory neurotransmitter in the mammalian brain (Meldrum, 2000). Following release from glutamatergic nerve terminals, it exerts its effects on three specific subtypes of ionotropic receptor in the postsynaptic membrane, designated according to their agonist specificities, α-amino-3-hydroxy-5-methyl-isoxazole-4-propionic acid (AMPA), kainic acid (kainate), and N-methyl-D-aspartate (NMDA) (Mayer & Armstrong, 2004). These receptors respond to glutamate binding by increasing cation conductance, resulting in neuronal depolarisation or excitation. The AMPA and kainate receptor subtypes are permeable to sodium ions and are involved in fast excitatory synaptic transmission. In contrast, the NMDA receptor is permeable to both sodium and calcium ions and, owing to a voltage-dependent blockade by magnesium ions at resting membrane potential, is only activated during periods of prolonged depolarisation, as might be expected during epileptiform discharges (Dingledine et al., 1999). Metabotropic glutamate receptors perform a similar function to $GABA_B$ receptors; they are G-protein coupled and act predominantly as auto-receptors on glutamatergic terminals, limiting glutamate release (Schoepp, 2001). Glutamate is removed from the synapse into nerve terminals and glial cells by a family of specific sodium-dependent transport proteins (EAAT1 – EAAT5) and is inactivated by the enzymes glutamine synthetase (glial cells only) and glutamate dehydrogenase (Daikhin & Yudkoff, 2000).

Other putative targets

In addition to these three principal classes of antiepileptic drug target, there are multiple proteins and processes involved in the regulation of the neuronal micro-environment and in maintaining the delicate balance between excitation and inhibition in the brain and which, theoretically at least, represent additional or secondary targets for antiepileptic drug action. These include the enzyme carbonic anhydrase and specific components of the synaptic vesicle release pathway, both of which will be discussed in more detail below.

■ Mechanisms of action of existing agents

Sodium channels

Blockade of voltage-gated sodium channels is the most common mechanism of action amongst currently available antiepileptic drugs (Ragsdale & Avoli, 1998; Rogawski & Löscher, 2004). The established agents phenytoin and carbamazepine are archetypal sodium channel blockers (Courtney & Etter, 1983; McLean & Macdonald, 1983), a mechanism they share with the newer drugs, lamotrigine, felbamate, topiramate, oxcarbazepine, zonisamide and rufinamide. There is also anecdotal evidence to suggest that sodium valproate and gabapentin have inhibitory effects on neuronal sodium channels (Kwan et al., 2001; Rogawski & Löscher, 2004). Voltage-gated sodium channels exist in one of three basic conformational states, resting, open, and inactivated. During a single round of depolarisation, channels cycle through these states in turn and the neurone is unable to respond to further depolarisations until sufficient numbers of voltage-gated sodium channels have returned to the resting state (Catterall, 1992). Antiepileptic agents with sodium channel blocking properties have highest affinity for the channel protein in the inactivated state and binding slows the otherwise rapid recycling process. As a result, these drugs produce a characteristic voltage- and frequency-dependent reduction in channel conductance, resulting in a limitation of repetitive neuronal firing, with little effect on the generation of single action potentials (Ragsdale et al., 1991).

Calcium channels

Voltage-gated calcium channels represent another important target for several antiepileptic agents (Stefani et al., 1997). The efficacy of ethosuximide and zonisamide in generalised absence epilepsy is believed to be mediated by blockade of the LVA T-type calcium channel in the dendrites of thalamocortical relay neurones (Coulter et al., 1989b; Suzuki et al., 1992). There is anecdotal evidence that sodium valproate may have a similar action (Kelly et al., 1990). Lamotrigine limits neurotransmitter release by blocking both N- and P/Q-types of the HVA calcium channel (Wang et al., 1996) and levetiracetam exerts a partial blockade of N-type calcium currents, suggesting a selective effect on an as yet unidentified sub-class of this particular channel type (Lukyanetz et al., 2002). Phenobarbital, felbamate, and topiramate are also believed to influence HVA calcium channel conductance, although their effects are less well characterised in terms of channel subtypes or interaction with specific protein subunits (Ffrench-Mullen et al., 1993; Stefani et al., 1996; Zhang et al., 2000). Finally, gabapentin and pregabalin also exert their effects via HVA calcium channels, but rather than interacting with a traditional channel sub-type such as N- or L-type, they appear to bind to an accessory subunit termed $\alpha_2\delta$-1, which can modulate the function of various native channels (Dooley et al., 2007). This subunit is known to be up-regulated in dorsal root ganglion cells of the spinal cord in response to nerve injury, with selective calcium channel blockade via the $\alpha_2\delta$-1 subunit explaining the efficacy of gabapentin and pregabalin in the treatment of neuropathic pain (Li et al., 2006).

$GABA_A$ receptors

Activation of the ionotropic $GABA_A$ receptor, resulting in an enhanced response to synaptically released GABA, is a significant antiepileptic drug mechanism. Phenobarbital and the benzodiazepines share this effect, but they bind to distinct sites on the receptor complex and differentially influence the opening of the chloride ion pore. Barbiturates increase the duration of chloride channel opening, while benzodiazepines increase the frequency of opening (Twyman et al., 1989). In addition, phenobarbital is capable of direct activation of the $GABA_A$ receptor in the absence of GABA, an effect which is believed to underlie its sedative properties (Rho et al., 1996). Felbamate and topiramate also modulate GABA responses at the $GABA_A$ receptor, with binding sites and effects on channel kinetics which are reported to be distinct from one another and from those observed with barbiturates and benzodiazepines (White et al., 1995; Rho et al., 1997). Finally, levetiracetam can indirectly influence $GABA_A$ receptor function by reducing the negative allosteric modulation of the receptor complex by β-carbolines and zinc (Rigo et al., 2002).

GABA turnover

Vigabatrin and tiagabine are modern antiepileptic agents which exert their actions by selective neurochemical effects at the inhibitory synapse, resulting in altered GABA turnover (Sills, 2003). Vigabatrin is an irreversible inhibitor of the mitochondrial enzyme GABA-transaminase which is responsible for the catabolism of GABA, whereas tiagabine prevents the removal of GABA from the synaptic cleft by blockade of GABA transport (Jung et al., 1977; Nielsen et al., 1991). These distinct mechanisms result in the global elevation of brain GABA concentrations and the temporarily prolonged presence of neuronally released GABA in the synapse, respectively. Although these drugs target both neurones and glial cells, vigabatrin has marginally higher affinity for neuronal GABA-T, whereas tiagabine is slightly more effective in reducing glial GABA uptake (Sills, 2003). Furthermore, tiagabine is selective for the GAT-1 GABA transporter and its pharmacological effects mirror the regional distribution of this protein, with a more pronounced action in hippocampus and neo-cortex (Ribak et al., 1996). Other antiepileptic agents, including sodium valproate, gabapentin and topiramate have also been reported to influence GABA turnover by increasing neurotransmitter synthesis and/or release (Löscher, 1999; Petroff et al., 1996; Petroff et al., 1999).

Glutamate receptors

None of the currently available antiepileptic agents exerts its effects solely by an action on the glutamate neurotransmitter system. Blockade of the NMDA subtype of glutamate receptor is, however, believed to contribute to the pharmacological profile of felbamate (Taylor et al., 1995) and topiramate is similarly distinguished by an inhibitory action on AMPA and kainate receptors, with a higher affinity for the latter (Gryder & Rogawski, 2003). Phenobarbital has also been reported to block AMPA receptors, albeit at concentrations towards the upper end of its clinical range (Kamiya et al., 1999). Although the literature contains reports that several antiepileptic drugs, most notably lamotrigine, can selectively reduce glutamate release (Teoh et al., 1995), this phenomenon is more likely related to an inhibitory action on pre-synaptic sodium and calcium channels than any direct effect on the glutamate system.

Synaptic vesicle protein 2A

Levetiracetam was developed for the treatment of epilepsy with no clear indication of how it worked at the cellular level. The recognition of a specific binding site for the drug in mammalian brain and its later identification as synaptic vesicle protein 2A (SV2A) has resulted in claims that levetiracetam represents the first in a new class of antiepileptic agents (Lynch et al., 2004; Klitgaard & Verdru, 2007). To some extent, this remains a speculative assertion. Despite intense investigation, the precise physiological role of SV2A is still unclear and important details of the interaction between drug and protein remain to be defined. Indeed, there is no still convincing evidence to suggest whether the interaction is facilitatory or inhibitory or if it results in altered packaging, trafficking, membrane fusion or recycling of synaptic vesicles within the nerve terminal (Janz et al., 1999). There is, however, credible evidence to support selective binding of levetiracetam to SV2A, with little or no affinity for other members of the same protein family, and an impressive correlation between SV2A binding affinity and the anticonvulsant efficacy of a series of levetiracetam analogues in audiogenic seizure sensitive mice (Lynch et al., 2004). Further characterisation of the SV2A-dependent effects of levetiracetam, and other structurally-related compounds which are currently in the development pipeline, is required.

Carbonic anhydrase

The acid-base balance and maintenance of local pH is critical to normal functioning of the nervous system. Various isoenzymes of carbonic anhydrase play an important role in this regard. They are responsible for catalysing the bi-directional conversion of carbon dioxide and water to bicarbonate and hydrogen ions ($CO_2 + H_2O \leftrightarrow HCO_3^- + H^+$). The forward reaction is rapid, whereas the rate of the reverse reaction is more modest. As a result, inhibition of carbonic anhydrase influences the latter more significantly, producing a localised acidosis and increased bicarbonate ion concentration (Millichap et al., 1955). This, in turn, attenuates excitatory neurotransmission by reducing NMDA receptor activity and enhances inhibitory neurotransmission by facilitating the responsiveness of $GABA_A$ receptors (Church and McLennan, 1989). Acetazolamide is a classical carbonic anhydrase inhibitor which has been employed as an antiepileptic agent with some success (Reiss & Oles, 1996). Topiramate and zonisamide share this mechanism, but are significantly less potent, and have greater selectivity for individual isoenzymes (topiramate selectively inhibits CA-II and CA-IV; Dodgson et al., 2000). Nevertheless, inhibition of carbonic anhydrase is believed to make a modest contribution to the overall antiepileptic action of both drugs.

■ Implications of mechanisms

While many antiepileptic drugs can be categorised according to a single, principal mechanism of action, it is increasingly recognised that several agents have multiple primary effects at therapeutic concentrations (Table I). Polypharmacology, or the possession of multiple mechanisms of action, is more common amongst modern antiepileptic agents than their traditional counterparts. One possible exception is sodium valproate, which is assumed to have multiple mechanisms of action on the basis that extensive laboratory investigations have failed to find a single foremost mechanism that would explain its spectra of clinical activity (Löscher, 1999). In the case of modern drugs, such as felbamate, topiramate, levetiracetam, and zonisamide, the evidence for multi-factorial pharmacology is considerably more direct and convincing.

Despite remarkable advances in our understanding of how antiepileptic drugs exert their effects at the cellular level, the value of mechanisms per se remains debatable. There is little or no consistent evidence to support the use of specific drugs in specific epilepsies on the basis of pharmacology alone. Nevertheless, it has been suggested that the use of antiepileptic drugs with multiple mechanisms of action may be more effective in patients with multiple seizure types and in circumstances, such as in drug resistant epilepsy, where polypharmacy may have previously been employed. Indeed, the use of a single drug with multiple but modest cellular effects may be an attractive proposition for all patients with epilepsy (Bourgeois, 2007). Such drugs cover all the pharmacological bases but have limited potential for overload on any given system. This may reduce the likelihood of both pharmacodynamic tolerance and adverse effects and increase the possibility of synergism between mechanisms. In addition, prescribing single drugs with multiple mechanisms of action can eliminate the difficulties associated with pharmacokinetic interaction between antiepileptic agents, simplify titration schedules, and promote ease of use amongst nonspecialists.

■ The need for new drugs

Despite the introduction of eleven new antiepileptic agents over the past twenty years, and an immeasurable improvement in our knowledge of how those drugs work at the cellular level, at least 30% of epilepsy patients continue to experience seizures on otherwise optimal therapy (Kwan & Brodie, 2000). Even amongst those patients who achieve seizure control, a significant proportion can expect dose-related adverse effects to impact upon their quality of life. For the most part, modern antiepileptic agents are associated with fewer and less severe side effects, they have simpler pharmacokinetics and fewer drug interactions, but they have largely failed to improve outcome, at least in terms of efficacy (Schmidt, 2002).

The list of possible reasons for this failure is lengthy. Some have suggested that the continued use of experimental seizure models such as the maximal electroshock test, first developed in the 1930s and employed in the identification of phenytoin, in modern screening protocols is to blame (Meldrum, 1997; Löscher, 1998). It is not unreasonable to suggest that "old models identify old drugs" and that, from a pharmacological perspective, using a limited number of traditional models as the primary screen for drug development may indeed favour certain mechanisms of action at the expense of novelty. The evidence, however, does not support this assertion. Prior to the development of modern AEDs, there were no compounds with selective effects on HVA calcium channels (such as gabapentin) or on GABA transporters (such as tiagabine). These are structurally novel antiepileptic drugs, with unique and selective pharmacological effects, that are active in at least one traditional seizure model (Rogawski & Porter, 1990; Rogawski, 2006). Thus, old models can identify new drugs. A more likely explanation is that the new generation of antiepileptic drugs share general pharmacological characteristics with their established counterparts. All tip the global excitation/inhibition balance in favour of the latter and most are relatively indiscriminate in terms of their anatomical distribution, cellular specificity, and functional consequences. The individual pharmacological details may differ, but the end result is essentially the same; an increase in GABAergic inhibition and/or reduction in glutamatergic excitation. Perhaps more significant, however, is the fact that none of the drugs in current use, whether established or modern, specifically targets the epileptic process. This is potentially their single biggest failing.

■ Drug development strategies

In order to understand why recent drug development in epilepsy has been relatively unsuccessful, it is important to review the strategies employed in each case. Starting with vigabatrin, which was first licensed in the UK in 1989, and ending with rufinamide, the most recent addition to the antiepileptic armamentarium, three principal approaches are evident; target-orientated design, structural modification, and random screening.

Amongst modern antiepileptic agents, vigabatrin and tiagabine are the sole products of target-orientated design, fulfilling their intended purpose of enhancing GABAergic neurotransmission by selective inhibition of GABA-transaminase and GABA re-uptake, respectively (Sills, 2003). Other new drugs are products of a structural modification strategy which is based on chemical adaptation of both exogenous and endogenous neuroactive compounds; gabapentin and pregabalin are analogues of GABA, whereas oxcarbazepine is a carbamazepine derivative, designed to bypass the epoxide metabolite believed to be responsible for many of the adverse effects of the parent compound (Tecoma, 1999). Finally, there are several new antiepileptic agents (such as topiramate, levetiracetam, zonisamide, and rufinamide) that have arisen from random screening of libraries of molecules. This category also includes lamotrigine, which might more accurately be defined as the product of a candidate screening programme, albeit one based on the incorrect assertion that anti-folate compounds possess antiepileptic activity (Reynolds et al., 1966).

Target-orientated design is likely to yield a single mechanism drug with high specificity which can be tailored to defects in the epileptic brain (where known), but one which may be inadequate for a heterogeneous disorder such as epilepsy (Löscher & Schmidt, 1994). To date, efforts at target-orientated drug design for epilepsy have foundered, most likely because targets were selected on the basis of a hypothesis rather than direct evidence.

Structural modification relies on the established activity of the parent molecule and provides an opportunity to improve on specific aspects of efficacy and/or tolerability. It could be argued that this approach is unlikely to change the spectrum of activity or to benefit those who are unresponsive to the medications upon which any novel compound is based and is employed predominantly to limit perceived commercial risk. Random screening has been the most successful drug development strategy in recent years, identifying several agents with a broad spectrum of clinical activity, but it is laborious and expensive. As far as screening is concerned, mechanism of action is largely irrelevant (and may remain undiscovered), with success dependent on the models employed in the screening protocol and genuine potential for useful compounds to be discarded prematurely.

In the past, antiepileptic drugs have been licensed and used clinically (often for many decades) long before their mechanisms of action were identified. Even in the development of new drugs, especially those arising from screening programmes, investigating cellular effects has been sidelined in favour of pursuing efficacy in preclinical models. Tackling the problem of drug resistance in epilepsy requires that pharmacology be a primary consideration. Previously, we have failed to adequately target antiepileptic agents to known molecular defects which distinguish epileptic brain from otherwise normal tissue, predominantly because our understanding of the causal and consequential pathophysiology of epilepsy was lacking. Today, however, we possess an unprecedented level of information about the epileptic process, derived from studies of resected human epileptic tissue, chronic animal models, and epilepsy genetics (Meldrum & Rogawski, 2007). Future antiepileptic drug development should focus primarily selecting appropriate pharmacological targets from this knowledge base, without discounting other biologically plausible candidates. New compounds should preferably possess multiple mechanisms of action, with a combination of both novel and traditional cellular effects, and undergo efficacy screening not just in established seizure models, but also in animal models of chronic recurrent seizures, and models of pharmacoresistant epilepsy (Rogawski, 2006).

Targets for novel antiepileptic drug development

As discussed above, our understanding of the pathophysiology of epilepsy has advanced remarkably in the past two decades and has resulted in the identification of multiple proteins and protein families involved in the generation of seizures or whose expression is modified in experimental and clinical epileptic tissue. Some of these potential drug targets, such as sodium channels and $GABA_A$ receptors, are familiar and novelty is represented by subtle variations of existing pharmacological approaches. Other targets, such as gap junctions, are entirely novel from the perspective of epilepsy treatment. The following list is not intended to be exhaustive, but rather to give a flavour of how antiepileptic drug pharmacology might evolve in the coming decades.

Voltage-gated sodium channels

Sodium channels belong to a superfamily of voltage-gated channels which are composed of multiple independent protein subunits and which form ion-selective pores in the cell membrane (Catterall, 1992). The native sodium channel comprises a single (α-subunit protein, which contains the pore-forming region and the voltage sensor, associated with one or more accessory β-subunit proteins which can modify the function of the α-subunit but which are not essential for basic channel activity (Catterall, 1992; Köhling, 2002).

There are four predominant sodium channel α-subunit genes expressed in mammalian brain, denoted SCN1A, SCN2A, SCN3A and SCN8A, which encode the channels $Na_v1.1$, $Na_v1.2$, $Na_v1.3$ and $Na_v1.6$, respectively (Yu & Catterall, 2003; Catterall et al., 2005).

To our knowledge, current antiepileptic drugs do not discriminate between these individual isoforms. These channels have different biophysical properties, with $Na_v1.1$ and $Na_v1.2$ predominantly responsible for fast inactivating currents and $Na_v1.6$ carrying a significant proportion of the persistent sodium current (Rogawski & Löscher, 2004; Stafstrom, 2007). They also have distinct anatomical distributions, with $Na_v1.2$ being the major isoform in seizure-prone brain regions, such as hippocampus and neo-cortex (Whitaker et al., 2000), and may be differentially expressed on the neuronal membrane, with different isoforms on dendrites, soma, axons, and nerve terminals (Meldrum & Rogawski, 2007). An intriguing but as yet unproven possibility is that different sodium channel isoforms might even be expressed on excitatory and inhibitory neurones (Prakriya & Mennerick, 2000). Thus, development of drugs which target specific isoforms of the sodium channel may be beneficial, in terms of improving efficacy and/or limiting adverse effects, by directing drugs to specific neurones, sub-cellular locations, or brain areas.

As discussed previously, voltage-gated sodium channels existing in one of three basic conformational states; resting, active, and inactivated. Current antiepileptic agents have greatest but not exclusive affinity for sodium channels in the inactivated state (Ragsdale et al., 1991; Catterall, 1992; Ragsdale & Avoli, 1998). Identifying compounds which bind solely to inactivated sodium channels may improve therapeutic indices by increasing the use-dependency of blockade, further sparing normal action potential generation in favour of limiting high frequency firing alone (Ilyin et al., 2006).

Evidence from chronic epilepsy models and human epileptic tissue suggests that the function of voltage-gated sodium channels can be disrupted by seizure activity, potentially leading to a reduction in pharmacological sensitivity (Remy et al., 2003a; Remy et al., 2003b). This is consistent with the so-called "altered target hypothesis" of pharmacoresistance discussed elsewhere in this volume by Professor Wolfgang Löscher. Whether this disruption is caused by a change in the subunit composition of individual channels, a localised alteration in the expression of specific sodium channel isoforms, or a change in the conformation or phosphorylation state of the protein remains to be determined. Whatever the cause, once elucidated, it offers a genuine opportunity for pharmacological exploitation of a known molecular defect associated with epilepsy.

$GABA_A$ receptors

The $GABA_A$ receptor is a ligand-gated ion channel, comprising five independent protein subunits arranged around a central chloride ion pore. Nineteen $GABA_A$ receptor subunits have been identified to date (α1-6, β1-3, γ1-3, δ, ε, θ, π, ρ1-2), any five of which could, in theory, form a functional channel (Barnard, 2001). In reality, only a handful of combinations are preferred. Typical benzodiazepine-sensitive $GABA_A$ receptors are composed of two α-subunits (α1, α2, α3 or α5), two β-subunits (β2 or β3), and a γ2 subunit (Johnson, 2005). Such receptors are termed "phasic" – they respond to GABA release from pre-synaptic nerve terminals by generating fast, transient, hyperpolarising currents in the post-synaptic cell membrane which rapidly desensitise (Rabow et al., 1995). Recent research efforts have also identified "tonic" $GABA_A$ receptors, which are observed at extra-synaptic sites and which are activated by ambient concentrations of GABA or the spill-over of synaptically released GABA (Kullmann et al., 2005). Tonic GABA$_A$ receptors preferentially contain α4 and α6 subunits, and invariably a δ-subunit in the place of γ2. They are benzodiazepine-insensitive, activated by neurosteroids, less readily desensitised, and may represent a novel class of antiepileptic drug target (Kullmann et al., 2005; Meldrum & Rogawski, 2007).

As with sodium channels, it is likely that GABA$_A$ receptors are subject to variable anatomical, cellular and sub-cellular distribution on the basis of subunit expression patterns. Development of subunit specific drugs may facilitate targeting of compounds, with resulting improvements of efficacy and/or tolerability profiles, and amelioration of the pharmacodynamic tolerance which has beset the use of traditional benzodiazepines in the chronic treatment of epilepsy. There is pharmacological precedence for this hypothesis; loreclezole is a selective agonist at β2- and β3-containing GABA$_A$ receptors and although effective in preventing seizures, its development as an antiepileptic agent was halted due to excessive sedation, most likely associated with a "phenobarbital-like" ability of the drug to activate the GABA$_A$ receptor complex in the absence of GABA itself (Groves et al., 2006). In contrast, experimental compounds, such as abecarnil and ELB139, are selective agonists at α3-containing receptors and appear to retain anticonvulsant and anxiolytic activity whilst being devoid of sedative properties (Turski et al., 1990; Langen et al., 2005). Abercarnil is also a partial agonist at α5-containing receptors and, as such, may have a reduced propensity for tolerance (Natolino et al., 1996). Full agonists at tonic GABA$_A$ receptors, which are not rapidly desensitised, are likely to share this characteristic (Reddy & Rogawski, 2000).

The expression of individual GABA$_A$ receptor subunits can be influenced by seizures, leading to a change in the pharmacological sensitivity of the receptor complex. Induction of spontaneous seizures in the pilocarpine model leads to a reduced expression of α1- and β1-subunits, and a corresponding increase in α4 and β3 (Brooks-Kayal et al., 1998). This, in turn, is associated with an elevation in the sensitivity to GABA, reduced augmentation by the α1-preferring compound zolpidem, and an enhanced block by zinc (Brooks-Kayal et al., 1998). This is, again, an example of the "altered target hypothesis" of drug resistant epilepsy. Detailed characterisation of GABA$_A$ receptor subunit changes associated with the development of seizures, derived from both experimental models and resected human tissue, has the potential to highlight novel targets associated with disease and, in doing so, help direct the development of novel subunit specific GABAergic agents.

Glutamate receptors

The glutamatergic neurotransmitter system has been a focal point for the development of novel neurotherapeutics for many years (Löscher & Rogawski, 2002). Much of this effort has, however, been in vain. In epilepsy, drugs which selectively target glutamate receptors, such as the competitive NMDA antagonist D-CPPene, have reached early clinical trials only to be promptly withdrawn due to a lack of efficacy at doses which precipitated intolerable adverse effects (Sveinbjornsdottir et al., 1993). As our understanding of the structure, function and pharmacological characteristics of glutamate receptors has evolved, it may be time to revisit this family of receptors which is so fundamental to excitatory neurotransmission in the mammalian brain.

The ionotropic glutamate receptors (AMPA, kainate, NMDA) are tetrameric assemblies of individual protein subunits which form a transmembrane, cation-selective pore, permeable to sodium (all receptors) and calcium ions (NMDA receptors alone) (Meldrum & Rogawski, 2007). AMPA receptor subunits are encoded by four discrete genes (GluR1 – GluR4), with five genes for kainate receptors (GluR5 – GluR7, KA1, KA2), and seven for NMDA (NR1, NR2A – NR2D, NR3A, NR3B (Mayer & Armstrong, 2004). As with all such multimeric receptor assemblies, subunit composition confers biophysical and pharmacological properties. AMPA receptors typically exist as either homotetramers of the GluR1 or GluR4 subunit or as symmetric dimers of GluR2/3 and either GluR1 or GluR4 (Meldrum and Rogawski, 2007). All NMDA receptors contain at least one NR1 subunit, which is responsible for binding of the co-agonist glycine, and two NR2 (or NR3) subunits which bind glutamate (Dingledine et al., 1999).

Alternative splicing and RNA editing aside, subunit heterogeneity of glutamate receptors is not as extensive as that of other ligand-gated ion channels, such as the $GABA_A$ receptor. As a result, the potential for developing subunit-specific treatments may be limited. Nevertheless, of the two existing antiepileptic agents which act, at least in part, by blocking glutamate receptors, topiramate is selective for GluR5-containing kainate receptors (Gryder & Rogawski, 2003), and felbamate targets NR2B-containing NMDA receptors (Harty & Rogawski, 2000). Thus, there is some pharmacological precedence, but whether there is sufficient heterogeneity in receptor composition or evidence of disease-related subunit expression remains to be determined.

Potassium channels

Voltage-gated potassium channels are responsible for the downstroke of the neuronal action potential and serve to limit excitability in the nervous system by promoting the repolarisation of neurones (Pongs, 1999). They exist as heteromeric assemblies of individual α-subunits, each one of which is akin to the principal, pore-forming α-subunit of the sodium channel. Potassium channels are the most diverse group of ion channels, with more than 70 α-subunit genes identified and around 40 expressed in the brain (Gutman et al., 2005). Four α-subunits, arranged around a central potassium ion-selective pore, are required to form functional channels and, again, subunit composition confers function and pharmacology (Pongs, 1999; Wickenden, 2002).

There are various families of potassium channels including voltage-gated (K_v), inward rectifier (K_{ir}), calcium-activated (K_{Ca}) and two-pore channels (K_{2P}). Within these families there are multiple sub-groups (e.g. K_v1 to K_v9), and within sub-groups, there are multiple protein subunits (e.g. $K_v1.1$ to $K_v1.8$), each encoded by an individual gene (Gutman et al., 2005). Of most relevance to epilepsy and the development of novel antiepileptic agents are the voltage-gated channels. These carry both the delayed rectifier current (I_K), which is responsible for repolarisation of the neuronal membrane following action potential generation, and also A- and M-currents, which play important roles in regulating the excitability of neurones in seizure-prone regions of brain, such as hippocampus and neo-cortex (Meldrum & Rogawski, 2007). The M-current is carried by channels containing subunits from the K_v7 sub-group (previously known as KCNQ) and is predominantly localised to the cell soma where it is involved in determining the threshold and rate of neuronal firing and in modulating the somatic response to dendritic inputs (Rogawski, 2000).

Voltage-gated potassium channels are an attractive target for antiepileptic drugs and the first clinically effective potassium channel activator is currently in the late stages of development for epilepsy (discussed in detail elsewhere in this volume). Retigabine was originally reported to be selective for $K_v7.2$- and $K_v7.3$-containing channels (Rundfeldt & Netzer, 2000; Wickenden et al., 2000) which contribute to the neuronal M-current, although it has subsequently been shown to activate channels containing all four K_v7 subunits expressed in brain ($K_v7.2$ – $K_v7.5$) (Tatulian et al., 2001). It has no activity at channels containing the $K_v7.1$ subunit which is responsible for the cardiac M-current (Tatulian et al., 2001). Retigabine causes a large hyperpolarising shift in the voltage-dependence of activation of these channels, leading to greater potassium conductance at resting membrane potentials, and a reduction in neuronal excitability (Meldrum & Rogawski, 2007). Development of further potassium channel openers is anticipated; the inward rectifying channel is a valid target, as are the various K_v1, K_v3, and K_v4 subunits which underpin the A-current (Wickenden, 2002).

Gap junctions

Gap junctions are responsible for the electrotonic coupling of both neurones and astrocytes in the central nervous system and provide a mechanism for rapid, non-synaptic communication between adjacent cells (Nakase & Naus, 2004; Nemani & Binder, 2005). They are believed to underlie the synchronisation of epileptiform activity and contribute to the high frequency (300-400 Hz) oscillations which precede the onset of ictal discharges in temporal lobe epilepsies (Timofeev & Steriade, 2004; Gigout et al., 2006). Gap junctions are formed from two hemichannels (connexons), one in the membrane of each cell, which are themselves comprised of six independent protein subunits (connexins) surrounding a central pore which is permeable to ions, second messengers and other small molecules (Nemani & Binder, 2005). Around twenty connexins have been identified in mammals, eleven of which are observed in brain tissue, with differential expression on the basis of cell type and stage of development. Cx43 is the major connexin in astrocytes, whereas Cx36 and Cx45 predominate in hippocampal and neo-cortical neurones (Venance et al., 2000; Nakase & Naus, 2004).

Experimental gap junction blockers, such as carbenoxolone, can suppress epileptiform discharges in the hippocampal slice preparation, including those evoked under zero Ca^{2+} conditions, supporting the involvement of gap junctions in non-synaptic transmission (Perez-Velazquez et al., 1994; Jahromi et al., 2002). Carbenoxolone is also effective when applied focally in the tetanus-toxin model (Nilsen et al., 2006) and against experimental absence seizures in both WAG/Rij rats and lethargic mice (Gareri et al., 2005). These observations and the biologically plausible role of gap junctions in the generation of epileptic discharges suggest that they represent important novel targets for antiepileptic drug development. Tonabersat is a gap junction blocker being developed for the treatment of migraine (Goadsby, 2007). It is an analogue of carabersat (SB-204269), whose development as an antiepileptic agent appears to have stalled as a result of formulation issues (Bialer et al., 2002). If these drugs share a similar pharmacodynamic profile, then investigation of gap junction blockers in epilepsy is clearly warranted.

HCN channels

Hyperpolarisation-activated, cyclic nucleotide-gated cation (HCN) channels are permeable to both sodium and potassium ions and participate in pacemaker currents in both neurones and cardiac cells (Herrmann et al., 2007). The neuronal current is termed I_h. HCN channels are opened by hyperpolarisation and modulated by the binding of cAMP, which shifts the threshold for activation to more positive potentials (Chen et al., 2002). They are similar in structure to potassium channels, comprising four independent protein subunits in homomeric or heteromeric tetramers surrounding a central ion pore. There are four known HCN channel subunits (HCN1 – HCN4) which display differential expression in brain, with HCN1 predominantly observed in hippocampus and neo-cortex and HCN2 in thalamus (Herrmann et al., 2007). This characteristic makes the HCN channel an attractive target for antiepileptic drug development, with the potential for HCN1-selective agents to be effective in limbic epilepsies and HCN2 compounds specific for absence seizures (Meldrum & Rogawski, 2007).

HCN2 knockout mice display an absence-seizure phenotype and the genetic WAG/Rij absence model has altered HCN1 expression in both thalamus and neo-cortex (Ludwig et al., 2003; Strauss et al., 2004; Budde et al., 2005). Changes in HCN subunit expression and I_h characteristics have also been observed in animal models of epileptogenesis (Chen et al., 2001; Shah et al., 2004), although whether these are causal or consequential remains unclear. Blockade of HCN channels by experimental compounds, such as ZD-7288, can limit spontaneous epileptiform discharges in the hippocampal slice preparation (Arias & Bowlby, 2005). Paradoxically, activation of dendritic I_h, leading to a modification of synaptic inputs to the soma, has been proposed to contribute to the antiepileptic actions of lamotrigine (Poolos et al., 2002). Dissecting the contributions of individual HCN channels to overall excitability on an anatomical, cellular and sub-cellular basis is required before the full potential of these proteins as a valid antiepileptic drug target can be realistically assessed.

Other targets

The foregoing is not intended as an exhaustive inventory of all potential targets for novel drug development in epilepsy. Many other proteins have appeal, particularly those whose expression can be definitively shown to be associated with seizure generation. These necessarily include both novel targets and new perspectives on traditional themes, such as voltage-gated calcium channel subunits which could, in theory, be up-regulated in the epileptic state, in a manner paralleling the increased expression of $\alpha_2\delta$-subunits in dorsal root ganglion cells in experimental pain models (Li et al., 2006; Dooley et al., 2007). Metabotropic receptors for both GABA and glutamate merit further investigation, particularly in light of their ability to modulate pre-synaptic neurotransmitter release (Alexander & Godwin, 2006; Bowery, 2006). Other neurotransmitters and neuromodulators, such as acetylcholine, serotonin and adenosine, also deserve consideration, despite the fact they have appeared on pharmacological wish-lists for epilepsy for many decades without any significant developments (Löscher et al., 2003; Boison, 2005; Pagonopolou et al., 2006; Bagdy et al., 2007). Drugs which target efflux transporters in the blood-brain barrier, recently implicated in the causation of pharmacoresistant epilepsy (Löscher & Potschka, 2005), have genuine promise as adjunctive or sensitising agents for the treatment of refractory epilepsy, even if they are not antiepileptic in their own right. In reality, no neurochemical process should be left unturned, and those in which subunit composition of receptors or ion channels influences pharmacological sensitivity or those which are associated with differential expression profiles on the basis of cell type and brain region should attract special attention.

Improving the likelihood of success

Identifying a successful new antiepileptic drug which benefits those patients living with drug resistant epilepsy is not simply dependent on target. The entire ethos of drug development in epilepsy should be re-evaluated.

Indiscriminate empirical screening of compound libraries has been a fruitful approach in the past, yielding topiramate, levetiracetam, and zonisamide, but this practice should cease, lest we require more garden-variety sodium channel blockers. Putting pharmacology first and selecting compounds on the basis of their pharmacodynamic profile is required. In doing so, we should focus our attention on those agents that have multiple cellular effects, and preferably a combination of novel and traditional mechanisms, in order to target drug resistant epilepsies but retain broad clinical utility. The inclusion of a traditional pharmacological mechanism should ensure at least minimal clinical effectiveness, thereby reducing commercial risk and avoiding the creation of a niche drug which may only be effective in a handful of patients and thus not economically viable. Where possible, types of target (voltage-gated ion channel, ligand-gated ion channel, metabotropic receptor, enzyme, transport protein) should be combined in order to improve spectrum of activity; experience suggests that drugs which target voltage-gated ion channels alone have a narrow spectrum of efficacy.

The practice of screening a series of structurally related compounds and selecting the most potent should, at the very least, be reviewed, given that drugs with modest effects on multiple targets are currently preferred from a clinical perspective. If nothing else, these agents can be employed with more confidence, particularly when the aetiology or diagnosis is unclear (Bourgeois, 2007). In contrast, more potent, single mechanism compounds may prove to have better utility if and when a clear and potentially rectifiable defect can be identified. Other characteristics which may improve the likelihood of success include structural novelty, efficacy in traditional seizure models and models of chronic and pharmacoresistant epilepsy, no drug interactions, protein binding or active metabolites, and a pharmacokinetic profile which demonstrates complete absorption at a moderate rate, renal excretion, and an elimination half-life of at least 12 hours (Steinhoff et al., 2003). If all of the above can be achieved in a single molecule, then it has a chance of being successful.

Conclusions

The pharmacological inadequacy of current antiepileptic agents is one of several emerging and entirely plausible hypotheses to explain drug resistance in epilepsy, a phenomenon which impacts at least 30% of all patients (Kwan & Brodie, 2000). Drug resistance is, by definition, a function of the availability of drugs, the mechanisms by which those drugs work, and the appropriateness of those mechanisms for the disease process. Until very recently, antiepileptic drug availability was limited and our naivety with regard to how those few drugs worked was surpassed only by our complete ignorance of the pathophysiology of epilepsy itself. The explosion in licensing of new antiepileptic agents throughout the 1990s and the early part of this century has been paralleled by remarkable advances in pharmacological knowledge and in our ability to investigate the cellular and molecular mechanisms underlying seizure generation.

It is now apparent that the antiepileptic drugs currently at our disposal exert their effects by blockade of voltage-gated sodium and calcium channels, allosteric activation of $GABA_A$ receptors, augmentation of GABA turnover, blockade of glutamate receptors, inhibition of carbonic anhydrase, and modulation of synaptic vesicles (Kwan *et al.*, 2001; Rogawski & Löscher, 2004). These mechanisms have arisen, through a degree of natural selection, from drug development programmes which were neither strategic nor evidence-based. Other than those drugs which demonstrate use-dependent blockade of sodium channels, none targets processes involved in or specifically associated with the generation of seizures. All influence normal physiological functions, as witnessed by their propensity for side effects, and all essentially shift the neurochemical balance in favour of inhibition over excitation.

The next generation of antiepileptic drugs should take advantage of new-found knowledge from animal models of chronic epilepsy, human epileptic tissue, and epilepsy genetics. They should be targeted to proteins which are known to be differentially expressed under epileptic conditions, such as specific ion channel and receptor subunits, or intimately involved in the generation of seizures, such as gap junctions. New drugs should possess multiple mechanisms of action, with a combination of traditional and novel cellular effects in order to achieve broad clinical utility and retain commercial viability. As our understanding of epilepsy improves, the entire ethos of drug development in epilepsy should be continually re-evaluated. The ultimate aim of future drug development in epilepsy will be to provide efficacy in epilepsies which are currently drug resistant, to retain broad-spectrum clinical activity, and to eliminate, or at least reduce, the burden of adverse effects. The necessary tools to achieve this objective are within our grasp.

References

Alexander GM, Godwin DW. Metabotropic glutamate receptors as a strategic target for the treatment of epilepsy. *Epilepsy Res* 2006; 71: 1-22.

Arias RL, Bowlby MR. Pharmacological characterization of antiepileptic drugs and experimental analgesics on low magnesium-induced hyperexcitability in rat hippocampal slices. *Brain Res* 2005; 1047: 233-44.

Bagdy G, Kecskemeti V, Riba P, Jakus R. Serotonin and epilepsy. *J Neurochem* 2007; 100: 857-73.

Barchi L. Ion channel mutations affecting muscle and brain. *Curr Opin Neurol* 1998; 11: 461-8.

Barnard EA. The molecular architecture of $GABA_A$ receptors. In: Möhler H (ed). *Pharmacology of GABA and glycine neurotransmission*. Handbook of Experimental Pharmacology 150. Berlin: Springer, 2001: 94-100.

Bialer M, Johannessen SI, Kupferberg HJ, Levy RH, Loiseau P, Perucca E. Progress report on new antiepileptic drugs: a summary of the Sixth Eilat Conference (EILAT VI). *Epilepsy Res* 2002; 51: 31-71.

Boison D. Adenosine and epilepsy: from therapeutic rationale to new therapeutic strategies. *Neuroscientist* 2005; 11: 25-36.

Bourgeois BFD. Broader is better: the ranks of broad-spectrum antiepileptic drugs are growing. *Neurology* 2007; 69: 1734-6.

Bowery NG. GABA$_B$ receptor: a site of therapeutic benefit. *Curr Opin Pharmacol* 2006; 6: 37-43.

Brodie MJ, Dichter MA. Antiepileptic drugs. *New Eng J Med* 1996; 334: 168-75.

Brooks-Kayal AR, Shumate MD, Jin H, Rikhter TY, Coulter DA. Selective changes in single cell GABA$_A$ receptor subunit expression and function in temporal lobe epilepsy. *Nat Med* 1998; 4: 1166-72.

Budde T, Caputi L, Kanyshkova T, et al. Impaired regulation of thalamic pacemaker channels through an imbalance of subunit expression in absence epilepsy. *J Neurosci* 2005; 25: 9871-82.

Catterall WA. Cellular and molecular biology of voltage-gated sodium channels. *Physiol Rev* 1992; 72: S15-S48.

Catterall WA, Goldin AL, Waxman SG. International Union of Pharmacology. XLVII. Nomenclature and structure-function relationships of voltage-gated sodium channels. *Pharmacol Rev* 2005; 57: 397-409.

Chen K, Aradi I, Santhakumar V, Soltesz I. H-channels in epilepsy: new targets for seizure control? *Trends Pharmacol Sci* 2002; 23: 552-7.

Chen K, Aradi I, Thon N, Eghbal-Ahmadi M, Baram TZ, Soltesz I. Persistently modified h-channels after complex febrile seizures convert the seizure-induced enhancement of inhibition to hyperexcitability. *Nat Med* 2001; 7: 331-7.

Church J, McLennan H. Electrophysiological properties of rat CA1 pyramidal neurones in vitro modified by changes in extracellular bicarbonate. *J Physiol* 1989; 415: 85-108.

Coulter DA, Huguenard JR, Prince DA. Calcium currents in rat thalamocortical relay neurones: kinetic properties of the transient low-threshold current. *J Physiol* 1989a; 414: 587-604.

Coulter DA, Huguenard JR, Prince DA. Characterization of ethosuximide reduction of low-threshold calcium currents in thalamic neurons. *Ann Neurol* 1989b; 25: 582-93.

Courtney KR, Etter EF. Modulated anticonvulsant block of sodium channels in nerve and muscle. *Eur J Pharmacol* 1983; 88: 1-9.

Daikhin Y, Yudkoff M. Compartmentation of brain glutamate metabolism in neurons and glia. *J Nutrition* 2000; 130: 1026S-1031S.

Dingledine R, Borges K, Bowie D, Traynelis SF. The glutamate receptor ion channels. *Pharmacol Rev* 1999; 51: 7-61.

Dodgson SJ, Shank RP, Maryanoff BE. Topiramate as an inhibitor of carbonic anhydrase isoenzymes. *Epilepsia* 2000; 41 (suppl 1): S35-S39.

Dooley DJ, Taylor CP, Donevan S, Feltner D. Ca^{2+} channel ($_2$(ligands: novel modulators of neurotransmission. *Trends Pharmacol Sci* 2007; 28: 75-82.

Ffrench-Mullen JM, Barker JL, Rogawski MA. Calcium current block by (-)-pentobarbital, phenobarbital, and CHEB but not (+)-pentobarbital in acutely isolated hippocampal CA1 neurons: comparison with effects on GABA-activated Cl$^-$ current. *J Neurosci* 1993; 13: 3211-21.

Gareri P, Condorelli D, Belluardo N, et al. Antiabsence effects of carbenoxolone in two genetic animal models of absence epilepsy (WAG/Rij rats and lh/lh mice). *Neuropharmacology* 2005; 49: 551-63.

Gigout S, Louvel J, Kawasaki H, et al. Effects of gap junction blockers on human neocortical synchronization. *Neurobiol Dis* 2006; 22: 496-508.

Goadsby PJ. Emerging therapies for migraine. *Nat Clin Prac Neurol* 2007; 3: 610-9.

Groves JO, Guscott MR, Hallett DJ, et al. The role of GABA$_A$β2 subunit-containing receptors in mediating the anticonvulsant and sedative effects of loreclezole. *Eur J Neurosci* 2006; 24: 167-74.

Gryder DS, Rogawski MA. Selective antagonism of GluR5 kainate-receptor-mediated synaptic currents by topiramate in rat basolateral amygdale neurons. *J Neurosci* 2003; 23: 7069-74.

Gutman GA, Chandy KG, Grissmer S, et al. International Union of Pharmacology. LIII. Nomenclature and molecular relationships of voltage-gated potassium channels. *Pharmacol Rev* 2005; 57: 473-508.

Harty TP, Rogawski MA. Felbamate block of recombinant N-methyl-D-aspartate receptors: selectivity for the NR2B subunit. *Epilepsy Res* 2000; 39: 47-55.

Herrmann S, Stieber J, Ludwig A. Pathophysiology of HCN channels. *Pflugers Arch – Eur J Physiol* 2007; 454: 517-22.

Hofmann F, Biel M, Flockerzi V. Molecular basis for Ca^{2+} channel diversity. *Ann Rev Neurosci* 1994; 17: 399-418.

Ilyin VI, Pomonis JD, Whiteside GT, et al. Pharmacology of 2-[4-(4-chloro-2-fluorophenoxy)phenyl]-pyrimidine-4-carboxamide: a potent, broad-spectrum state-dependent sodium channel blocker for treating pain states. *J Pharmacol Exp Ther* 2006; 318: 1083-93.

Jahromi SS, Wentlandt K, Piran S, Carlen PL. Anticonvulsant actions of gap junctional blockers in an *in vitro* seizure model. *J Neurophysiol* 2002; 88: 1893-902.

Janz R, Goda Y. Geppert M, Missler M, Sudhof TC. SV2A and SV2B function as redundant Ca^{2+} regulators in neurotransmitter release. *Neuron* 1999; 24: 1003-16.

Johnson GAR. $GABA_A$ receptor channel pharmacology. *Curr Pharmaceut Des* 2005; 11: 1867-85.

Jung MJ, Lippert B, Metcalf B, Böhlen P, Schechter PJ. γ-Vinyl GABA (4-amino-hex-5-enoic acid), a new irreversible inhibitor of GABA-T: effects on brain GABA metabolism in mice. *J Neurochem* 1997; 29: 797-802.

Kamiya Y, Andoh T, Furuya R, et al. Comparison of the effects of convulsant and depressant barbiturate stereoisomers on AMPA-type glutamate receptors. *Anesthesiology* 1999; 90: 1704-13.

Kelly KM, Gross RA, Macdonald RL. Valproic acid selectively reduces the low-threshold (T) calcium current in rat nodose neurons. *Neurosci Lett* 1990; 116: 233-8.

Klitgaard H, Verdru P. Levetiracetam: the first SV2A ligand for the treatment of epilepsy. *Exp Opin Drug Discov* 2007; 2: 1537-45.

Köhling R. Voltage-gated sodium channels in epilepsy. *Epilepsia* 2002; 43: 1278-95.

Kullmann DM, Ruiz A, Rusakov DM, Scott R, Semyanov A, Walker MC. Presynaptic, extrasynaptic and axonal GABAA receptors in the CNS: where and why? *Prog Biophys Mol Biol* 2005; 87: 33-46.

Kwan P, Brodie MJ. Early identification of refractory epilepsy. *N Engl J Med* 2000; 342: 314-9.

Kwan P, Sills GJ, Brodie MJ. The mechanisms of action of commonly used antiepileptic drugs. *Pharmacol Ther* 2001; 90: 21-34.

Langen B, Egerland U, Bernöster K, Dost R, Unverferth K, Rundfeldt C. Characterization in rats of the anxiolytic potential of ELB139 [1-(4-chlorophenyl)-4-piperidin-1-yl-1,5-dihydro-imidazol-2-on], a new agonist at the benzodiazepine binding site of the $GABA_A$ receptor. *J Pharmacol Exp Ther* 2005; 314: 717-24.

Li C-Y, Zhang X-L, Matthews EA, et al. Calcium channel $\alpha_2\delta_1$ subunit mediates spinal hyperexcitability in pain modulation. *Pain* 2006; 125: 20-34.

Löscher W. New visions in the pharmacology of anticonvulsion. *Eur J Pharmacol* 1998; 342: 1-13.

Löscher W. Valproate: a reappraisal of its pharmacodynamic properties and mechanisms of action. *Prog Neurobiol* 1999; 58: 31-59.

Löscher W, Potschka H. Drug resistance in brain diseases and the role of drug efflux transporters. *Nat Rev Neurosci* 2005; 6: 591-602.

Löscher W, Rogawski MA. Epilepsy. In: Lodge D, Danysz W, Parsons CG (eds). *Ionotropic glutamate receptors as therapeutic targets*. Johnson City, Tennessee: F.P. Graham Publishing Co., 2002: 91-132.

Löscher W, Schmidt D. Strategies in antiepileptic drug development: is rational drug design superior to random screening and structural variation? *Epilepsy Res* 1994; 17: 95-134.

Löscher W, Potschka H, Wlaz P, Danysz W, Parsons CG. Are neuronal nicotinic receptors a target for antiepileptic drug development? Studies in different seizure models in mice and rats. *Eur J Pharmacol* 2003; 466: 99-111.

Ludwig A, Budde T, Stieber J, et al. Absence epilepsy and sinus dysrhythmia in mice lacking the pacemaker channel HCN2. *EMBO J* 2003; 22: 216-24.

Lukyanetz EA, Shkryl VM, Kostyuk PG. Selective blockade of N-type calcium channels by levetiracetam. *Epilepsia* 2002; 43: 9-18.

Lynch BA, Lambeng N, Nocka K, Kensel-Hammes P, Bajjalieh SM, Matagne A, et al. The synaptic vesicle protein SV2A is the binding site for the antiepileptic drug levetiracetam. *Proc Natl Acad Sci USA* 2004; 101: 9861-6.

Mayer ML, Armstrong N. Structure and function of glutamate receptor ion channels. *Ann Rev Physiol* 2004; 66: 161-81.

McLean MJ, Macdonald RL. Multiple actions of phenytoin on mouse spinal cord neurons in cell culture. *J Pharmacol Exp Ther* 1983; 227: 779-89.

Meldrum BS. Identification and preclinical testing of novel antiepileptic compounds. *Epilepsia* 1997; 38 (suppl 9): S7-S15.

Meldrum BS. Glutamate as a neurotransmitter in the brain: review of physiology and pathology. *J Nutrition* 2000; 130: 1007S-1015S.

Meldrum BS, Rogawski MA. Molecular targets for antiepileptic drug development. *Neurotherapeutics* 2007; 4: 18-61.

Millichap JG, Woodbury DM, Goodman LS. Mechanism of the anticonvulsant action of acetazoleamide, a carbonic anhydrase inhibitor. *J Pharmacol Exp Ther* 1955; 115: 251-8.

Nakase T, Naus CC. Gap junctions and neurological disorders of the central nervous system. *Biochim Biophys Acta* 2004; 1662: 149-58.

Natolino F, Zanotti A, Contarino A, Lipartiti M, Guisti P. Abecarnil, a β-carboline derivative, does not exhibit anticonvulsant tolerance or withdrawal effects in mice. *Naunyn-Schmiedebergs Arch Pharmacol* 1996; 354: 612-7.

Nemani VM, Binder DK. Emerging role of gap junctions in epilepsy. *Histol Histopathol* 2005; 20: 253-9.

Nielsen EB, Suzdak PD, Andersen KE, Knutsen LJS, Sonnewald U, Braestrup, C. Characterization of tiagabine (NO-328), a new potent and selective GABA uptake inhibitor. *Eur J Pharmacol* 1991; 196: 257-66.

Nilsen KE, Kelso ARC, Cock HR. Antiepileptic effect of gap-junction blockers in a rat model of refractory focal cortical epilepsy. *Epilepsia* 2006; 47: 1169-75.

Olsen RW, Avoli M. GABA and epileptogenesis. *Epilepsia* 1997; 38: 399-407.

Pagonopolou O, Efthimiadou A, Asimakopoulos B, Nikolettos NK. Modulatory role of adenosine and its receptors in epilepsy: possible therapeutic approaches. *Neurosci Res* 2006; 56: 14-20.

Perez-Velazquez JL, Valiante TA, Carlen PL. Modulation of gap junctional mechanisms during calcium-free induced field burst activity: a possible role for electrotonic coupling in epileptogenesis. *J Neurosci* 1994; 14: 4308-17.

Petroff OAC, Rothman DL, Behar KL, Lamoureux D, Mattson RH. The effect of gabapentin on brain γ-aminobutyric acid in patients with epilepsy. *Ann Neurol* 1996; 39: 95-9.

Petroff OAC, Hyder F, Mattson RH, Rothman DL. Topiramate increases brain GABA, homocarnosine, and pyrrolidinone in patients with epilepsy. *Neurology* 1999; 52: 473-8.

Pongs O. Voltage-gated potassium channels: from hyperexcitability to excitement. *FEBS Lett* 1999; 452: 31-5.

Poolos NP, Migliore M, Johnston D. Pharmacological upregulation of h-channels reduces the excitability of pyramidal neuron dendrites. *Nat Neurosci* 2002; 5: 767-74.

Prakriya M, Mennerick S. Selective depression of low-release probability excitatory synapses by sodium channel blockers. *Neuron* 2000; 26: 671-82.

Rabow LE, Russek SJ, Farb DH. From ion currents to genomic analysis: recent advances in $GABA_A$ receptor research. *Synapse* 1995; 21: 189-274.

Ragsdale DS, Avoli M. Sodium channels as molecular targets for antiepileptic drugs. *Brain Res Rev* 1998; 26: 16-28.

Ragsdale DS, Scheuer T, Catterall WA. Frequency and voltage-dependent inhibition of type IIA Na$^+$ channels, expressed in a mammalian cell line, by local anesthetic, antiarrhythmic, and anticonvulsant drugs. *Mol Pharmacol* 1991; 40: 756-65.

Reddy DS, Rogawski MA. Chronic treatment with the neuroactive steroid ganaxolone in the rat induces anticonvulsant tolerance to diazepam but not to itself. *J Pharmacol Exp Ther* 2000; 295: 1241-8.

Reiss WG, Oles KS. Acetazolamide in the treatment of seizures. *Ann Pharmacother* 1996; 30: 514-9.

Remy S, Gabriel S, Urban BW, et al. A novel mechanism underlying drug resistance in chronic epilepsy. *Ann Neurol* 2003a; 53: 469-79.

Remy S, Urban BW, Elger CE, Beck H. Anticonvulsant pharmacology of voltage-gated Na$^+$ channels in hippocampal neurons of control and chronically epileptic rats. *Eur J Neurosci* 2003b; 17: 2648-58.

Reynolds EH, Milner G, Matthews DM, Chanarin I. Anticonvulsant therapy, megaloblastic haemopoiesis and folic acid metabolism. *QJM* 1966; 35: 521-37.

Rho JM, Donevan SD, Rogawski MA. Direct activation of GABA$_A$ receptors by barbiturates in cultured rat hippocampal neurons. *J Physiol* 1996; 497: 509-22.

Rho JM, Donevan SD, Rogawski MA. Barbiturate-like actions of the propanediol dicarbamates felbamate and meprobamate. *J Pharmacol Exp Ther* 1997; 280: 1383-91.

Ribak C, Tong WM, Brecha NC. GABA plasma membrane transporters, GAT-1 and GAT-3, display different distributions in the rat hippocampus. *J Comp Neurol* 1996; 367: 595-606.

Rigo JM, Hans G, Nguyen L, et al. The anti-epileptic drug levetiracetam reverses the inhibition by negative allosteric modulators of neuronal GABA- and glycine-gated currents. *Br J Pharmacol* 2002; 136: 659-72.

Rogawski MA. KCNQ2/KCNQ3 K$^+$ channels and the molecular pathogenesis of epilepsy: implications for therapy. *Trends Neurosci* 2000; 23: 393-98.

Rogawski MA. Molecular targets versus models for new antiepileptic drug discovery. *Epilepsy Res* 2006; 68: 22-8.

Rogawski MA, Löscher W. The neurobiology of antiepileptic drugs. *Nat Rev Neurosci* 2004; 5: 553-64.

Rogawski MA, Porter RJ. Antiepileptic drugs: pharmacological mechanisms and clinical efficacy with consideration of promising developmental stage compounds. *Pharmacol Rev* 1990; 42: 223-86.

Rundfeldt C, Netzer R. The novel anticonvulsant retigabine activates M-currents in Chinese hamster ovary-cells transfected with human KCNQ2/3 subunits. *Neurosci Lett* 2000; 282: 73-6.

Schachter SC. Currently available antiepileptic drugs. *Neurotherapeutics* 2007; 4: 4-11.

Schmidt D. The clinical impact of new antiepileptic drugs after a decade of use in epilepsy. *Epilepsy Res* 2002; 50: 21-32.

Schmidt D, Löscher W. Drug resistance in epilepsy: putative neurobiologic and clinical mechanisms. *Epilepsia* 2005; 46: 858-77.

Schoepp DD. Unveiling the functions of presynaptic metabotropic glutamate receptors in the central nervous system. *J Pharmacol Exp Ther* 2001; 299: 12-20.

Shah MM, Anderson AE, Leung V, Lin X, Johnston D. Seizure-induced plasticity of h channels in entorhinal cortical layer III pyramidal neurons. *Neuron* 2004; 44: 495-508.

Sills GJ. Pre-clinical studies with the GABAergic compounds vigabatrin and tiagabine. *Epileptic Disord* 2003; 5: 51-6.

Stafstrom CE. Persistent sodium current and its role in epilepsy. *Epilepsy Curr* 2007; 7: 15-22.

Stefani A, Calabresi P, Pisani A, Mercuri NB, Siniscalchi A, Bernardi G. Felbamate inhibits dihydropyridine-sensitive calcium channels in central neurons. *J Pharmacol Exp Ther* 1996; 277: 121-7.

Stefani A, Spadoni F, Bernardi G. Voltage-activated calcium channels: targets of antiepileptic drug therapy? *Epilepsia* 1997; 38: 959-65.

Steinhoff BJ, Hirsch E, Mutani R, Nakken KO. The ideal characteristics of antiepileptic therapy: an overview of old and new AEDs. *Acta Neurol Scand* 2003; 107: 87-95.

Strauss U, Kole MHP, Bräuer AU, et al. An impaired neocortical I_h is associated with enhanced excitability and absence epilepsy. *Eur J Neurosci* 2004; 19: 3048-58.

Suzuki S, Kawakami K, Nishimura S, et al. Zonisamide blocks T-type calcium channels in cultured neurons of rat cerebral cortex. *Epilepsy Res* 1992; 12: 21-7.

Sveinbjornsdottir S, Sander JWAS, Upton D, et al. The excitatory amino acid antagonist D-CPPene (SDZ EAA 494) in patients with epilepsy. *Epilepsy Res* 1993; 16: 165-74.

Tatulian L, Delmas P, Abogadie FC, Brown DA. Activation of expressed KCNQ potassium currents and native neuronal M-type potassium currents by the anti-convulsant drug retigabine. *J Neurosci* 2001; 21: 5535-45.

Taylor LA, McQuade RD, Tice MA. Felbamate, a novel antiepileptic drug, reverses N-methyl-D-aspartate/glycine-stimulated increases in intracellular Ca^{2+} concentration. *Eur J Pharmacol* 1995; 289: 229-33.

Tecoma ES. Oxcarbazepine. *Epilepsia* 1999; 40 (suppl 5): S37-S46.

Teoh H, Fowler LJ, Bowery NG. Effect of lamotrigine on the electrically-evoked release of endogenous amino acids from slices of dorsal horn of the rat spinal cord. *Neuropharmacology* 1995; 34: 1273-8.

Timofeev I, Steriade M. Neocortical seizures: initiation, development and cessation. *Neuroscience* 2004; 123: 299-336.

Turski L, Stephens DN, Jensen LH, et al. Anticonvulsant action of the beta-carboline abecarnil: studies in rodents and baboon, *Papio papio*. *J Pharmacol Exp Ther* 1990; 253: 344-52.

Twyman RE, Rogers CJ, Macdonald RL. Differential regulation of (-aminobutyric acid receptor channels by diazepam and phenobarbital. *Ann Neurol* 1989; 25: 213-20.

Venance L, Rozov A, Blatow M, Burnashev N, Feldmeyer D, Monyer H. Connexin expression in electrically coupled postnatal rat brain neurons. *Proc Natl Acad Sci USA* 2000; 97: 10260-5.

Wang SJ, Huang CC, Hsu KS, Tsai JJ, Gean PW. Inhibition of N-type calcium currents by lamotrigine in rat amygdalar neurones. *Neuroreport* 1996; 7: 3037-40.

Whitaker WRJ, Clare JJ, Powell AJ, Chen YH, Faull RLM, Emson PC. Distribution of voltage-gated sodium channel alpha-subunit and beta-subunit mRNAs in human hippocampal formation, cortex, and cerebellum. *J Comp Neurol* 2000; 422: 123-9.

Wickenden AD. Potassium channels as anti-epileptic drug targets. *Neuropharmacology* 2002; 43: 1055-60.

Wickenden AD, Yu W, Zou A, Jegla T, Wagoner PK. Retigabine, a novel anticonvulsant, enhances activation of KCNQ2/Q3 potassium channels. *Mol Pharmacol* 2000; 58: 591-600.

White HS, Brown D, Skeen GA, Wolf HH, Twyman RE. The anticonvulsant topiramate displays a unique ability to potentiate GABA-evoked chloride currents. *Epilepsia* 1995; 36 (suppl 3): S39-S40.

Yu FH, Catterall WA. Overview of the voltage gated sodium channel family. *Genome Biol* 2003; 4: 207.1-207.7.

Zhang X, Velumian AA, Jones OT, Carlen PL. Modulation of high-voltage-activated calcium channels in dentate granule cells by topiramate. *Epilepsia* 2000; 41 (suppl 1): S52-S60.

Antiepileptic drugs in development with a real potential

Emilio Perucca

Institute of Neurology IRCCS C. Mondino Foundation and Clinical Pharmacology Unit, Department of Internal Medicine and Therapeutics, University of Pavia, Pavia, Italy

---

When second generation antiepileptic drugs (AEDs) started to be introduced in the early nineties, there was widespread hope that these agents could decrease substantially the burden of drug-resistant epilepsy. In fact, many of these medications offer advantages in terms of better tolerability and a lower interaction potential, and they allow physicians to better tailor drug choice to the need of the individual patient (Perucca, 2001). However, only less than 10-15% of patients refractory to older AEDs achieve complete seizure freedom with the new medications (Walker & Sander, 1996; Perucca et al., 2006). This justifies continuing efforts into the discovery of newer agents with an improved potential. The recent approval by the European Medicines Agency (EMEA) of stiripentol as adjunctive therapy to clobazam and valproic acid for severe myoclonic epilepsy in infancy (Chiron et al., 2009) and of rufinamide as adjunctive therapy of Lennox-Gastaut syndrome (Hakimian et al., 2007), demonstrates that there is also scope for developing newer medications targeted for specific, highly refractory epileptic syndromes.

The increasing cost of drug development and the realization that controlling drug-refractory seizures is a more challenging goal than initially thought has reduced somewhat investment into discovery of newer AEDs. However, there are also major incentives to develop better medications for epilepsy, not least the fact that a well tolerated drug with efficacy superior to that of existing agents could easily capture a large fraction of the market (Perucca et al., 2007). Moreover, many drugs initially marketed for epilepsy are subsequently found to have additional indications in other therapeutic areas, both in neurology and in psychiatry.

A recent review of the drug development scenario in epilepsy listed over 20 compounds which are being studied in healthy subjects or in patients with seizure disorders (Perucca et al., 2007). The present article will focus particularly on five agents which are in advanced development, have been described in sufficient detail in the published literature, and may become commercially available in the next few years. Other promising compounds for which extensive preclinical and clinical data have been obtained will not be discussed here in detail, either because information on these agents is mostly unpublished, or because to the author's knowledge their clinical development is not being actively pursued at the time of writing.

■ Brivaracetam

Brivaracetam (UCB 34714), or (2S)-2-[(4R)-2-oxo-4-propylpyrolidinyl] butanamide, is a 2-pyrrolidone derivative with a structure closely related to levetiracetam. The finding that levetiracetam acts by binding to synaptic vesicle protein 2A (SV2A) (Lynch et al., 2004) stimulated UCB S.A. to set up a drug discovery programme aimed at identifying analogues with higher affinity for SV2A than levetiracetam. Brivaracetam emerged from a primary screening of approximately 12,000 compounds in vitro, a secondary screening of 900 compounds in mice with audiogenic seizures, and a tertiary screening of 30 drug candidates in the kindling model (Kenda et al., 2004, White et al., 2008). Brivaracetam has been assessed in randomized double-blind placebo-controlled trials in patients with epilepsy, and is currently in advanced Phase III development.

Activity in preclinical models and mechanisms of action

Compared to levetiracetam, brivaracetam shows a 10-fold higher affinity for SV2A and a slightly broader spectrum of activity in animal models, including protection against seizures induced by maximal electroshock (MES) and pentylenetetrazole (PTZ) (Kenda et al., 2004). Brivaracetam is also more potent than levetiracetam in protecting against the acquisition of kindling and occurrence of secondarily generalized motor seizures in the corneal kindling model in mice, in inhibiting behavioral seizures and electrographic afterdischarges in amygdala kindled rats, in suppressing audiogenic seizures in genetically susceptible mice, and in abolishing spike-wave discharges in the genetic absence rat from Strasbourg (GAERS) (Matagne et al., 2003; Von Rosenstiel, 2007). Brivaracetam also possesses more potent antiseizure and antimyoclonic activity than levetiracetam in an established rat model of cardiac arrest-induced post-hypoxic myoclonus (Tai & Truong, 2007), and reduces dose-dependently the cumulative duration of active seizures in the acute model of partially drug resistant self-sustaining status epilepticus (SSSE) induced by perforant path stimulation in adult male rats (Wasterlain et al., 2005). Overall, these results suggest that brivaracetam may have broad spectrum antiepileptic efficacy against both partial seizures and a variety of primarily generalized seizures. Anticonvulsant effects in animals models are obtained at lower doses than those causing neurotoxic manifestations (von Rosenstiel, 2007).

Differences between brivaracetam and levetiracetam have also been reported in neurophysiological experiments in vitro. In particular, brivaracetam has been shown to be more potent that levetiracetam in suppressing high potassium-low calcium-induced epileptiform bursting in hippocampal slices, as well as spontaneous bursts occurring in the CA3 area (Margineanu et al., 2003).

The actions of brivaracetam appear to be mediated, at least to a large extent, by its interaction with SV2A (Kenda et al., 2004, Gillard et al., 2007; Von Rosenstiel, 2007; White et al., 2008). Although levetiracetam also binds at the same site, the precise molecular events which are triggered by the binding have not been fully elucidated, and the possibility exists that brivaracetam interaction with SV2A differs not only quantitatively, in terms of affinity, but also qualitatively, in terms of pharmacodynamic effects. This could explain the broader anticonvulsant activity of brivaracetam in animal models, although it is also possible that properties unrelated to SV2A binding contribute to differences in activity between brivaracetam and levetiracetam (White et al., 2008). In particular, there is evidence that brivaracetam may cause a modest inhibition of voltage-gated sodium channels (Zona et al., 2004).

Pharmacokinetic properties

After single oral doses up to 1,400 mg and multiple doses up to 800 mg/day in healthy subjects, brivaracetam is rapidly and almost completely absorbed from the gastrointestinal tract, with a median time to peak concentration occurring at 0.5 to 1.25 hours in most dose groups (Malawska and Kulig, 2005; Sargentini-Maier et al., 2007a; Von Rosenstiel, 2007). Plasma drug levels increase proportionally with dose up to single doses of 600 mg. A high-fat meal has no effect on the area under the serum concentration curve (AUC), but it reduces the peak concentration and delays time to peak to about 3 hours (Sargentini-Maier et al., 2007a). In these studies, apparent oral clearance (CL/F) was estimated to be about 0.8 to 1.0 ml min^{-1} kg^{-1}, while apparent oral volume of distribution (Vd/F) was around 0.6 l/kg^{-1}. In healthy subjects, the half-life of brivaracetam is in the range of 6 to 11 hours, with an average value of 7.7 hours (Malawska and Kulig, 2005; Sargentini-Maier et al., 2007). Plasma protein binding is low ($\leq 20\%$).

Less than 10% of an orally administered dose of brivaracetam is excreted unchanged in urine (Sargentini-Maier et al., 2007). Brivaracetam is eliminated primarily by biotransformation. The main metabolic pathways include hydrolysis of the acetamide group, CYP2C8-mediated hydroxylation, and a combination of these pathways (Sargentini-Maier et al., 2007b; Von Rosenstiel, 2007). No pharmacological activity of the resulting metabolites has been shown.

Brivaracetam CL/F is reduced by 24%, 32% and 35% in subjects with relatively mild, moderate and severe hepatic impairment, respectively (Von Rosenstiel, 2007). The half-life in these subjects (14.2, 16.4 and 17.4 hours, respectively) is longer than in healthy volunteers. The pharmacokinetics of brivaracetam in the elderly and in renally impaired subjects are similar to those reported in healthy subjects (Von Rosenstiel, 2007).

Drug interactions

In a population pharmacokinetics analysis of data from adjunctive therapy, brivaracetam CL/F was estimated to be 5.15 l/h in the presence of enzyme inducing AEDs compared with 3.63 l/h in the absence of enzyme inducers (Lacroix et al., 2007). Based on these results, enzyme inducing AEDs are expected to reduce serum brivaracetam concentrations by about 30%.

In vitro studies have shown that brivaracetam exerts an inhibitory action on epoxide hydrolase and, to a lesser extent, on the cytochrome P450 (CYP) enzymes CYP3A4 and CYP2C19. In addition, it may induce weakly CYP3A4 (Von Rosenstiel, 2007).

In adjunctive therapy trials in patients with epilepsy, brivaracetam at doses ranging from 5 to 150 mg/day did not appear to modify the serum concentrations of lamotrigine, levetiracetam, the mono-hydroxy-derivative of oxcarbazepine, valproic acid and topiramate (Otoul et al., 2007). In healthy subjects, administration of brivaracetam 200 mg b.i.d., which is above the dose expected to be required in patients with epilepsy, resulted in a

13% reduction in the serum levels of concurrently administered carbamazepine and a 2.5-fold increase in the levels of carbamazepine-10,11-epoxide (Von Rosenstiel, 2007). When brivaracetam at doses up to 400 mg/day was added on to carbamazepine in patients with epilepsy, a dose-dependent increase in serum carbamazepine-10,11-epoxide and, at 400 mg/day, a slight reduction in serum carbamazepine levels were confirmed. However, the carbamazepine-10,11-epoxide/carbamazepine ratio remained within the range reported in patients not treated with brivaracetam (Von Rosenstiel, 2007). In another study in healthy subjects, brivaracetam (400 mg/day for 10 days) caused a slight reduction in the peak serum phenytoin concentration and AUC after a single dose of phenytoin (Von Rosenstiel, 2007). In a small group of patients exposed to brivaracetam 20 and 50 mg/day, however, a mean 25% increase in serum phenytoin concentration was reported after addition of brivaracetam, though it was unclear whether this reflected a drug interaction or a chance finding (Otoul et al., 2007).

At the high dosage of 400 mg/day, brivaracetam has been found to decrease moderately the estrogen and progestagen components of a steroid oral contraceptive (Von Rosenstiel, 2007).

Efficacy and tolerability data

A single-blind placebo-controlled trial assessed the effect of brivaracetam on the photosensitive EEG response in patients with epilepsy (Kasteleijn-Nolst Trenité et al., 2007a). Of the 18 evaluable patients, none achieved complete suppression of photosensitivity on placebo, whereas 14 showed complete suppression after single doses of brivaracetam ranging from 10 to 80 mg. The response was rapid in onset (about 0.5 hours), and its duration was twice as long after an 80 mg dose (59.5 hours) than after lower doses.

In a first exploratory double-blind adjunctive-therapy trial, 157 patients with refractory partial seizures were randomized to placebo, brivaracetam 25 mg b.i.d. and brivaracetam 75 mg b.i.d. (Van Paesschen & Von Rosenstiel, 2007; Van Paesschen et al., 2007). Although no difference was found in the primary end-point (percent reduction in seizure frequency over placebo during the 7-week maintenance period), the median percent reduction in seizure frequency compared with baseline was greater in both the 50 mg/day group (-38.2%, $p < 0.02$) and the 150 mg/day group (-30.0%, $p < 0.02$) than in the placebo group (-18.9%). Responder rates (defined as proportions of patients with at least 50% reduction in seizure frequency compared with baseline) were 23.1% for placebo, 39.6% for brivaracetam 50 mg/day and 33.3% for brivaracetam 150 mg/day (Figure 1A).

A second double-blind adjunctive-therapy trial was completed in 208 patients with refractory partial seizures, who were randomized to receive either placebo or one of three doses of brivaracetam (5, 20 or 50 mg/day, each dosed b.i.d. without titration) for 7 weeks (French et al., 2007). Of the 208 randomized patients, 197 completed the study. Reductions in weekly partial-onset seizure frequency over placebo were 9.8% at 5 mg/day ($p = 0.24$), 14.9% at 20 mg/day ($p = 0.06$) and 22.1% at 50 mg/day ($p = 0.004$). Responder rates were 16.7% in the placebo group, and 32.0%, 44.2% and 55.8% in the groups assigned to receive 5, 20 and 50 mg/day brivaracetam, respectively (Figure 1B). Large phase III placebo-controlled studies in partial epilepsy and other syndromes, including progressive myoclonic epilepsies, are ongoing.

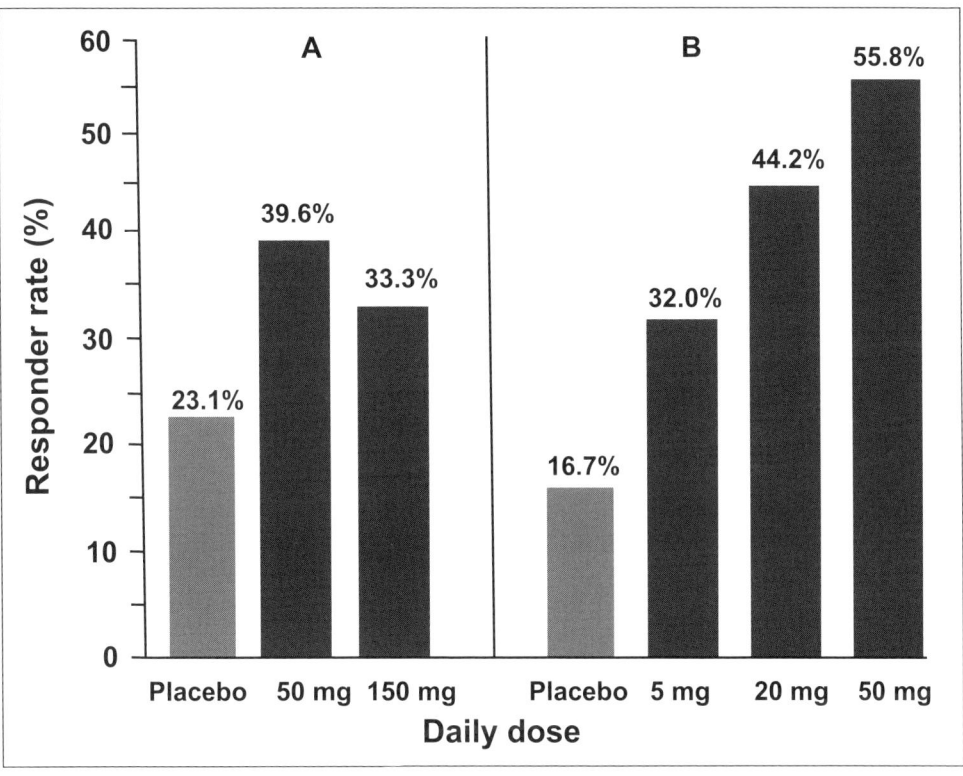

Figure 1. Responder rates (proportion of patients with at least 50% reduction in seizure frequency during the maintenance phase compared with baseline) in two double-blind placebo-controlled adjunctive-therapy trials of brivaracetam in patients with refractory partial seizures. The total number of patients randomized was 157 in trial A (Van Paesschen et al., 2007) and 208 in trial B (French & Von Rosenstiel, 2007). For details and statistical significances, see text.

In healthy subjects and epilepsy patients, brivaracetam was well tolerated after single oral doses up to 1,000 mg and multiple doses up to 800 mg/day, given on a *b.i.d.* basis. Treatment emergent adverse events were generally mild and mostly CNS-related, the most common being somnolence and dizziness (Kasteleijn-Nolst Trenité *et al.*, 2007a; Sargentini-Maier *et al.*, 2007a; Von Rosenstiel, 2007). In the two placebo-controlled trials in refractory partial epilepsy, adverse event profiles at all brivaracetam doses were similar to those reported for the placebo group (French *et al.*, 2007; Van Paesschen & Von Rosenstiel, 2007).

Critical assessment

Brivaracetam is quite promising because of its high responder rates, particularly in the study that explored doses in the lower range, and its excellent tolerability without dose titration. These results, however, should be regarded as preliminary, since efficacy data are only available from trials with short duration (7 weeks). Given its structural similarity to levetiracetam, the key question is in what way brivaracetam differs from its predecessor. Pharmacokinetically, brivaracetam shows no clear advantages, and it has a greater potential for drug interactions than levetiracetam. More data are needed to determine whether this compound brings any improvement in efficacy or tolerability over levetiracetam, and whether it retains efficacy in patients who failed to respond to levetiracetam.

■ Carisbamate

Carisbamate (RWJ-333369, S-2-O-carbamoyl-1-o-chlorophenylethanol) is a monocarbamate derivative which resembles somewhat in its structure the dicarbamate felbamate (Rogawski, 2006). However, carisbamate has only one carbamate group and only two carbons in its side chain, which prevents the formation of α,β unsaturated aldehydes considered to be responsible for the severe idiosyncratic reactions associated with felbamate (Thomson et al., 2006). Carisbamate shows a broad range of activities in animal models, and is being investigated clinically in a number of indications, including epilepsy, neuralgia and neuropathic pain (Kulig & Malawska, 2007).

Activity in preclinical models and mechanisms of action

Carisbamate displays broad spectrum activity in experimental models of seizures and epilepsy, with ED50 values generally in the range of 5 to 60 mg/kg, which are below the neurotoxic doses (Novak et al., 2007). In addition to protection against seizures induced by MES, PTZ, bicuculline and picrotoxin, effectiveness has been demonstrated in mice with audiogenic seizures, in the corneal and hippocampal kindling model of partial epilepsy in rats, and in rats with spontaneous recurrent seizures following kainate-induced status epilepticus (Grabenstatter & Dudek, 2004; White et al., 2006, François et al., 2007). In the amygdala kindling model, carisbamate not only suppresses fully kindled seizures, but it also delays the acquisition of kindling (Klein et al., 2007). Carisbamate is also effective in the GAERS model, which is predictive of efficacy against absence epilepsy (François et al., 2007), and suppresses seizure activity in two models of refractory epilepsy, the 6-Hz psychomotor seizure model, and the lamotrigine-resistant amygdala-kindled rat (White et al., 2006). In the lithium and pilocarpine model of status epilepticus in rats, carisbamate can prevent the onset of status, terminate fully established status (White et al., 2006) and protect against status-induced neuronal damage and the onset of post-status spontaneous seizures (François et al., 2005). Evidence for a suppressing effect of carisbamate on seizure activity and epileptogenesis was also obtained in an *in vitro* model which evaluates the expression of spontaneous recurrent epileptiform discharges after a low Mg^{2+}-induced status epilepticus-like injury in cultured rat hippocampal neurons (Deshpande et al., 2007). No evidence for a neuroprotective effect, however, was found in a rat model of traumatic brain injury (Keck et al., 2007).

Carisbamate prevents kindling-induced mechanical allodynia in rats (White et al., 2007) and displays activity in models of neuropathic pain (Cood et al., 2007). These findings led to initiation of clinical studies in diabetic neuropathy (Kulig & Malawska, 2007).

The mechanism of action of carisbamate is unknown (Bialer et al., 1977). Although the compound has been described as a "neuromodulator" (White et al., 2006; Kulig & Malawska, 2007; Novak et al., 2007), its molecular interactions causing reduced seizure susceptibility have not been determined.

Pharmacokinetic properties

Carisbamate is absorbed rapidly from the gastrointestinal tract, peak plasma concentrations being obtained at 1 to 3 hours post-dose after single and multiple dosing (Yao et al., 2006; Bialer et al., 2007). Oral bioavailability is virtually complete and is not affected by food intake to a clinically significant extent. Binding to plasma proteins is about 44% and concentration independent. Vd/F in adults is about 50 l. In healthy adults, average values for carisbamate CL/F are in the order of 3.4 to 4.2 l/h, and mean half-lives are in the order of 10.6 to 12.8 hours (Yao et al., 2006; Bialer et al., 2007). Carisbamate pharmacokinetics are similar after single and multiple doses, and do not deviate substantially from linearity after single doses ranging from 100 to 750 mg and multiple doses ranging from 200 to 1,500 mg/day in two divided daily administrations (Yao et al., 2006).

Carisbamate is negligibly excreted unchanged in urine and its elimination is dependent primarily on metabolism. The main identified metabolic pathways include O-glucuronidation (44% of the dose), and carbamate ester hydrolysis followed by oxidation of the aliphatic side chain (36% of the dose) (Mannens et al., 2007). Minor pathways include chiral inversion to the R-enantiomer followed by O-glucuronidation, and hydroxylation of the aromatic ring followed by sulfation. Only traces of (pre) mercapturic acid conjugates (each < 0.3% of the dose) are detected in urine, suggesting a low potential for formation of reactive metabolites.

In a study that assessed the pharmacokinetics of carisbamate after single and multiple doses (up to 500 mg b.i.d.) in subjects aged 18 to 55, 65 to 74 and > 75 years respectively, no apparent differences in pharmacokinetic parameters were found among the three age groups (Ragueneau-Majlessi et al., 2007).

Drug interactions

In studies in healthy subjects, the pharmacokinetics of carisbamate were not influenced by concomitant administration lamotrigine (100 mg/day) or valproic acid (1,000 mg/day) (Chien et al., 2007). Carbamazepine (600 mg/day), however, reduced serum carisbamate concentrations by 37% on average, presumably by inducing carisbamate metabolism (Chien et al., 2006). It is reasonable to assume that phenytoin and barbiturates can affect carisbamate pharmacokinetics similarly to carbamazepine, but these interactions have not been reported to date. Serum carisbamate concentrations can be reduced by about 20-30% by concomitant intake of an oral contraceptive containing 0.035 mg ethinylestradiol and 1 mg noretindrone (Novak et al., 2007), probably due to stimulation of carisbamate glucuronidation by the estrogenic component of the contraceptive.

In clinical pharmacology studies, carisbamate at doses up 500 mg b.i.d. had only minimal influences on the activity of the drug metabolizing enzymes CYP2C9, CYP2D6 and CYP3A4, as assessed by the clearance of the probe substrates tolbutamide, desipramine and midazolam, respectively (Novak et al., 2007). Carefully conducted studies in healthy subjects showed that carisbamate 500 mg b.i.d. does not affect the serum levels of carbamazepine (Chien et al., 2006) and decreases only to a minor extent the serum levels of valproic acid (-15% on average) and lamotrigine (-20% on average) (Chien et al., 2007).

Carisbamate had no significant effect on the pharmacokinetics of an oral contraceptive containing 0.035 mg ethinylestradiol and 1 mg noretindrone (Novak et al., 2007).

Efficacy and tolerability data

A non-randomized, single-blind, placebo-controlled proof-of-concept study evaluated the effect of single doses of carisbamate (250 to 1,000 mg) on the photosensitive EEG response in 18 patients with epilepsy (Kasteleijn-Nolst Trenité et al., 2007b). Photosensitivity was assessed at hourly intervals for up to 8 hours after administration of placebo on day 1, carisbamate on day 2 and placebo again on day 3. In the 13 evaluable patients, a dose-dependent inhibition of the photosensitive response was observed, with abolishment of the response in 3 patients and a clinically significant reduction in 7 additional patients. The effect was already present before or near the time of the peak concentration of carisbamate in serum and its duration was dose-related, with inhibition of photosensitivity for up to 32 h after doses of 750 or 1,000 mg.

A phase IIB randomized double-blind placebo-controlled parallel-group adjunctive-therapy study has been completed in 537 adults with refractory partial seizures (Faught et al., 2007). In this 16-week trial (including 4-week titration), carisbamate was evaluated at maintenance doses of 100, 300, 800 and 1,600 mg/day, given in two divided daily administrations. Median percent reduction in partial seizure frequency during the 16-week treatment compared with baseline was 6.2% for placebo, 15.4% for 100 mg/day, 24.0% for 300 mg/day, 20.9% for 800 mg/day and 28.6% for 1,600 mg/day ($p < 0.01$ vs. placebo for all doses except 100 mg/day). Responder rates were 10.1% on placebo and 12.4%, 23.6%, 18.5% and 24.8% for 100, 300, 800 and 1,600 mg/day, respectively ($p < 0.01$ vs placebo for 300 and 1,600 mg/day) (*Figure 2*). Fewer subjects discontinued the trial due to adverse events in the 100 mg (5%) and 300 mg (6%) groups than for placebo (8%).

Large phase III placebo-controlled adjunctive-therapy studies in refractory epilepsy are nearing completion.

In studies conducted to date, adverse events associated with carisbamate were reported mostly at dosages ≥ 1000 mg/day and include headache, dizziness, somnolence and nausea. In the phase IIB trial, doses of 200 to 400 mg/day were well tolerated in the first week, suggesting that no or minimal dose titration is needed at these doses (Novak et al., 2007).

Critical assessment

Among the drugs discussed in this article, carisbamate is the one for which making predictions about therapeutic potential is most difficult, mainly because its mode of action is unknown and efficacy and tolerability data are very limited at this stage. Favourable features of carisbamate include a modest interaction potential except for susceptibility to enzyme induction and a high probability, based on preclinical data, that clinical efficacy may extend to generalized epilepsy syndromes. In the only trial reported to date, however, efficacy rates in patients with refractory partial seizures have not been impressive. A large development programme is ongoing and results are expected to be available in the near future.

■ Eslicarbazepine acetate

Eslicarbazepine acetate (S-licarbazepine acetate, BIA 2-093) corresponds chemically to S-(-)-10-acetoxy-10,11-dihydro-5H-dibenzo/b,f/azepine-5-carboxamide, and therefore it is structurally related to both carbamazepine and oxcarbazepine (Benes et al., 1999).

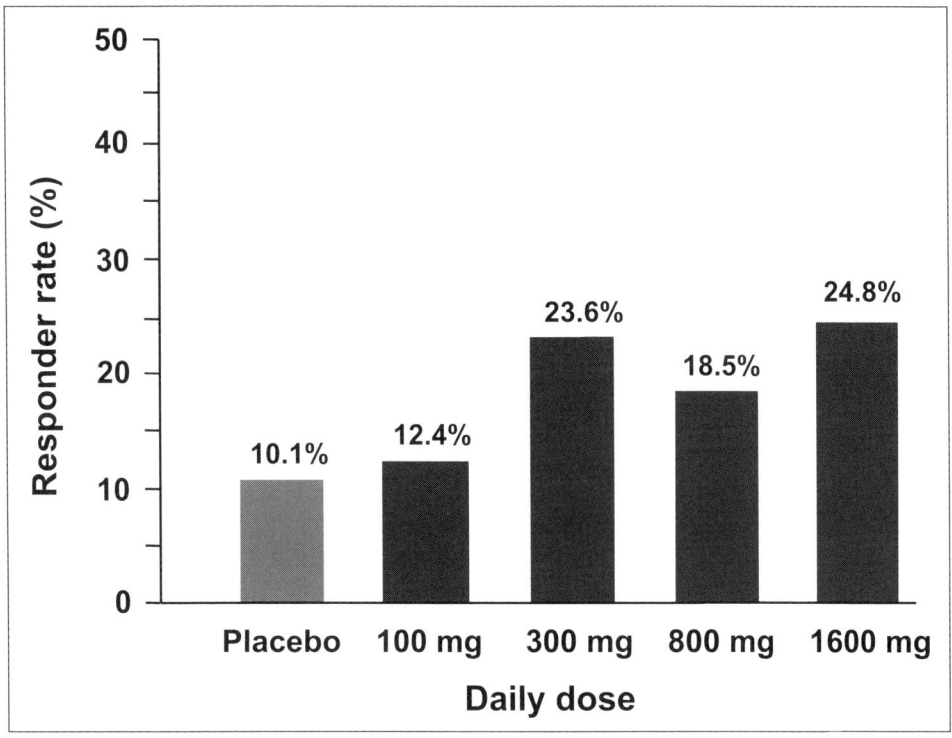

Figure 2. Responder rates (proportion of patients with at least 50% reduction in seizure frequency during the 16-week treatment compared with baseline) in a double-blind placebo-controlled adjunctive-therapy trial of carisbamate in 537 patients with refractory partial seizures (Faught et al., 2007). For details and statistical evaluation, see text.

Eslicarbazepine acetate resulted from a drug discovery programme aimed at identifying a compound with a pharmacokinetic and, possibly, pharmacodynamic profile superior to that of oxcarbazepine.

Activity in preclinical models and mechanisms of action

As discussed below, eslicarbazepine acetate is primarily a pro-drug of S-licarbazepine (eslicarbazepine), which identifies chemically with the S-enantiomer of the active monohydroxy derivative of oxcarbazepine (Benes et al., 1999; Hainzl et al., 2001). Given these structural similarities, it is not suprising that eslicarbazepine acetate resembles carbamazepine and oxcarbazepine in experimental models of seizures and epilepsy (Ambrosio et al., 2002). Eslicarbazepine acetate is effective against MES-induced seizures and seizures induced by amygdaloid kindling in rats, whereas it is inactive against clonic seizures induced by PTZ (Benes et al., 1999). Effectiveness has also been shown against seizures induced by picrotoxin (Sierra-Paredes et al., 2006) and latrunculin A (Sierra-Paredes et al., 2007) microdialysis in the rat hippocampus. Both eslicarbazepine acetate and licarbazepine have been shown to delay the development of corneal kindling in rats (Potschka et al., 2007). Compared with carbamazepine, eslicarbazepine acetate shows a lower neurotoxic potential, resulting in a superior protective index in classical seizure models (Benes et al., 1999; Ambrosio et al., 2000). Whether major differences occur in pharmacological activity between S-licarbazepine, the metabolite primarily responsible for the clinical effects of eslicarbazepine acetate, and R-licarbazepine (a metabolite which contributes clinically to the action of oxcarbazepine) is unclear. In the MES test, S-licarbazepine is more potent than R-licarbazepine, but it also shows greater neurotoxicity (Benes et al., 1999).

Eslicarbazepine does not bind to receptors for benzodiazepines, (γ-aminohydroxybutyric acid (GABA), and glutamate (Ambrosio et al., 2001, 2002). The primary mechanism of action of eslicarbazepine acetate and S-licarbazepine is blockade of voltage-dependent sodium channels (Benet et al., 199; Ambrosio et al., 2001, 2002; Almeida & Soares-da-Silva, 2007). The affinity of S-licarbazepine for the inactivated state of the sodium channel is similar to that of carbamazepine, but its affinity for the resting state of the channel is 3-fold lower (Bonifacio et al., 2001). Similarly to other voltage-sensitive sodium channel blockers, S-licarbazepine inhibits the sodium-dependent release of neurotransmitters, with a potency comparable to that of carbamazepine and oxcarbazepine (Ambrosio et al., 2001; Parada and Soares-da-Silva, 2002).

Pharmacokinetic properties

After single and multiple oral doses in healthy subjects and in patients with epilepsy, the serum concentrations of unchanged eslicarbazepine acetate are generally undetectable (< 10 ng/ml) (Almeida and Soares-da-Silva, 2003, 2004; Almeida et al., 2005). The compound is rapidly hydrolyzed in vivo to S-licarbazepine (eslicarbazepine). S-licarbazepine, in turn, undergoes minor chiral conversion to (R)-licarbazepine, the concentration of which in serum is only about 5% of the concentration of S-licarbazepine (Hainzl et al., 2001; Almeida et al., 2005). By contrast, after administration of oxcarbazepine, the serum concentration of (R)-licarbazepine is about 20 to 25% of the S-licarbazepine concentration (Volosov et al., 1999).

After oral administration of single doses of eslicarbazepine acetate ranging between 20 and 1,200 mg or multiple doses ranging from 200 mg b.i.d. to 2,400 mg once daily, absorption is rapid and peak serum concentrations of licarbazepine (sum of the S- and R-enantiomers) are achieved at 0.75 to 4 hours (Almeida and Soares-da-Silva, 2003, 2004; Vaz-da-Silva et al., 2005). In these studies, the relationship between serum licarbazepine concentrations and dose did not deviate from linearity to a major extent (Almeida & Soares-da-Silva, 2007). The AUC of licarbazepine after intake of eslicarbazepine acetate is about 16% greater than after an equimolar dose of oxcarbazepine (Bialer et al., 2005). Food has no major influence on the pharmacokinetic profile of licarbazepine (Maia et al., 2005a). A suspension formulation has been found to be bioequivalent to the tablet formulation (Fontes-Ribeiro et al., 2005).

The binding of S-licarbazepine to plasma proteins is about 30% (Almeida and Soares-da-Silva, 2007). The half-life of licarbazepine is in the range of 8-17 hours after single doses and 9-13 hours after multiple dosing (Almeida & Soares-da-Silva, 2003, 2004; Almeida et al., 2005). During repeated dosing, steady-state licarbazepine concentrations are reached within 4-5 days with once or twice daily administration (Almeida & Soares-da-Silva, 2004; Vaz-da-Silva et al., 2005), leading to the suggestion that the "effective" half-life of licarbazepine is in the order of 17-24 hours (Almeida & Soares-da-Silva, 2004, 2007; Almeida et al., 2005).

Licarbazepine is eliminated in urine in free form and as a glucuronide-conjugate. About 20% and 40% of an orally administered dose are recovered in urine in the next 12 and 24 hours, respectively (Almeida & Soares-da-Silva, 2004). Oxcarbazepine has been also identified as a minor metabolite (Almeida & Soares-da-Silva, 2003).

The pharmacokinetics of S-licarbazepine after administration of multiple doses of eslicarbazepine acetate are similar in males and females (Falcão et al., 2007). After administration of eslicarbazepine acetate in children aged 2 to 17 years, S-licarbazepine CL/F was higher in younger than in older children, and there was an inverse relationship between CL/F and age (Nunes et al., 2007a). No age or gender-related differences in the serum levels of (R)- and (S)-licarbazepine were found in a study that compared the pharmacokinetics of eslicarbazepine acetate after single (600 mg) and multiple doses (600 mg once daily for 8 days) in 12 young (mean age 30 years, range 18-38) and 12 elderly (mean age 70 years, range 65-80) healthy subjects (Almeida et al., 2005). The pharmacokinetics of eslicarbazepine acetate and its metabolites in subjects with moderate liver impairment is similar to that reported in subjects with normal liver function (Almeida et al., 2007). The CL/F of S-licarbazepine and other metabolites of eslicarbazepine acetate is, however, significantly reduced in patients with impaired renal function (Maia et al., 2007).

Drug interactions

Since enzyme inducing AEDs are known to increase the clearance of licarbazepine derived from oxcarbazepine (May et al., 2003), it is reasonable to assume that the same interaction may affect licarbazepine derived from eslicarbazepine acetate.

There is insufficient information on the influence of eslicarbazepine acetate on the serum levels of concomitantly administered AEDs. Preliminary findings suggest that eslicarbazepine acetate does not affect the serum levels of valproic acid, but it may reduce the serum levels of topiramate (Almeida & Soares-da-Silva, 2007). Evidence on a possible lowering effect of eslicarbazepine acetate on serum lamotrigine levels is equivocal (Almeida & Soares-da-Silva, 2007; Nunes et al., 2007b).

In in vitro studies, S-licarbazepine had no significant effect on the activity of CYP1A2, CYP2A6, CYP2B6, CYP2C19, CYP2D6, CYP2E1, CYP3A4, CYP4A9/11, epoxide hydrolase and the uridine glucurunosyl transferase (UGT) enzyme UGT1A6 in human liver microsomes (Almeida & Soares-da-Silva, 2007). The same studies identified a modest inhibition of CYP2C9-mediated tolbutamide 4-hydroxylation, and a mild activation of UGT1A1-mediated ethinylestradiol glucuronidation.

Phase II interaction studies in vivo have been conducted to determine whether eslicarbazepine acetate affects the pharmacokinetics of warfarin, steroid oral contraceptives and digoxin. At a dosage of 1,200 mg/day given once daily, eslicarbazepine acetate caused a mean 23% decrease in the serum levels of the active S-enantiomer of warfarin (Almeida & Soares-da-Silva, 2007). This effect was associated with only a minor change in international normalized ratio (INR) and was not considered clinically significant. In another study, administration of eslicarbazepine acetate (1,200 mg/day once daily) together with a steroid oral contraceptive resulted in a mean 24% decrease in the AUC of levonorgestrel and a mean 32% decrease in the AUC of ethinylestradiol (Almeida & Soares-da-Silva, 2007). At a dose of 1,200 mg/day, eslicarbazepine acetate did not affect the pharmacokinetics of digoxin to a clinically significant extent (Maia et al., 2005).

Efficacy and tolerability data

Eslicarbazepine acetate has been assessed in a double-blind placebo-controlled parallel-group adjunctive-therapy study in 143 patients with refractory partial seizures (Elger *et al.*, 2007). Patients on carbamazepine and oxcarbazepine were excluded from the study. Eslicarbazepine acetate was administered at escalating doses of 400, 800 and 1,200 mg/day, each for 4-week periods, with a once daily schedule in one group and a twice daily schedule in another. The responder rate assessed over the entire 12-week treatment period was significantly higher in the once daily group than in the placebo group (54% vs 28%, p < 0.01), whereas the responder rate in the twice daily group (41%) did not differ significantly from placebo *(Figure 3)*. Discontinuation rates for adverse events were 6% in the once daily group, 9% in the twice daily group, and 8% in the placebo group. The most

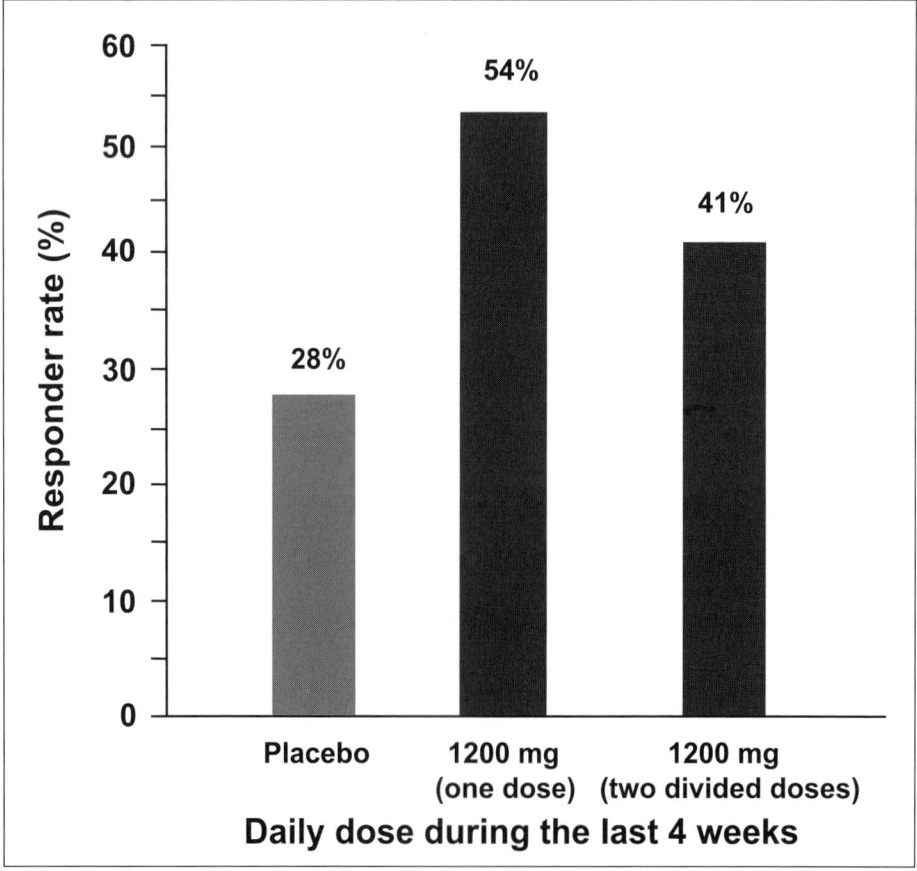

Figure 3. Responder rates (proportion of patients with at least 50% reduction in seizure frequency compared with baseline) in a 12-week double-blind placebo-controlled adjunctive-therapy trial of eslicarbazepine acetate in 143 patients with refractory partial seizures (Elger *et al.*, 2007). Daily dosage was 400 mg during weeks 1-4, 800 mg during weeks 5-8, and 1,200 mg in the last 4 weeks. Responder rates are calculated over the entire treatment period. For details and statistical significance, see text.

common adverse events were headache, nausea/vomiting, dizziness and somnolence, each occurring in less than 10% in any of the groups. Overall, adverse events rates in both eslicarbazepine acetate groups were comparable to those reported in the placebo group.

Three additional placebo-controlled adjunctive therapy studies in refractory partial seizures are ongoing, together with adjunctive therapy studies in children, monotherapy studies in adults with partial seizures, phase II studies in acute mania and recurrence prevention trials in bipolar disorder (Almeida & Soares-da-Silva, 2007).

Critical assessment

Eslicarbazepine acetate is a pro-drug which closely resembles oxcarbazepine, the primary difference being that the circulating active moiety is almost exclusively S-licarbazepine in subjects treated with eslicarbazepine acetate and a mixture of about 20% S-licarbazepine and 20% R-licarbazepine in subjects treated with oxcarbazepine. Based on this, it is very likely that eslicarbazepine acetate will be an efficacious and well tolerated agent. The key question on whether it will be any different from oxcarbazepine cannot be answered at present because there are insufficient experimental data on the comparative activities of S- and R-licarbazepine, and there have been no head-to-head comparisons with oxcarbazepine. An interesting feature of eslicarbazepine acetate is that its is being developed with a once daily dosing schedule, which distinguishes it from many other AEDs. The observation that in the exploratory trial once daily dosing had superior efficacy and at least as good tolerability compared with twice daily dosing is intriguing in view of the relatively short half-life of S-licarbazepine.

■ Lacosamide

Lacosamide (SPM 927), also formerly known as harkoseride, is the R-enantiomer of 2-acetamido-N-benzyl-3-methoxypropionamide and, therefore, is structurally unrelated to existing AEDs. Lacosamide has already undergone an extensive Phase III programme as adjunctive therapy for patients with refractory partial seizures, and also as monotherapy for patients with painful diabetic neuropathy.

Activity in preclinical models and mechanisms of action

Lacosamide displays anticonvulsant activity in a wide variety of rodent models of seizures and epilepsy, mostly in the dose range of 1 to 30 mg/kg i.p. (Beyreuther et al., 2007a). Seizure suppressing effects have been demonstrated against audiogenic seizures in Frings mice, MES-induced tonic extension seizures in mice and rats, N-methyl-D-aspartate (NMDA)-induced seizures in mice, and behavioural seizures and afterdischarges in the hippocampal kindled rat model of partial epilepsy (Duncan et al., 2005; Beyreuther et al., 2007; Stöhr et al., 2007a). At a dosage of 10 mg/kg, lacosamide delays amygdala kindling acquisition in rats (Brandt et al., 2006). Lacosamide is also effective in the 4-aminopyridine model of epileptiform bursting (Lees et al., 2006), and in the 6 Hz psychomotor seizure model of pharmacoresistant epilepsy (Beyreuther et al., 2007; Stöhr et al., 2007a). In the latter model, it shows supra-additive anticonvulsant effects when combined with other AEDs (Stöhr et al., 2007b).

Lacosamide does not block the tonic-clonic seizures induced by picrotoxin and bicuculline, nor the clonic seizures induced by PTZ in mice and rats. However, it increases the threshold for minimal seizures induced by intravenous PTZ infusions in mice (Beyreuther et *al.*, 2007a). Lacosamide is effective in reducing cumulative seizure duration in the perforant path model of SSSE in rats, and a reduction of SSSE-induced hippocampal damage has been demonstrated in this model (Beyreuther *et al.*, 2007a). A possible neuroprotective effect is suggested by a number of experimental findings. In particular, lacosamide decreases infarct volume in the rat middle cerebral artery occlusion model of ischemia when administered 15 min before occlusion and for four hours post-infusion, and produces a concentration-dependent block of glutamate- and oxygen-glucose deprivation-induced apoptosis in organotypic rat hippocampal slice cultures (White *et al.*, 2008). However, lacosamide does not prevent brain damage or functional deficits in a rat model of traumatic brain injury (White *et al.*, 2008).

Lacosamide is effective in various animal models of chronic pain (Beyreuther *et al.*, 2006, 2007a-d; Hao *et al.* 2006; Stöhr *et al.*, 2006).

Lacosamide does not appear to share modes of actions identified for other AEDs (Errington *et al.*, 2006). Its anticonvulsant and analgesic effects appear to be mediated by a dual mode of action (Heers *et al.*, 2007). The first is a selective enhancement of slow inactivation of voltage-gated sodium channels, without apparent interaction with fast inactivation gating (Errington *et al.*, 2008). The second is a functional interaction with collapsin-response mediator protein 2 (CRMP-2 alias DRP-2) (Freitag *et al.*, 2007), a protein which has been implicated in both epileptogenesis and the pathogenesis of neuropathic pain (Beyreuther *et al.*, 2007).

Pharmacokinetic properties

Lacosamide is well absorbed from the gastrointestinal tract, peak serum concentrations being obtained at 1 to 4 hours after dosing (Doty *et al.*, 2007). Its oral bioavailability is virtually complete (Kropeit *et al.*, 2004; Rosenfeld *et al.*, 2005; Biton *et al.*, 2007), and is not affected by food (Cawello *et al.*, 2004; Doty *et al.*, 2007). Serum lacosamide concentrations are linearly related to dose after single oral doses up to 800 mg and intravenous doses up to 300 mg (Horstmann *et al.*, 2002; Rosenfeld *et al.*, 2004, Doty *et al.*, 2007).

Lacosamide shows minimal (< 15%) binding to plasma proteins (Doty *et al.*, 2007) and is eliminated with a half-life of 12 to 16 hours (Doty *et al.*, 2007; White *et al.* 2008). Approximately 40% of an orally administered dose is recovered unchanged in urine, and another 30% is recovered in the form of the inactive O-demethyl-metabolite SPM 12809 (Bialer *et al.*, 2004; Schiltmeyer *et al.*, 2004). The CYP2C19 genotype seems to have no major influence on serum lacosamide levels, but serum SPM 12809 levels are markedly reduced in poor CYP2C19 metabolizers, suggesting that CYP2C19 contributes to lacosamide demethylation (Kropeit *et al.*, 2005).

After normalization for dose and differences in body weight, serum lacosamide concentrations are comparable in males and females. Steady-state lacosamide concentrations in 23 subjects over 65 years of age (age range not stated) were about 10-35% higher than those observed in non-elderly adults (Schiltmeyer *et al.*, 2004).

Drug interactions

In drug interaction studies, serum lacosamide concentrations were not affected by concomitant treatment with carbamazepine 400 mg/day or valproic acid 600 mg/day (Horstmann *et al.*, 2002; Kropeit *et al.*, 2005; Doty *et al.*, 2007).

In vitro, lacosamide shows no or low potential to inhibit CYP1A1, CYP1A2, CYP2B6, CYP2C8, CYP2C9, CYP2C19, CYP2D6, CY2E1, CYP3A4 and CYP3A5 in human hepatocytes or recombinant human enzymes (Beyreuther *et al.*, 2007a; Doty *et al.*, 2007). Since the inhibitory concentrations on these enzymes are more than 15- to 30-fold higher than the clinically occurring serum lacosamide levels, these data suggest that lacosamide is unlikely to inhibit the metabolism of concurrently administered CYP substrates. At therapeutic concentrations, lacosamide was also devoid of enzyme inducing effects on CYP1A2, CYP2B6, CYP2C9, CYP2C19 and CYP3A4 in human hepatocytes (Beyreuther *et al.*, 2007a).

In clinical studies, lacosamide has been found not to affect the plasma concentrations of carbamazepine, carbamazepine-10,11-epoxide, phenytoin, valproic acid, lamotrigine, monohydroxycarbazepine, topiramate, zonisamide, levetiracetam, gabapentin, metformin, digoxin, omeprazole, ethinylestradiol and levonorgestrel (Kropeit *et al.*, 2005; Jatuzis *et al.*, 2005; Ben-Menachem *et al.*, 2007; Doty *et al.*, 2007; Thomas *et al.*, 2007).

Efficacy and tolerability data

Following pilot open label studies (Fountain *et al.*, 2000; Sachdeo *et al.*, 2003), three large randomized adjunctive-therapy trials have been completed in patients with refractory partial seizures. Each trial involved a titration period, during which lacosamide was increased up to the target dose in 100 mg/day weekly increments, and a 12-week maintenance period (Doty *et al.*, 2007). Lacosamide was always given on a *b.i.d.* basis.

In the first trial, 418 patients stabilized on one or two AEDs were randomized to receive placebo or target lacosamide doses of 200, 400 or 600 mg/day (Ben-Menachem *et al.*, 2007). Responder rates during the maintenance period compared with baseline (with efficacy data carried forward for patients who discontinued during the titration period) were 22%, 33%, 41% and 38% for placebo, lacosamide 200, 400 and 600 mg/day, respectively. The difference over placebo was statistically significant ($p < 0.02$) for the high and the intermediate dose (*Figure 4A*). Discontinuation rates for adverse events were 5% in the placebo group and 11%, 19% and 30% in the 200, 400 and 600 mg/day lacosamide groups, respectively. The most common dose-related adverse events were dizziness (55% in the highest dose group versus 10% on placebo), nausea, fatigue, ataxia and visual disturbances. In all lacosamide dose groups, proportions of patients reporting somnolence were remarkably similar to the placebo rate. Lacosamide produced a small, dose-related increase in ECG PR interval.

In the second trial, 485 patients receiving up to three AEDs were randomized to placebo or target lacosamide doses of 200 or 400 mg/day (Halasz *et al.*, 2006; Bialer *et al.*, 2007). The median percent reductions in seizure frequency were 35%, and 36% for lacosamide 200 and 400 mg/day ($p < 0.05$ vs placebo for both doses), respectively, compared with 21% for placebo. Responder rates were 26%, 35%, and 41% for placebo, lacosamide 200 and 400 mg/day, respectively ($p < 0.01$ for the 400 mg/day group) (*Figure 4B*). Dizziness and headache were the most commonly reported adverse events in this trial (Doty *et al.*, 2007).

The third trial, conducted in 405 patients also receiving up to three AEDs, investigated target doses of 400 or 600 mg/day (Chung *et al.*, 2007). Both lacosamide doses were significantly superior to placebo ($p < 0.001$), with responder rates of 38.3% at 400 mg/day and 41.2% at 600 mg/day compared with 18.3% on placebo (*Figure 4C*). The most common adverse events ($\geq 10\%$ in any lacosamide group) were dizziness, nausea, diplopia, blurred vision, vomiting, headache, tremor, abnormal coordination, somnolence and nystagmus.

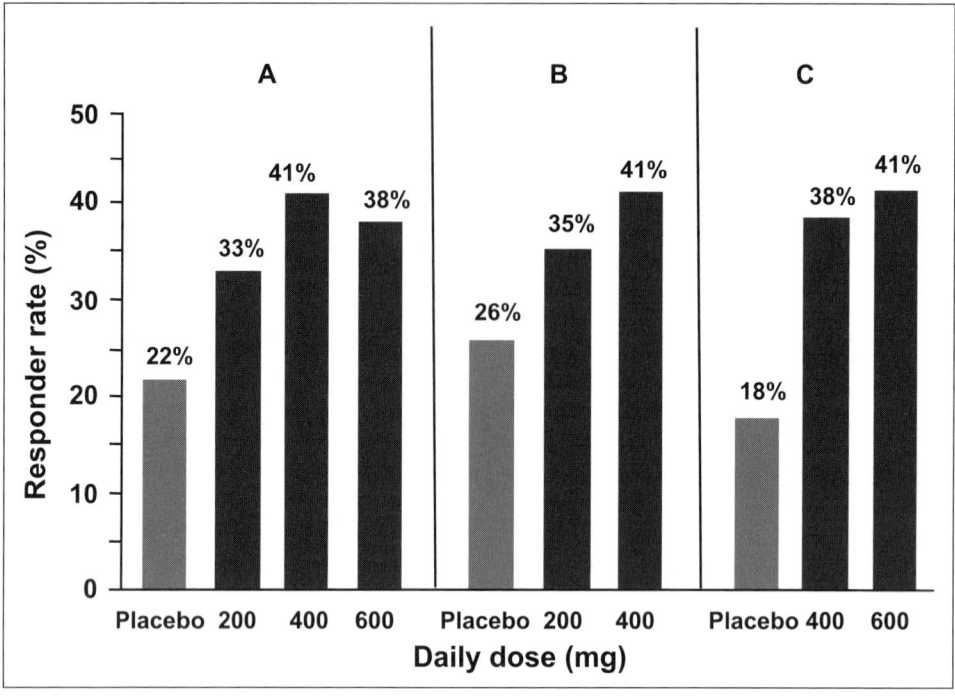

Figure 4. Responder rates (proportion of patients with at least 50% reduction in seizure frequency during the maintenance phase compared with baseline) in three double-blind placebo-controlled adjunctive-therapy trials of lacosamide in patients with refractory partial seizures. For patients who discontinued before the maintenance period, efficacy data were carried forward from the titration period. The total number of patients randomized was 418 in trial A (Ben-Menachem et al., 2007), 485 in trial B (Halasz et al., 2007; Bialer et al., 2007) and 405 in trial C (Chung et al., 2007). For details and statistical significances, see text.

An intravenous formulation of lacosamide has been developed as replacement therapy for patients temporarily unable to continue on oral therapy. In healthy subjects, infusions of 200 mg lacosamide over periods of 15, 30 and 60 min were as well tolerated as the ingestion of a 200 mg tablet (Kropeit et al., 2004). Intravenous 30- to 60-min infusions (up to 300 mg b.i.d. for two days) given as replacement therapy in patients with epilepsy also showed a comparable tolerability profile to oral lacosamide (Biton et al., 2007).

Lacosamide has been investigated in randomized placebo-controlled double-blind trials in patients with neuropathic pain attributed to distal diabetic neuropathy (Wymer et al., 2005; Ziegler et al., 2005; Rauck et al., 2007). Overall, results of these studies suggests that lacosamide may be efficacious in attenuating pain associated with peripheral neuropathy at doses up to 400 mg/day. A 600 mg/day dose was also tested but it did not appear to confer additional benefit, and was less tolerated.

Critical assessment

Interesting features of lacosamide in epilepsy include a novel mode of action, relatively high responder rates, the availability of an intravenous formulation, a low potential for drug-drug-interactions, and lack of sedative effects. Apparent drawbacks include the need for gradual titration, and a rather narrow effective dose range with a relatively high intolerance rate at 600 mg/day. The clinical usefulness of lacosamide will be influenced by the feasibility of dose optimization to minimize adverse effects, and by determination of whether its efficacy, so far demonstrated only in partial seizures, also extends to generalized epilepsy syndromes.

Retigabine

Retigabine (D23129) corresponds chemically to N-[2-amino-4-(4-fluorobenzylamino)-phenyl]carbamic acid ethyl ester. Retigabine was discovered by an *in vivo* screening programme driven by pharmacophore modeling, aimed at identifying compounds with potent activity in seizure models and mechanisms of action different from those of existing AEDs (Porter *et al.*, 2007a). This programme used as starting point for structural optimization flupirtine, an analgesic with anticonvulsant properties which underwent some clinical testing in the '80s.

Activity in preclinical models and mechanisms of action

Retigabine displays broad-spectrum protective activity against seizures induced by electrical (MES) and chemical stimuli (PTZ, picrotoxin, penicillin, kainate and i.c.v. administered NMDA) (Kapetanovic & Rundfeldt, 1996; Rostock *et al.*, 1996; Plosker & Scott, 2006; Porter *et al.*, 2007a; White *et al.*, 2008). It is also effective in genetic epilepsy models, including the genetically epilepsy prone rats (GEPR) and the audiogenic seizure-susceptible DBA/J2 mice (Tober *et al.*, 1994; Dailey *et al.*, 1995). Retigabine blocks the expression of behavioral seizures and decreases the duration of electrographic afterdischarges in amygdaloid kindled rats (Tober *et al.*, 1996), and inhibits the acquisition of kindling in this model (Porter *et al.*, 2007a). Activity is also observed in the hippocampal kindling model in rats, and corneal kindling model in mice (Porter *et al.*, 2007a; Rowley *et al.*, 2007). Retigabine differs from most other anticonvulsants because it is more potent in kindling models than in other seizure models. In the amygdala kindled rats, for example, an increase in the threshold for induction of afterdischarges is found at doses as low as 0.01 mg/kg, and seizure severity and duration are reduced at 5 mg/kg, which is a nontoxic dose in these animals (Tober *et al.* 1996).

Retigabine is also effective in blocking epileptiform activity in various *in vitro* models. In particular, it suppresses magnesium-induced late recurrent discharges (Armand *et al.*, 2000), and 4-amino-pyridine-induced discharges (Armand *et al.*, 1999) in the entorhinal cortex, blocks carbamazepine- and phenytoin-resistant spontaneous bursting in entorhinal cortex slices from rats pretreated with kainate (Smith *et al.*, 2007), and inhibits different discharge patterns in cortical epileptic tissue resected from patients with epilepsy (Straub *et al.*, 2001).

Potentially useful properties of retigabine in non-epilepsy indications are suggested by demonstration of analgesic activity in two models of neuropathic pain (Porter *et al.*, 2007a), antidystonic effects in a mutant hamster model (Richter *et al.*, 2006), activity in a rodent model of mania (Dencker *et al.*, 2008), antagonisms of the excitatory responses induced by cocaine and other psychostimulants in rats (Hansen *et al.*, 2007), and reversal of the functional abnormalities caused by mutations of the *KCNQ2* gene in a patient with peripheral nerve excitability (Wuttke *et al.*, 2007). There is also evidence suggesting potential usefulness in the treatment of urinary incontinence and irritable bowel syndrome (Porter *et al.*, 2007a). Finally, retigabine shows neuroprotective activity in models of ischemic brain damage (Porter et al., 2007a) and oxidative stress (Boscia et al., 2006). A protective effect has been also demonstrated against neuronal damage caused by sustained kainic acid-induced status epilepticus (Porter et al., 2007a).

The primary mechanism of action of retigabine consists in stabilization of the neuronal membrane through specific enhancement of the M-type potassium current, which is carried by the Kv7 channel, previously known as the KCNQ channel (Rundfeldt, 1997; Rundfeldt & Netzer, 2000a; Lawrence et al., 2006; Rivera-Arconada & Lopez-Garcia et al., 2006). The effects of retigabine on the Kv7 channel appear to be mediated by an action on isoforms 2/3 and, possibly, also 3/5 (Plosker & Scott, 2006). Retigabine appears to reduce excitability by shifting the activation of Kv7 current to more hyperpolarized potentials and by slowing the deactivation and increasing the activation phase (Tatulian et al., 2001, 2003). Interestingly, a mutation in Kv7 channel subunits is known to be etiologically linked to benign familial convulsions, an autosomal dominant epilepsy syndrome, and retigabine can reverse the functional deficit associated with this mutation (Porter et al., 2007a).

Additional pharmacological properties of retigabine include an increase in GABA-mediated currents in cortical neurons (Rundfeldt & Netzer, 2000a,b; Otto et al., 2002), blockade of 4-amino-pyridine-induced neosynthesis of neuroactive aminoacids, stimulation of GABA synthesis in hippocampal slices (Kapetanovic et al., 1995), and very weak blocking effects on neuronal sodium and mixed calcium currents (Rundfeldt & Netzer, 2000a). These effects are recorded at higher concentrations than those required to block the M-current, and their potential contribution to the clinical effects of retigabine is unclear.

Pharmacokinetic properties

Retigabine is rapidly absorbed from the gastrointestinal tract, peak serum concentration being recorded 1-2 hours following single and multiple dosing (Ferron et al., 2002). In healthy subjects, oral bioavailability is about 60% (Herman et al., 2003). Exposure to retigabine was not modified by intake with a high-fat meal, although time to peak concentration was slightly delayed by food intake (Porter et al., 2007a). The pharmacokinetics of retigabine are linear and dose-proportional after single doses up to 700 mg in healthy subjects (Ferron et al., 2002) and multiple doses up to 1200 mg/day in patients with epilepsy (Plosker & Scott, 2006).

Retigabine is about 80% bound to plasma proteins. Vd/F values ranged from 6.2 to 8.8 L/kg after single doses, and from 5.1 to 7.4 L/kg after multiple doses (Ferron et al., 2002). The pharmacokinetics of retigabine show some diurnal variation, with trough serum concentrations at steady-state being approximately 35% lower in the evening than in the morning. The half-life of retigabine is in the order of 5 to 9 hours after single and multiple doses, while CL/F is estimated at 0.5-0.7 L/h/kg (Ferron et al., 2002). After normalizing for body weight, retigabine CL/F and Vd/F were 25% and 30% lower, respectively, in black than in white subjects (Ferron et al., 2002). There are no major gender-related differences in retigabine CL/F. In a group of subjects aged 66 to 81 years, retigabine CL/F was found to on average 30% lower than in non-elderly adults (Hermann et al., 2003).

Retigabine is eliminated by N-glucuronidation, N-acetylation and, to a lesser extent, by renal excretion in unchanged form (Hempel et al., 1999). The primary N-acetyl metabolite retains some pharmacological activity and is found in serum at concentrations similar to those of the parent drug (Ferron et al., 2002). Two distinct inactive N-glucuronides have also been identified, the formation of which is catalized by UGT1A1, UGT1A9 and UGT1A4 (McNeilly et al., 1997; Borlak et al., 2006) and may contribute to the entero-hepatic circulation of the drug (McNeilly et al., 1997; Hiller et al., 1999).

The pharmacokinetics of retigabine are unaltered in patients with Gilbert's syndrome, in subjects with N-acetyltransferase 2 (NAT2) slow acetylator status, and in carriers of both variants. However, exposure to N-acetyl-retigabine is about 30% higher in rapid acetylators than in slow acetylators (Hermann et al., 2006).

Drug interactions

Serum retigabine concentrations are unaltered by concomitantly administered valproic acid or topiramate (Ferron et al., 2001a). An increase in retigabine CL/F by about 30% is observed in patients comedicated with carbamazepine or phenytoin, presumably due to induction of retigabine metabolism (Ferron et al., 2001a). Phenobarbital, on the other hand, was not found to alter retigabine pharmacokinetics, an intriguing finding in view of the enzyme inducing effects of barbiturates (Ferron et al., 2003). A slight decline (13%) in retigabine CL/F has been reported in subjects who received a very low dose of lamotrigine (25 mg/day) for 8 days, and was interpreted as being due to competition for renal elimination rather than competition for glucuronidation (Hermann et al., 2003). Whether a more marked interaction occurs in patients receiving therapeutic doses of lamotrigine is unknown.

Retigabine has been reported not to affect to an important extent the serum concentration of concomitantly administered carbamazepine, phenytoin, valproic acid, phenobarbital, and topiramate (Ferron et al., 2001a, 2003; Sachdeo et al., 2001). At a dosage of 600 mg/day, retigabine has been found to cause a moderate (22%) increase in lamotrigine clearance (Hermann et al., 2003).

In an interaction study, a very short course of retigabine (150 mg t.i.d. on days 10-14) in women taking a low-dose oral contraceptive did not affect the pharmacokinetics of ethinylestradiol and levonorgestrel (Ferron et al., 2001b).

Efficacy and tolerability data

An initial open-label dose-finding study in 60 patients with refractory epilepsy established the maximally tolerated dose at 1,200 mg/day using either a b.i.d. or a t.i.d. regimen (Sachdeo et al., 2005). Dizziness and somnolence were the most common adverse effects that were dose limiting. A separate small-scale double-blind study explored different titration rates, and dose increments of 150 mg every 7 days were found to be associated with fewer discontinuations than increments every 2 or 4 days (Abou-Khalil et al., 2005; Plosker & Scott, 2006).

The first large double-blind adjunctive-therapy efficacy trial of retigabine was conducted in 399 patients with refractory partial seizures (Porter et al., 2007b). After an 8-week baseline, patients were randomized to 16-week treatment (8-week forced titration and 8-week maintenance) with placebo or retigabine, at target dosages of 600, 900 and 1200 mg/day given in three divided daily administrations. The median percent reduction in seizure frequency from baseline (primary end-point) was 13% for placebo and 23% for 600 mg/day, 29% for 900 mg/day and 35% for 1,200 mg/day ($p < 0.001$ for differences across all treatment arms). Responder rates calculated over the entire treatment period compared with baseline were 15.6% for placebo, 23.2% for 600 mg/day, 31.6% for 900 mg/day (p = 0.021) and 33.0% for 1,200 mg/day (p = 0.016) *(Figure 5A)*. Responder rates calculated over the maintenance period were 27.7% for 600 mg/day, 40.5% for 900 mg/day and 41.2% for 1,200 mg/day versus 25.6% for placebo. The most common dose-related adverse events were somnolence, confusion, dizziness, speech disorder and vertigo, which occurred in 14 to 22% of patients in the highest dose group compared with 0-6% in the placebo group. Proportion of patients withdrawing for adverse events were 17%, 20% and 29% in the 600, 900 and 1,200 mg/day groups respectively, compared with 12.5% in the placebo group.

A second double-blind parallel-group adjunctive-therapy trial was completed recently in North and Latin America in a total of 306 patients with refractory partial seizures (Little, 2008). The trial, which has only been reported in summarized form, compared a target dose of 1,200 mg/day given in three divided daily administrations with placebo. The design included an 8-week baseline, a 6-week titration phase, a 12-week maintenance phase and an 8-week transition to open-label treatment. The median percent reduction in partial seizure frequency from baseline (primary end-point for the FDA-driven analysis) was 17.5% for placebo and 44.3% for retigabine (p < 0.0001). Responder rates during the entire treatment period compared with baseline were 18% for placebo and 45% for retigabine (p < 0.0001) *(Figure 5B)*. Responder rates during the maintenance period (primary end-point for the EMEA-driven analysis) were 22.6% for placebo and 55.5% for retigabine (p < 0.0001). Overall, 26.8% of patients discontinued for adverse events in the retigabine group, compared with 8.6% in the placebo group.

An additional double-blind randomized adjunctive-therapy placebo-controlled trial designed to investigate lower doses in patients with refractory partial seizures is in progress (Porter *et al.*, 2007a).

Critical assessment

An attractive feature, and a source of uncertainty, for retigabine is its highly innovative mode of action. Since there is no clinical experience with potassium channel openers, it is difficult to predict what impact a drug acting by this mechanism could have in the treatment of the epilepsies. Moreover, the preclinical studies conducted with retigabine in seizure and epilepsy models do not allow reliable predictions about its potential usefulness in generalized epilepsies. The first placebo-controlled efficacy trial in refractory partial seizures showed moderate efficacy at 900 mg/day, and a relatively high discontinuation rate for adverse events at 1200 mg/day. The second trial showed more robust efficacy at 1200 mg/day, although again a quarter of patients discontinued for adverse events. The results of the ongoing trial exploring doses below 1200 mg/day are eagerly awaited. A three times daily schedule is not optimal in terms of convenience, and a sustained-release formulation might allow less frequent dosing with, possibly, improved tolerability (Perucca, 2006).

■ Other compounds in clinical development

A non-exhaustive list of additional compounds at different stages of development is provided in *Table I*. For more information on these agents and other molecules at earlier stages of development, the reader is referred to recent reviews (Bialer *et al.*, 2004, 2007; Rogawski, 2006; Perucca, 2007, Rogawski, 2006).

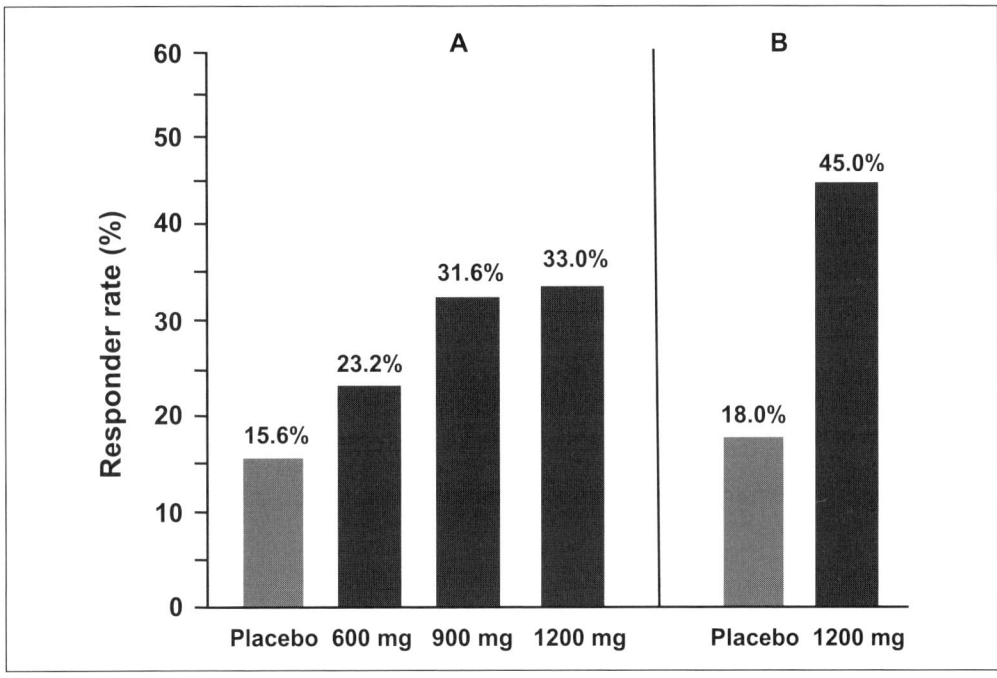

Figure 5. Responder rates (proportion of patients with at least 50% reduction in seizure frequency during the entire treatment period compared with baseline) in two double-blind placebo-controlled adjunctive-therapy trial of retigabine in patients with refractory partial seizures. The total number of patients randomized was 399 in trial A (Porter et al., 2007b) and 306 patients in trial B (Little, 2008). For details and statistical significance, see text.

Table I. Other potential antiepileptic drugs in clinical development

Compound	Brief description	Primary mechanisms of action	Key references
E-2007	A novel agent in early development as adjunctive therapy in partial epilepsy.	Noncompetitive AMPA* receptor antagonist	Bialer et al., 2007
Fluorofelbamate	A felbamate derivative designed to avoid conversion to toxic metabolites considered to mediate bone marrow and liver toxicity	Probably similar to felbamate	Mazarati et al., 2002; Parker et al., 2005; Bialer et al., 2007
Ganaxolone (CCD 1042)	A neurosteroid in early clinical development for a number of epilepsy syndromes and for other indications.	Positive allosteric modulator of GABA-A receptors	Carter et al., 1997; Kerrigan et al., 2000; Laxer et al., 2000; Wohlfarth et al., 2002; Bialer et al., 2007
Huperzine A	An alkaloid herbal derivative which is approved in China for the treatment of Alzheimer's disease, and is undergoing pilot exploratory studies in epilepsy.	Acetylcholinesterase inhibitor and NMDA antagonist	Zangara et al., 2003; Zhang et al., 2002; White et al., 2005; Bialer et al., 2007

JZP-4	A structural analogue of lamotrigine undergoing Phase I evaluation.	Blockade of voltage-dependent sodium channels and of high-voltage N, L, P/Q calcium channels	Bialer et al., 2007
Losigamone (AO33)	A β-methoxy-butenolide comprising two enantiomers with different pharmacokinetic and pharmacodinamic properties, which has been already assessed in two double-blind trials in partial epilepsy.	Probably multiple, including inhibition of persistent sodium currents	Zhang et al., 1992; Jones & Davis, 1999; Bauer et al., 2001; Kimber-Trojnar et al., 2003; Baulac et al., 2003; White et al., 2008
NS 1209 (SPD 502)	A racemic compound endowed with anticonvulsant, neuroprotective and analgesic activity in animal models, undergoing exploratory clinical testing in refractory *status epilepticus*.	Competitive AMPA receptor antagonist	Nielsen et al., 1999; Ben-Menachem et al., 2003; Bialer et al., 2007
Safinamide	An α-aminoamide derivative with potential in Parkinson's disease, epilepsy and restless leg syndrome, primarily investigated in Parkinson's disease	Sodium and calcium channel blocker and MAO-B inhibitor	Marzo et al., 2004; Chazot, 2007; Fariello, 2007
Seletracetam (UCB 44212)	A pyrrolidone derivative with much greater potency than levetiracetam in animal models, undergoing early clinical studies in refractory epilepsies.	An SV2A ligand, and a blocker of N- and Q-type high-voltage activated calcium channels	Matagne et al., 2005; Pisani et al., 2005; Rigo et al., 2005; Bialer et al., 2007
Talampanel (GYKI 53773, LY300164)	A 2,3-benzodiazepine derivative already assessed in two double-blind trials in refractory partial seizures.	Noncompetitive AMPA receptor antagonist	Vizi et al., 1996; Andrasi, 2001; Chappell et al., 2002; Langan et al., 2003; Bialer et al., 2007; White et al., 2008
T2000	A non-sedating barbiturate, being developed primarily in essential tremor	Related to other barbiturates?	Melmed et al., 2007
Tonabersat (SB220243)	A benzopyran with anticonvulsant, antimigraine and antiinflammatory properties, being primarily developed in migraine	Gap junction blocker and inhibitor of NO release	Parsons et al., 2001, Tvedskov et al., 2004; Goadsby, 2007
Valrocemide (TV 1901, SPD-493)	A valproic acid derivative undergoing early evaluation in refractory epilepsy.	Probably similar to valproic acid	Hovinga, 2004; Bialer et al., 2007
YKP3089	A novel agent with anticonvulsant, anxiolytic and analgesic activity in animal models, currently entering clinical development	Unknown	

* AMPA: α-amino-2,3-dihydro-5-methyl-3-oxo-4-isoxazolepropionic acid.

Many of the compounds listed in *Table I* have not yet undergone randomized controlled trials in patients with epilepsy, and available data are insufficient to make reliable predictions on their potential therapeutic usefulness. For other compounds, such as losigamone and talampanel, results of clinical studies have been published in detail (Bauer et al., 2001; Chappell et al., 2002; Baulac et al., 2003), but the development of these agents does not seem to be pursued actively at the present time. It should be noted that a sponsor's decision to proceed with development is influenced by many factors, for example general investment strategies and prioritization in resource allocation, and may bear little or no relation with the intrinsic properties of a given product. In fact, it is not uncommon for agents which have been in a dormant state for years to re-enter active development and reach the market, as shown most recently for rufinamide (Hakimian et al., 2007).

Conclusions

Newer AEDs with an improved tolerability profile and/or the ability to produce seizure freedom in patients refractory to available treatments are sorely needed. To address these needs, efforts are ongoing within academia and the pharmaceutical industry to understand better the mechanisms of epileptogenesis and ictogenesis, to unravel the causes of drug resistance, and to identify new strategies for drug discovery (Bialer et al., 2007).

Ideal requirements for a successful AED include robust efficacy, broad spectrum of activity against partial and generalized seizure types, excellent tolerability, favorable pharmacokinetics and little or no drug-drug interactions. A novel mode of action will make a candidate AED more attractive, but it may not translate into clinical success: in fact, some second generation drugs with non-innovative modes of actions such as oxcarbazepine have been far more successful clinically than drugs with unique mechanisms such as tiagabine and vigabatrin. Effectiveness in non-epileptic disorders may contribute to the commercial success of an AEDs (Perucca et al., 2007), though it may have drawbacks if it causes shifting of resources away from development in epilepsy.

Spectrum of activity against different seizure types, pharmacokinetic properties and drug interaction potential can be predicted with relative reliability based on preclinical models and early studies in healthy subjects (Perucca et al., 2007). Conversely, large randomized studies are required to determine efficacy and tolerability, and their relationship with dose and dosing schedules (Arroyo et al., 2004). As discussed in this article, some compounds have progressed sufficiently in their development to allow some cautious predictions about their therapeutic potential. However, determination of their actual usefulness and safety, including potential efficacy in less common epilepsy syndromes, will have to await the results of further studies and postmarketing experience (Perucca et al., 2000).

Clearly, the "magic bullet" capable of rendering all patients seizure-free without major adverse effects is not in sight. Many compounds in current development, however, have promising features, and they may eventually reach the market and prove to be preferable options in selected groups of patients. Indeed, any new antiepileptic medication represents an incremental gain in the possibility of tailoring drug choice to the characteristics of the individual. At the same time, however, an ever enlarging pharmacological armamentarium for epilepsy will require physicians to acquire more specific knowledge and expertise in order to use each drug safely and effectively. This is a challenge that physicians treating people with epilepsy must be prepared to address.

Summary

About one third of patients with epilepsy fail to achieve seizure freedom with currently available medications, and a substantial proportion of those who achieve seizure freedom do so at a price of significant adverse effects. To address these shortcomings, major efforts are ongoing within academia and the pharmaceutical industry in order to understand better the mechanisms of epileptogenesis and ictogenesis, to unravel the causes of drug resistance, and to discover new antiepileptic drugs with improved efficacy and tolerability. About 20 potential antiepileptic molecules have reached various stages of clinical development. The present article will focus on five compounds (brivaracetam, carisbamate, eslicarbazepine acetate, lacosamide and retigabine) which are in more advanced active development and have been described in considerable detail in the published literature. For each of these agents, mechanisms of action, pharmacokinetic properties, drug interaction potential, efficacy and tolerability data are reviewed. A number of additional investigational agents are also briefly discussed. Clearly, the "magic bullet" capable of rendering all patients seizure-free without major adverse effects is not in sight. Many compounds in current development, however, have promising features, and after reaching the market they may prove to be a preferred option in selected groups of patients. In this respect, any new medication represents an incremental gain in the possibility of tailoring drug choice to the characteristics of the individual. At the same time, however, an ever enlarging pharmacological armamentarium for epilepsy will require physicians to acquire more specific knowledge and expertise in order to use each drug safely and effectively. This is a challenge that physicians treating people with epilepsy must be prepared to address.

References

Abou-Khalil B, Porter R, Nohria V. Safety and tolerability of different titration rates of the novel antiepileptic drug retigabine. 59th Annual Meeting of the American Epilepsy Society, Washington DC, December 2-6, 2005. Poster presented at the Valeant Pharmaceuticals Scientific Exhibit.

Almeida L, Soares-da-Silva P. Safety, tolerability and pharmacokinetic profile of BIA 2-093, a novel putative antiepileptic agent, during first administration to humans. *Drugs RD* 2003; 4: 269-84.

Almeida L, Soares-da-Silva P. Safety, tolerability, and pharmacokinetic profile of BIA 2-093, a novel putative antiepileptic, in a rising multiple-dose study in young healthy humans. *J Clin Pharmacol* 2004; 44: 906-18.

Almeida L, Soares-da-Silva P. Eslicarbazepine acetate (BIA 2-093). *Neurotherapeutics* 2007; 4: 88-96.

Almeida L, Silveira P, Vaz-da-Silva M, Soares-da-Silva P. Pharmacokinetic profile of BIA 2-093, a putative new antiepileptic drug, during single and multiple administration in human healthy volunteers. *Epilepsia* 2002; 43 (suppl 8): 146-7.

Almeida L, Falcão A, Maia J, Mazur D, Gellert M, Soares-da-Silva P. Single-dose and steady-state pharmacokinetics of eslicarbazepine acetate (BIA 2-093) in healthy elderly and young subjects. *J Clin Pharmacol* 2005; 45: 1062-6.

Almeida L, Maia J, Potgieter H, Soares-da-Silva M. Effect of moderate liver impairment on the eslicarbazebine acetate pharmacokinetics. *Epilepsia* 2007; 48 (suppl 6): 339.

Ambrosio AF, Silva AP, Araujo I, Malva JO, Soares-da-Silva AP, Carvalho CM. Neurotoxic/neuroprotective profile of carbamazepine, oxcarbazepine and two new putative antiepileptic drugs, BIA 2-093 and BIA 2-024. *Eur J Pharmacol* 2000; 46: 191-201.

Ambrosio AF, Silva AP, Malva JO, Soares-da-Silva P, Carvalho AP, Carvalho CM. Inhibition of glutamate release by BIA 2-093 and BIA 2-024, two novel derivatives of carbamazepine, due to blockade of sodium but not calcium channels. *Biochem Pharmacol* 2001; 61: 1271-5.

Ambrosio AF, Soares-da-Silva P, Carvalho CM, Carvalho AP. Mechanisms of action of carbamazepine, oxcarbazepine, BIA-2-093, and BIA-2-024. *Neurochem Res* 2002; 27: 121-30.

Andrasi F. Talampanel. *Drugs Fut* 2001; 26: 754-6.

Armand V, Rundfeldt C, Heinemann U. Effects of retigabine (D-23129) on different patterns of epileptiform activity induced by 4-aminopyridine in rat entorhinal cortex hippocampal slices. *Arch Pharmacol* 1999; 359: 33-9.

Armand V, Rundfeldt C, Heinemann U. Effects of retigabine (D-23129) on different patterns of epileptiform activity induced by low magnesium in rat entorhinal cortex hippocampal slices. *Epilepsia* 2000; 41: 28-33.

Arroyo S, Chadwick DW, Frencj J, Mattson RH, Perucca E. Epilepsies and convulsive disorders. In: Du Souich P, Erill S, Orme M (eds). *The IUPHAR Compendium of Basic Principles for Pharmacological Research in Humans*. Irvine, CA: IUPHAR, 2004: 165-82.

Bauer J, Dienel A, Elger CE. Losigamone add-on therapy in partial epilepsy: a placebo-controlled study. *Acta Neurol Scand* 2001; 103: 226-30.

Benes J, Parada A, Figueiredo AA, et al. Anticonvulsant and sodium channel-blocking properties of novel 10,11-dihydro-5H-dibenz[b,f]azepine-5-carboxamide derivatives. *J Med Chem* 1999; 42: 2582-7.

Ben-Menachem E. 2003. NS1209: A neuroprotective AMPA antagonist with pronounced anticonvulsive and aniepileptogenic effect in preclinical models. *Epilepsia* 2003; 44 (suppl 9): 258.

Ben-Menachem E, Biton V, Jatuzis D, Abou-Khalil B, Doty P, Rudd GD. Efficacy and safety of oral lacosamide as adjunctive therapy in adults with partial-onset seizures. *Epilepsia* 2007; 48: 1308-17.

Beyreuther B, Callizot N, Stöhr T. Antinociceptive efficacy of lacosamide in a rat model for painful diabetic neuropathy. *Eur J Pharmacol* 2006; 539: 64-70.

Beyreuther BK, Freitag J, Heers C, Krebsfänger N, Scharfenecker U, Stöhr T. Lacosamide: a review of preclinical properties. *CNS Drug Rev* 2007a; 13: 21-42.

Beyreuther BK, Callizot N, Brot MD, Feldman R, Bain SC, Stöhr T. Antinociceptive efficacy of lacosamide in rat models for tumor- and chemotherapy-induced cancer pain. *Eur J Pharmacol* 2007b; 565: 98-104.

Beyreuther BK, Geis C, Stöhr T, Sommer C. Antihyperalgesic efficacy of lacosamide in a rat model for muscle pain induced by TNF. *Neuropharmacology* 2007c; 52: 1312-7.

Beyreuther B, Callizot N, Stöhr T. Antinociceptive efficacy of lacosamide in the monosodium iodoacetate rat model for osteoarthritis pain. *Arthritis Res Ther* 2007d; 9: R14.

Bialer M, Johannessen SI, Kupferberg HJ, Levy RH, Perucca E, Tomson T. Progress report on new antiepileptic drugs: a summary of the Seventh Eilat Conference (EILAT VII). *Epilepsy Res* 2004; 61: 1-48.

Bialer M, Johannessen SI, Kupferberg HJ, Levy RH, Perucca E, Tomson T. Progress report on new antiepileptic drugs: A summary of the Eighth Eilat Conference (EILAT VIII). *Epilepsy Res* 2007; 73: 1-52.

Biton V, Rosenfeld WE, Whitesides J, Fountain NB, Vaiciene N, Rudd GD. Intravenous lacosamide as replacement for oral lacosamide in patients with partial-onset seizures. *Epilepsia* 2007.

Bonifacio MJ, Sheridan RD, Parada A, Cunha RA, Patmore L, Soares-da-Silva P. Interaction of the novel anticonvulsant, BIA 2-093, with voltage-gated sodium channels: comparison with carbamazepine. *Epilepsia* 2001; 42: 600-8.

Borlak J, Gasparic A, Locher M, Schupke H, Hermann R. N-Glucuronidation of the antiepileptic drug retigabine: results from studies with human volunteers, heterologously expressed human UGTs, human liver, kidney, and liver microsomal membranes of Crigler-Najjar type II. *Metabolism* 2006; 55: 711-21.

Boscia F, Annunziato L, Taglialatela M. Retigabine and flupirtine exert neuroprotective actions in organotypic hippocampal cultures. *Neuropharmacology* 2006; 51: 283-94.

Brandt C, Heile A, Potschka H, StöhrT, Löscher W. Effects of the novel antiepileptic drug lacosamide on the development of amygdala kindling in rats. *Epilepsia* 2006; 47: 1803-9.

Carter RB, Wood PL, Wieland S, et al. Characterization of the anticonvulsant properties of ganaxolone (CCD 1042; 3-alpha-hydroxy-3beta-methyl-5alpha-pregnan-20-one), a selective, high-affinity, steroid modulator of the gamma-aminobutyric acid (A) receptor. *J Pharmacol Exp Ther* 1997; 280: 1284-95.

Cawello W, Kropeit D, Schiltmeyer B, Hammes W, Horstmann R. Food does not affect the pharmacokinetics of SPM927. *Epilepsia* 2004; 45 (suppl 7): 307.

Chappell AS, Sander JW, Brodie MJ, et al. A crossover, add-on trial of talampanel in patients with refractory partial seizures. *Neurology* 2002; 58: 1680-2.

Chazot PL. Safinamide for the treatment of Parkinson's disease, epilepsy and restless legs syndrome. *Curr Opin Investig Drugs* 2007; 8: 570-9.

Chien S, Bialer M, Solanki B, et al. Pharmacokinetic interaction study between the new antiepileptic and CNS drug RWJ-333369 and carbamazepine in healthy adults. *Epilepsia* 2006; 47: 1830-40.

Chien S, Yao C, Mertens A, et al. An interaction study between the new antiepileptic and CNS drug carisbamate (RWJ-333369) and lamotrigine and valproic acid. *Epilepsia* 2007; 48: 1328-38.

Chiron C. Stiripentol. *Neurotherapeutics* 2007; 4: 123-5.

Chung SS, Sperling M, Biton V, Krauss G, Beaman M, Hebert D. Lacosamide: Efficacy and safety as oral adjunctive treatment for partial-onset seizures. *Epilepsia* 2007; 48 (suppl 6): 321.

Dailey JW, Cheong JH, Ko KH, Adam-Curtis LE, Jobe PC. Anticonvulsant properties of D-20443 in genetically epilepsy-prone rats: prediction of clinical response. *Neurosci Lett* 1995; 195: 77-80.

Dencker D, Dias R, Pedersen ML, Husum H. Effect of the new antiepileptic drug retigabine in a rodent model of mania. *Epilepsy Behav* 2008; 12: 49-53.

Despande LS, Nagarkatti N, Sombati S, DeLorenzo RJ. Antiepileptic and antiepileptogenic effects of carisbamate (RWJ333369) in an *in vitro* model of epilepsy. *Epilepsia* 2007; 48 (suppl 6): 125.

Doty P, Rudd GD, Stöhr T, Thomas D. Lacosamide. *Neurotherapeutics* 2007; 4: 145-8.

Duncan GE, Kohn H. The novel antiepileptic drug lacosamide blocks behavioral and brain metabolic manifestations of seizure activity in the 6 Hz psychomotor seizure model. *Epilepsy Res* 2005; 67: 81-7.

Elger C, Bialer M, Cramer JA, Maia J, Almeida L, Soares-da-Silva P. Eslicarbazepine acetate: a double-blind, add-on, placebo-controlled exploratory trial in adult patients with partial-onset seizures. *Epilepsia* 2007; 48: 497-504.

Errington AC, Coyne L, Stöhr T, Selve N, Lees G. Seeking a mechanism of action for the novel anticonvulsant lacosamide. *Neuropharmacology* 2006; 50: 1016-29.

Errington AC, Stöhr T, Heers C, Lees G. The investigational anticonvulsant lacosamide selectively enhances slow inactivation of voltage-gated sodium channels. *Mol Pharmacol* 2008; 73: 157-69.

Falcão A, Maia J, Almeida L, Mazur D, Gellert M, Soares-da-Silva P. Effect of gender on the pharmacokinetics of eslicarbazepine acetate (BIA 2-093), a new voltage-gated sodium channel blocker. *Biopharm Drug Dispos* 2007; 28: 249-56.

Fariello RG. Safinamide. *Neurotherapeutics* 2007; 4: 110-6.

Faught E, Rosenfeld W, Holmes GL, et al. A double-blind, placebo-controlled, dose-ranging study to evaluate the efficacy and tolerability of carisbamate (RWJ-333369) as adjunctive therapy in patients with refractory partial seizures. Poster presented at the Annual Meeting of the American Epilepsy Society, Philadelphia, December 1-4, 2007. Abstract in *Epilepsia* 2007; 48 (suppl 6): 330.

Ferron GM, Sachdeo R, Pardot A, Fritz T, Althouse S, Troy S. Pharmacokinetic interaction between valproic acid, topiramate, phenytoin or carbamazepine and retigabine in epileptic patients. *Clin Pharm Ther* 2001a; 69: 18.

Ferron GM, Paul J, Richards L, Getsy J, Troy S. Retigabine does not alter the pharmacokinetics of a low dose oral contraceptive in women. *Neurology* 2001b; 56 (suppl 3): P05.052.

Ferron GM, Paul J, Fruncillo R, *et al.* Multiple-dose, linear, dose-proportional pharmacokinetics of retigabine in healthy volunteers. *J Clin Pharmacol* 2002; 42: 175-82.

Ferron GM, Patat A, Parks V, Rolan P, Troy SM. Lack of pharmacokinetic interaction between retigabine and phenobarbitone at steady-state in healthy subjects. *Br J Clin Pharmacol* 2003; 56: 39-45.

Fontes-Ribeiro C, Nunes T, Falcão A, *et al.* Eslicarbazepine acetate (BIA 2-093): Relative bioavailability and bioequivalence of 50 mg/mL oral suspension and 200 mg and 800 mg tablet formulations. *Drugs R D* 2005; 6: 253-60.

Fountain NB, French JA, Privitera MD. Harkoseride: safety and tolerability of a new antiepileptic drug in patients with refractory partial seizures. *Epilepsia* 2000; 41 (suppl 7): 169.

François J, Ferrandon A, Koning E, Nehlig A. A new drug RWJ-333369 protects limbic areas in the lithium-pilocarpine model (li-pilo) of epilepsy and delays or prevents the occurrence of spontaneous seizures. *Epilepsia* 2005; 46 (suppl 8): 269-70.

François J, Boehrer A, Nehlihg A. Effects of carisbamate (RWJ-333369) in two models of genetically determined generalized epilepsy, the GAERS and the audiogenic Wistar AS. *Epilepsia* 2007 Epub ahead of print

Freitag J, Beyreuther B, Heers C, Stöhr T. Lacosamide modulates collapsin response mediated protein 2 (CRMP-2). *Epilepsia* 2007; 48 (suppl 6): 320.

French JA, Brodsky A, Von Rosenstiel P on behalf of the Brivaracetam N1193 Study Group. Efficacy and tolerability of 5, 20 and 50 mg/day brivaracetam (UCB 34714) as adjunctive treatment in adults with refractory partial-onset epilepsy. *Epilepsia* 2007; 48 (suppl 6): 400.

Gillard M, Fuks B, Lambeng N, Chatelain P, Matagne A. Binding characteristics of brivaracetam, a novel antiepileptic drug candidate. *Epilepsia* 2007; 48 (suppl 6): 317.

Goadsby PJ. Emerging therapies for migraine. *Nat Clin Pract Neurol* 2007; 3: 610-9.

Grabenstatter HL, Dudek FE. The use of chronic models in antiepileptic drug discovery: The effect of RWJ-333369 on spontaneous motor seizures in rats with kainite-induced epilepsy. *Epilepsia* 2004; 45 (suppl 7): 197.

Hainzl D, Parada A, Soares-da-Silva P. Metabolism of two new antiepileptic drugs and their principal metabolites S(+)- and R(-)-10,11-dihydro-10-hydroxy carbamazepine. *Epilepsy Res* 2001; 44: 197-206.

Hakimian S, Cheng-Hakimian A, Anderson GD, Miller JW. Rufinamide: a new anti-epileptic medication. Expert Opin Pharmacother 2007; 8: 1931-40.

Halasz P, Kalviainen R, Mazurkiewicz-Beldzinska M, Rosenow F, Doty P, Sullivan T. Lacosamide: efficacy and safety as oral adjunctive therapy in adults with partial seizures. *Epilepsia* 2006; 47 (suppl 4): 3.

Hansen HH, Ebbesen C, Mathiesen C, *et al.* The KCNQ channel opener retigabine inhibits the activity of mesencephalic dopaminergic systems of the rat. *J Pharmacol Exp Ther* 2006; 318: 1006-19.

Hao JX, Stöhr T, Selve N, Wiesenfeld-Hallin Z, Xu XJ. Lacosamide, a new anti-epileptic, alleviates neuropathic pain-like behaviors in rat models of spinal cord or trigeminal nerve injury. *Eur J Pharmacol* 2006; 553: 135-40.

Heers C, Beyreuther BK, Freitag J, Lees G, Errington A, Stöhr T. Novel dual mechanism of action of the antiepileptic drug lacosamide. 27th International Epilepsy Congress, Singapore, 8-12 July 2007, abstract p. 236.

Hempel R, Schupke H, McNeilly PJ, *et al.* Metabolism of retigabine (D-23129), a novel anticonvulsant. *Drug Metab Dispos* 1999; 27: 613-22.

Hermann R, Ferron GM, Erb K, *et al*. Effects of age and sex on the disposition of retigabine. *Clin Pharmacol Ther* 2003; 73: 61-70.

Hermann R, Borlak J, Munzel U, *et al*. The role of Gilbert's syndrome and frequent NAT2 slow acetylation polymorphisms in the pharmacokinetics of retigabine. *Pharmacogenomics J* 2006; 6: 211-9.

Hiller A, Nguyen N, Strassburg CP, *et al*. Retigabine N-glucuronidation and its potential role in enterohepatic circulation. *Drug Metab Dispos* 1999; 27: 605-12.

Horstmann R, Bonn R, Cawello W, Doty P, Rudd D. Basic clinical pharmacological investigations of the new antiepileptic drug SPM 927. *Epilepsia* 2002; 43 (suppl 7): 188.

Hovinga CA. Valrocemide (Teva/Acorda). *Curr Opin Investig Drugs* 2004; 5: 101-6.

Jatuzis D, Biton V, Ben-Menachem E, *et al*. Evaluation of the effect of oral lacosamide on concomitant AED plasma concentrations in patients with partial seizures. *Epilepsia* 2005; 46 (suppl 8): 170.

Jones FA, Davies JA. The anticonvulsant effects of the enantiomers of losigamone. *Br J Pharmacol* 1999; 128: 1223-8.

Kapetanovic IM, Rundfeldt C. D 23129: A new anticonvulsamt compound. *CNS Drug Rev* 1996; 2: 308-21.

Kapetanovic IM, Yonekawa WD, Kupferberg HJ. The effects of D 23129, a new experimental anticonvulsant drug, on neurotransmitter aminoacids in the rat hippocampus *in vitro*. *Epilepsy Res* 1995; 22: 167-73.

Kasteleijn-Nolst Trenité DG, Genton P, Parain D, *et al*. Evaluation of brivaracetam, a novel SV2A ligand, in the photosensitivity model. *Neurology* 2007a; 69: 1027-34.

Kasteleijn-Nolst Trenité DG, French JA, Hirsch E, *et al*. Evaluation of carisbamate, a novel antiepileptic drug, in photosensitive patients: an exploratory, placebo-controlled study. *Epilepsy Res* 2007b; 74: 193-200.

Keck CA, Thompson HJ, Pitkänen A, *et al*. The novel antiepileptic agent RWJ-333369-A, but not its analog RWJ-333369, reduces regional cerebral edema without affecting neurobehavioral outcome or cell death following experimental traumatic brain injury. *Restor Neurol Neurosci* 2007; 25: 77-90.

Kenda BM, Matagne AC, Talaga PE, *et al*. Discovery of 4-substituted pyrrolidone butanamides as new agents with significant antiepileptic activity. *J Med Chem* 2004; 47: 530-49.

Kerrigan JF, Shields WD, Nelson TY, *et al*. Ganaxolone for treating intractable infantile spasms: a multicenter, open-label, add-on trial. *Epilepsy Res* 2000; 42: 133-9.

Klein B, Smith MD, White HS. The novel neuromodulator carisbamate delays the acquisition of rat amygdala kindling and mantains acute antiepileptic activity when evaluated in post-kindled rats. *Epilepsia* 2007; 48 (suppl 6): 367-8.

Kropeit D, Schiltmeyer B, Cawello W, Hammes W, Horstmann R. Bioequivalence of short-time infusions compared to oral administration of SPM 927. *Epilepsia* 2004; 45 (suppl 7): 123-4.

Kropeit D, Scharfenecker U, Schiltmeyer B, *et al*. Lacosamide has low potential for drug-drug interaction. 59th Annual Meeting of the American Epilepsy Society, Washington DC, December 2-6, 2005. Poster presented at the Schwarz Biosciences, Inc. Scientific Exhibit.

Kulig K, Malawska B. Carisbamate, a new carbamate for the treatment of epilepsy. *IDrugs* 2007; 10: 720-7.

Lacroix B, Von Rosenstiel P, Sargentini-Maier ML. Population pharmacokinetics of brivaracetam in patients with partial epilepsy. *Epilepsia* 2007; 48 (suppl 6): 333-4.

Langan YM, Lucas R, Jewell H, *et al*. Talampanel, a new antiepileptic drug: single- and multiple-dose pharmacokinetics and initial 1-week experience in patients with chronic intractable epilepsy. *Epilepsia* 2003; 44: 46-53.

Lawrence JJ, Saraga F, Churchill JF, *et al*. Somatodendritic Kv7/KCNQ/M channels control interspike interval in hippocampal interneurons. *J Neurosci* 2006; 26: 12325-38.

Laxer K, Blum D, Abou-Khalil BW, *et al.* Assessment of ganaxolone's anticonvulsant activity using a randomized, double-blind, presurgical trial design. Ganaxolone Presurgical Study Group. *Epilepsia* 2000; 41: 1187-94.

Lees G, Stohr T, Errington AC. Stereoselective effects of the novel anticonvulsant lacosamide against 4-AP induced epileptiform activity in rat visual cortex in vitro. *Neuropharmacology* 2006; 50: 98-110.

Leppik IE, De Rue K, Edrich P, Perucca E. Measurement of seizure freedom in adjunctive therapy studies in refractory partial epilepsy: The levetiracetam experience. *Epileptic Disorders* 2006; 8: 118-30.

Little LW. Valeant Pharmaceuticals reports positive Phase III results for retigabine in Restore 1. Press Release, Valeant Pharmaceuticals, Aliso Viejo, California, 12 February 2008.

Lynch BA, Lambeng N, Nocka K, *et al.* The synaptic vesicle protein SV2A is the binding site for the antiepileptic drug levetiracetam. *Proc Natl Acad Sci U S A* 2004; 101: 9861-6.

Maia J, Vaz-da-Silva M, Almeida L, *et al.* Effect of food on the pharmacokinetic profile of eslicarbazepine acetate (BIA 2-093). *Drugs R D* 2005a; 6: 201-6.

Maia J, Almeida L, Vaz-da-Silva M, *et al.* Effect of eslicarbazebine acetate on steady-state pharmacokinetics of digoxin. *Epilepsia* 2005b; 46 (suppl 8): 191.

Maia J, Almeida L, Potgieter H, Soares-da-Silva M. Effect of renal impairment on the pharmacokinetics of eslicarbazebine acetate. *Epilepsia* 2007; 48 (suppl 6): 337.

Malawska B, Kulig K. Brivaracetam UCB. *Curr Opin Invest Drugs* 2005; 6: 740-6.

Mannens GSJ, Hendrickx J, Janssen CGM, *et al.* The absorption, metabolism and excretion of the novel neuromodulator RWJ-333369 in man. *Drug Metab Disp* 2007; 35: 554-65.

Margineanu D-G, Kenda BM, Michel P, Matagne A, Klitgaard HV. ucb 34714, a new pyrrolidone derivative: comparison with levetiracetam in hippocampal slice epilepsy models in vitro. *Epilepsia* 2003; 44 (suppl 9): 261.

Marzo A, Dal Bo L, Monti NC, *et al.* Pharmacokinetics and pharmacodynamics of safinamide, a neuroprotectant with antiparkinsonian and anticonvulsant activity. *Pharmacol Res* 2004; 50: 77-85.

Matagne A, Kenda BM, Michel P, Klitgaard HV. ucb 34714, a new pyrrolidone derivative: Comparison with levetiracetam in animal models of chronic epilepsy in vivo. *Epilepsia* 2003; 44 (suppl 9): 260.

Matagne A, Margineanu DG, Michel P, Kenda BM. Seletracetam (ucb 44212), a new pyrrolidone derivative, reveals potent activity in in vitro and in vivo models of epilepsy. *J Neurol Sci* 2005; 238 (suppl 1): S133.

Mazarati AM, Sofiam RD, Wasterlain CG. Anticonvulsant and antiepileptogenic effects of fluorofelbamate in experimental status epilepticus. *Seizure* 2002; 11: 423-30.

May TW, Korn-Merker E, Rambeck B. Clinical pharmacokinetics of oxcarbazepine. *Clin Pharmacokinet* 2003; 42: 1023-42.

Melmed C, Moros D, Rutman H. Treatment of essential tremor with the barbiturate T2000 (1,3-dimethoxymethyl-5,5-diphenyl-barbituric acid). *Mov Disord* 2007; 22: 723-7.

McNeilly PJ, Torchin CD, Anderson LW, Kapetanovic IM, Kupferberg HJ, Strong JM. In vitro glucuronidation of D-23129, a new anticonvulsant, by human liver microsomes and liver slices. *Xenobiotica* 1997; 27: 431-41.

Nehlig A, Rigoulot M-A, Boehrer A. A new drug, RWJ-333369, displays potent antiepileptic properties in genetic models of absence and audiogenic epilepsy. *Epilepsia* 2005; 46 (suppl 8): 215.

Nielsen EØ, Varming T, Mathiesen C, *et al.* SPD 502: a water-soluble and in vivo long-lasting AMPA antagonist with neuroprotective activity. *J Pharmacol Exp Ther* 1999; 289: 1492-501.

Novak GP, Kelley M, Zannikos P, Klein B. Carisbamate (RWJ-333369). *Neurotherapeutics* 2007; 4: 106-9.

Nunes T, Minciu I, Almeida L, et al. Pharmacokinetics of eslicarbazepine acetate in children and adolescents with epilepsy. 27th International Epilepsy Congress, Singapore, 8-12 July 2007a, abstract p. 071.

Nunes T, Maia J, Almedia L, Soares-da-Silva P. Pharmacokinetic interaction between eslicarbazepine acetate and lamotrigine in healthy subjects. *Epilepsia* 2007b; 48 (suppl 6): 339-40.

Otoul C, Von Rosenstiel P, Stockis A. Evaluation of the pharmacokinetic interaction of brivaracetam on other antiepileptic drugs in adults with partial-onset seizures. *Epilepsia* 2007; 48 (suppl 6): 334.

Otto JF, Kimball MM, Wilcox KS. Effects of the anticonvulsant retigabine on cultured cortical neurons: changes in electroresponsive properties and synaptic transmission. *Mol Pharmacol* 2002; 61: 921-7.

Parada A, Soares-da-Silva P. The novel anticonvulsant BIA 2-093 inhibits transmitter release during opening of voltage-gated sodium channels: a comparison with carbamazepine and oxcarbazepine. *Neurochem Int* 2002; 40: 435-40.

Parker RJ, Hartman NR, Roecklein BA, et al. Stability and comparative metabolism of selected felbamate metabolites and postulated fluorofelbamate metabolites by postmitochondrial suspensions. *Chem Res Toxicol* 2005; 18: 1842-8.

Parsons AA, Bingham S, Raval P, Read S, Thompson M, Upton N. Tonabersat (SB-220453) a novel benzopyran with anticonvulsant properties attenuates trigeminal nerve-induced neurovascular reflexes. *Br J Pharmacol* 2001; 132: 1549-57.

Perucca E. The clinical pharmacology and therapeutic use of the new antiepileptic drugs. *Fund Clin Pharmacol* 20001; 15: 405-17.

Perucca E. Retigabine in partial seizures. A viewpoint. *CNS Drugs* 2006; 20: 609-10.

Perucca E, Beghi E, Shorvon S, Tomson T. Assessing risk to benefit ratio in antiepileptic drug therapy. *Epilepsy Res* 2000; 41: 107-39.

Perucca E, French J, Bialer M. Development of new antiepileptic drugs: Challenges, incentives, and recent advances. Lancet Neurol 2007; 6: 793-804.

Pisani A, Bonsi P, Martella G, Cuomo D, Klitgaard HV, Margineanu D-G. Seletracetam (ucb 44212), a nes pyrrolidone derivative, inhibits high-voltage-activated Ca2+ currents and intracellular [Ca2+] increase in rat cortical neurons in vitro. *Epilepsia* 2005; 46 (suppl 8): 119.

Plosker GL, Scott LJ. Retigabine in partial seizures. *CNS Drugs* 2006; 20: 601-8.

Porter RJ, Nohria V, Rundfeldt C. Retigabine. *Neurotherapeutics* 2007; 4: 149-54.

Porter RJ, Partiot A, Sachdeo R, Nohria V, Alves WM; 205 Study Group. Randomized, multicenter, dose-ranging trial of retigabine for partial-onset seizures. *Neurology* 2007b; 68: 1197-204.

Potschka H, Pekcec A, Soares-da-Silva P. Inhibition of kindling progression by eslicarbazepine acetate and licarbazepine. 27th International Epilepsy Congress, Singapore, 8-12 July 2007, abstract p. 071.

Raguenau-Malessi I, Levy R, Solanki B, Zannikos P, Novak G. Pharmacokinetics, safety, and tolerability of the new antiepileptic drug carisbamate (RWJ-333369) in elderly adults. *Epilepsia* 2007; 48 (suppl 6): 326.

Richter A, Sander SE, Rundfeldt C. Antidystonic effects of Kv7 (KCNQ) channel openers in the dt sz mutant, an animal model of primary paroxysmal dystonia. *Br J Pharmacol* 2006; 149: 747-53.

Rigo JM, Nguyen L, Hans G, et al. Seletracetam (ucb 44212): Effect on inhibitory and excitatory neurotransmission. *Epilepsia* 2005; 46 (suppl 8): 110.

Rivera-Arconada I, Lopez-Garcia JA. Retigabine-induced population primary afferent hyperpolarisation in vitro. *Neuropharmacology* 2006; 51: 756-63.

Rogawski MA. Diverse mechanisms of antiepileptic drugs in the development pipeline. *Epilepsy Res* 2006; 69: 273-94.

Rowley NM, Hart L, White HS. Anticonvulsant drug efficacy in the mouse corneal kindled model correlates with efficacy in the hippocampal kindled rat model of partial epilepsy. *Epilepsia* 2007; 48 (suppl 6): 292.

Rosenfeld W, Biton V, Mameniskiene R, et al. Pharmacokinetics and safety of lacosamide administered as replacement for adjunctive oral lacosamide in patients with partial-onset seizures. *Epilepsia* 2005; 46 (suppl 8): 184.

Rostock A, Tober C, Rundfeldt C, Bartsch R, Engel J, Polymeropoulos EE, et al. D-23129: a new anticonvulsant with a broad spectrum activity in animal models of epileptic seizures. *Epilepsy Res* 1996; 23: 211-23.

Rundfeldt C. The new anticonvulsant retigabine (D-23129) acts as an opener of K+ channels in neuronal cells. *Eur J Pharmacol* 1997; 336: 243-9.

Rundfeldt C, Netzer R. The novel anticonvulsant retigabine activates M-currents in Chinese hamster ovary-cells tranfected with human KCNQ2/3 subunits. *Neurosci Lett* 2000a; 282: 73-6.

Rundfeldt C, Netzer R. Investigations into the mechanism of action of the new anticonvulsant retigabine. Interaction with GABAergic and glutamatergic neurotransmission and with voltage gated ion channels. *Arzneimittelforschung* 2000b; 50: 1063-70.

Sachdeo RC, Ferron GM, Partiot AM, Nohria, V, Alves WM, 205 Study Group. An early determination of drug-drug interactions between valproic acid, phenytoin, carbamazepine or topiramate and retigabine in epileptic patients. *Neurology* 2001; 56: A331-A332.

Sachdeo R, Montouris G, Beydoun A. An open-label, maximum tolerated dose trial to evaluate oral SPM 927 as adjunctive therapy in patients with partial seizures, *Neurology* 2003; 60 (suppl 1): A433.

Sachdeo R, Porter R, Biton V, Rosenfeld W, Alves W, Nohria V. Dose-finding study of retigabine (a novel antiepileptic drug) in patients with epilepsy. *Epilepsia* 2005; 46 (suppl 8): 185.

Sargentini-Maier ML, Rolan P, Connell J, et al. The pharmacokinetics, CNS pharmacodynamics and adverse event profile of brivaracetam after single increasing oral doses in healthy males. *Br J Clin Pharmacol* 2007a; 63: 680-8.

Sargentini-Maier ML, Espie P, Coquette A, Stockis A. Pharmacokinetics and metabolism of 14C-brivaracetam, a novel SV2A ligand, in healthy subjects. *Drug Metab Dispos* 2007b Oct 1; [Epub ahead of print].

Schiltmeyer B, Cawello W, Kropeit D, Hammes W, Horstmann R. Pharmacokinetics of the new antiepileptic drug SPM 927 in human subjects with different age and gender. *Epilepsia* 2004; 45 (suppl 7): 313.

Sierra-Paredes G, Núñez-Rodriguez A, Vázquez-López A, Oreiro-García T, Sierra-Marcuño G. Anticonvulsant effect of eslicarbazepine acetate (BIA 2-093) on seizures induced by microperfusion of picrotoxin in the hippocampus of freely moving rats. *Epilepsy Res* 2006; 72: 140-6.

Sierra-Paredes G, Oreiro-García MT, Vázquez-Illanes MD, Sierra-Marcuño G. Effect of eslicarbazepine acetate (BIA 2-093) on latrunculin A-induced seizures and extracellular amino acid concentrations in the rat hippocampus. *Epilepsy Res* 2007; 77: 36-43.

Silveira P, Falcão A, Almeida L, Maia J, Soares-da-Silva P. BIA 2-093 pharmacokinetics in healthy elderly subjects. *Epilepsia* 2004; 45 (suppl 3): 157.

Smith MD, Adams AC, Saunders GW, White HS, Wilcox KS. Phenytoin- and carbamazepine-resistant spontaneous bursting in rat entorhinal cortex is blocked by retigabine in vitro. *Epilepsy Res* 2007; 74: 97-106.

Stöhr T, Krause E, Selve N. Lacosamide displays potent antinociceptive effects in animal models for inflammatory pain. *Eur J Pain* 2006; 10: 241-9.

Stöhr T, Kupferberg HJ, Stables JP, et al. Lacosamide, a novel anti-convulsant drug, shows efficacy with a wide safety margin in rodent models for epilepsy. *Epilepsy Res* 2007a; 74: 147-54a.

Stöhr T, Shandra P, Kashenko O, Shandra A. Synergism of lacosamide and first-generation and novel antiepileptic drugs in the 6 Hz seizure model in mice. *Epilepsia* 2007; 48 (suppl 6): 367-8.

Straub H, Kohling R, Hohling J, et al. Effects of retigabine on rhytmic synchronous activity of human neocortical slides. *Epilepsy Res* 2001; 44: 155-65.

Tai KK, Truong DD. Brivaracetam is superior to levetiracetam in a rat model of post-hypoxic myoclonus. *J Neural Transm* 2007; 114: 1547-51.

Tatulian L, Delmas P, Abogadie FC, Brown DA. Activation of expressed KCNQ potassium currents and native neuronal M-type potassium currents by the anti-convulsant drug retigabine. *J Neurosci* 2001; 21: 5535-45.

Tatulian L, Brown DA. Effect of the KCNQ potassium channel opener retigabine on single KCNQ2/3 channels expressed in CHO cells. *J Physiol* 2003; 549 (Pt 1): 57-63.

Thomas D, Scharfenecker U, Nickel B, Doty P, Cawello W, Horstmann R. Low potential for drug-drug interaction of lacosamide. 27th International Epilepsy Congress, Singapore, 8-12 July 2007, abstract p. 235.

Thompson CD, Kinter MT, Macdonald TL. Synthesis and in vitro reactivity of 3-carbamoyl-2-phenylopropionaldehyde and 2-phenylopropenal: putative reactive metabolites of felbamate. *Chem Res Toxicol* 1996; 9: 1225-9.

Tober C, Rundfeldt C, Rostock A, Bartsch R. The phenyl carbamic acid ester D-23129 is highly effective in epilepsy models for generalized and focal seizures at nontoxic doses. *Abstr Soc Neurosci* 1994; 20: 1641.

Tober C, Rostock A, Rundfeldt C, Bartsch R. D-23129: a potent anticonvulsant in the amygdala kindling model of complex partial seizures. *Eur J Pharmacol* 1996; 303: 163-9.

Tvedskov JF, Iversen HK, Olesen J. A double-blind study of SB-220453 (Tonerbasat) in the glyceryltrinitrate (GTN) model of migraine. *Cephalalgia* 2004; 24: 875-82.

Van Paesschen W, Von Rosenstiel P. Efficacy and tolerability of brivaracetam as adjunctive treatment for adults with refractory partial-onset epilepsy. 27th International Epilepsy Congress, Singapore, 8-12 July 2007, abstract 63.

Van Paesschen W, Brodski A on behalf of Brivaracetam N1114 Study Group. Efficacy and tolerability of 50 and 150 mg/day brivaracetam (UCB 34714) as adjunctive treatment in adults with refractory partial-onset epilepsy. *Epilepsia* 2007; 48 (suppl 6): 329.

Vaz-da-Silva M, Nunes T, Soares E, et al. Eslicarbazebine acetate pharmacokinetics after single and repeated doses in healthy subjects. *Epilepsia* 2005; 46 (suppl 8): 191.

Vizi ES, Mike A, Tarnawa I. 2,3-Benzodiazepines (GYKI 52466 and analogs): Negative allosteric modulators of AMPA receptors. *CNS Drug Rev* 1996; 2: 91-126.

Volosov A, Xiaodong S, Perucca E, Yagen B, Sintov A, Bialer M. Enantioselective pharmacokinetics of 10-hydroxycarbazepine after oral administration of oxcarbazepine to healthy Chinese subjects. *Clin Pharmacol Ther* 1999; 66: 547-53.

Von Rosenstiel P. Brivaracetam (UCB 34714). *Neurotherapeutics* 2007; 4: 84-7.

Walker MC, Sander JW. The impact of new antiepileptic drugs on the prognosis of epilepsy: seizure freedom should be the ultimate goal. *Neurology* 1996; 46: 912-4.

Wasterlain CG, Suchomelova L, Matagne AC, et al., Brivaracetam is a potent anticonvulsant in experimental status epilepticus, *Epilepsia* 46 (2005) (suppl 8), 219.

White HS, Schachter S, Lee D, Xiaoshen J, Eisenberg D. Anticonvulsant activity of Huperzine A, an alkaloid extract of Chinese club moss (Huperzia serrata). *Epilepsia* 2005; 46 (suppl 8): 220.

White HS, Sirvastava, Klein B, Zhao B, Choi YM, Lee SJ. The novel investigational neuromodulator RWJ-333369 displays a broad-spectrum anticonvulsant profile in rodent seizure and epilepsy mosles. *Epilepsia* 2006; 47 (suppl 4): 200-1.

White HS, Klein BD, Smith MD. Amygdala-kindled rats develop mechanical allodynia that is attenuated by the novel neuromodulator carismabate. *Epilepsia* 2007; 48 (suppl 6): 371-2.

White S, Perucca E, Privitera M. Investigational drugs. In: Engel J Jr, Pedley TA, Aicardi J, Dichter MA, Perucca E, et al. (eds). *Epilepsy. A Comprehensive Textbook*. Philadelphia: Lippincott, Williams & Wilkins, 2008: 1721-40.

Wohlfarth KM, Bianchi MT, Macdonald RL. Enhanced neurosteroid potentiation of ternary GABA(A) receptors containing the delta subunit. *J Neurosci* 2002; 22: 1541-9.

Wuttke TV, Jurkat-Rott K, Paulus W, Garncarek M, Lehmann-Horn F, Lerche H. Peripheral nerve hyperexcitability due to dominant-negative KCNQ2 mutations. *Neurology* 2007; 69: 2045-53.

Wymer J, Garrison C, Simpson J, Koch B. A multicenter, randomised, double-blind, placebo-controlled trial to assess the efficacy and safety of lacosamide in subjects with painful distal diabetic neuropathy. 59th Annual Meeting of the American Epilepsy Society, Washington DC, December 2-6, 2005. Poster presented at the Schwarz Biosciences, Inc. Scientific Exhibit.

Yao C, Chien S, Doose DR, Novak G, Bialer M. Pharmacokinetics of the new antiepileptic and CNS drug RWJ-333369 following single and multiple dosing to humans. *Epilepsia* 2006; 47: 1822-9.

Zangara A. The psychopharmacology of huperzine A: an alkaloid with cognitive enhancing and neuroprotective properties of interest in the treatment of Alzheimer's disease. *Pharmacol Biochem Behav* 2003; 75: 675-86.

Zhang CL, Chatterjee SS, Stein U, Heinemann U. Comparison of the effects of losigamone and its isomers on maximal electroshock induced convulsions in mice and on three different patterns of low magnesium induced epileptiform activity in slices of the rat temporal cortex. *Naunyn Schmiedebergs Arch Pharmacol* 1992; 345: 85-92.

Zhang YH, Zhao XY, Chen XQ, Wang Y, Yang HH, Hu GY. Spermidine antagonizes the inhibitory effect of huperzine A on [3H]dizocilpine (MK-801) binding in synaptic membrane of rat cerebral cortex. *Neurosci Lett* 2002; 319: 107-10.

Ziegler D, Bongardt S, Koch B, Thierfelder S. Efficacy and safety of lacosamide in the treatment of neuropathic pain attributed to distal diabetic neuropathy. 59th Annual Meeting of the American Epilepsy Society, Washington DC, December 2-6, 2005. Poster presented at the Schwarz Biosciences, Inc. Scientific Exhibit.

Zona C, Pieri M, Klitgaard HV, Margineanu D-G. UCB 34714, a new pyrrolidone derivative, inhibits Na+ currents in rat cortical neurons in culture. *Epilepsia* 2004; 45 (suppl 7): 146.

How many patients with drug-resistant epilepsy become seizure-free *because* of surgery?

Dieter Schmidt

Epilepsy Research Group, Berlin, Germany

Resective surgery is standard of care for eligible patients with drug resistant epilepsy (Engel et al., 2003). The best seizure outcome has been reported for patients with mesial temporal lobe epilepsy, particularly those with a structural lesion in the MRI (Téllez-Zenteno et al., 2005). The compelling evidence base for the efficacy and safety of epilepsy surgery includes many clinical observations and the only controlled trial of temporal lobe surgery versus medical treatment in non-operated patients (Wiebe et al., 2001; Téllez-Zenteno et al., 2005). While earlier studies traditionally focused on surgical outcome alone, epilepsy centers are now reporting long-term outcomes in cohorts of surgical patients with epilepsy and in nonrandomized controls, for example in patients who have ineligible for surgery or are on a waiting list for surgery (Bien et al., 2006). In addition, new evidence has suggested that a change in antiepileptic drug (AED) regimens is improving seizure freedom in as many as 20% of apparently drug-resistant patients (Luciano & Shorvon, 2007; Callaghan et al., 2007). A significant minority of patients (16.6%) is rendered seizure-free by addition of newly administered AEDs even after failure of two to five past antiepileptic drugs (Schiller & Najar, 2008). In support of this observation, long-term seizure outcome of non- surgical candidates has been reported to better than previously thought (Selwa et al., 2003). Given that epilepsy is drug resistant in as many as one in three newly diagnosed patients (Kwan & Brodie, 2000; Schmidt & Löscher, 2005), uncertainty about the long-term evidence for comparative efficacy for surgery and AEDs, the two commonly used treatment for chronic epilepsy, is a strategic problem. Clearly, the most compelling evidence that patients become seizure-free *because* of surgery is to show that more surgical patients become seizure-free compared to non-operated patients. Two questions are briefly addressed here:

1. *Does surgery eliminate drug resistance of epilepsy and need for AED treatment more often than a change of AEDs in non-operated patients? And, if so:*
2. *What are the putative mechanisms underlying the effect of surgery on drug resistance?*

Long-term seizure outcome of surgery in drug-resistant epilepsy

Long-term studies of clinical experience suggest that following temporal lobe surgery a median of 66% of patients become seizure free with continued medical treatment (Tellez-Zenteno et al., 2005). In a series of 165 patients with mesial temporal lobe epilepsy showing hippocampal sclerosis undergoing surgery, ILAE class I outcome (no seizures, no auras after surgery) was noted in 87 of 165 patients (52.7%) at one year after surgery, in 19 of 35 patients (54.3%) available for review or 19 of all 165 patients (11.5%) 8 years after surgery (Özkara et al., 2008) *(Figure 1)*.

In a series of patients initially seizure-free after temporal lobe surgery, the proportion of patients dropped from 76 of 88 patients (86%) at 3 months after surgery to 9 of 12 patients (50%) available for review after 9 years or 9 of 88 (10%) of all patients initially seizure free (Jutila et al., 2005). In a study of surgical patients with mostly temporal lobe epilepsy, who had been seizure free (allowing for simple partial seizures) 5 years after surgery, the proportion of seizure-free patients dropped from 100% at 5 years to approximately 50% at 15 years after surgery (Sperling et al., 2007). In a report of long-term seizure outcome of 48 patients undergoing temporal lobe surgery from a single center, 27 of 48 patients (56%) were seizure-free after 1 year, and 25 of 48 (52%) after 10 years (Kelley & Theodore, 2005). In a study of long-term follow-up of temporal lobe surgery in 37 children, at 1 year 75% (27/36) were classified as Engel Class I, at 5 years, 82% (29/35) were class I, and at

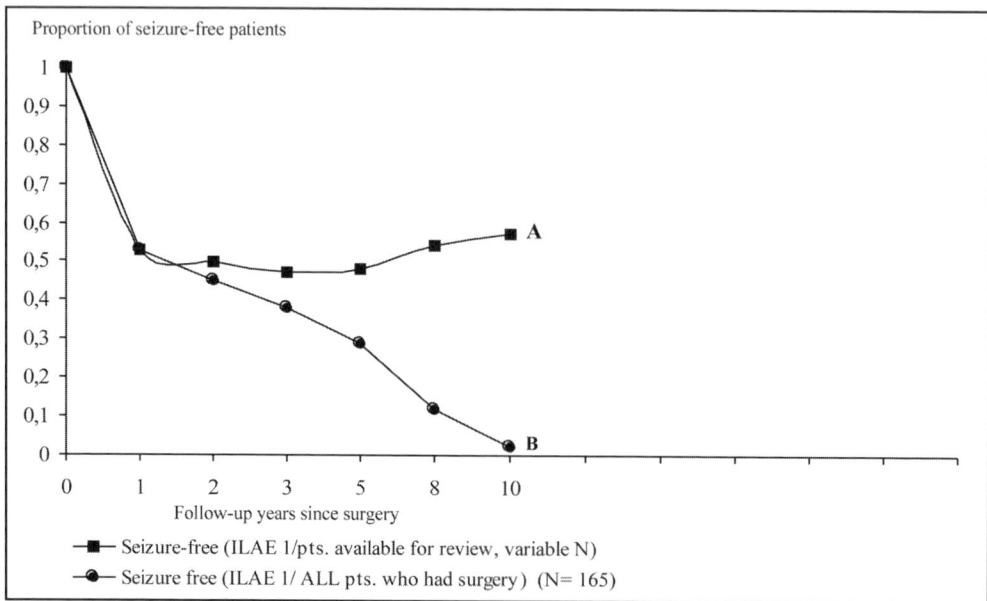

Figure 1. Seizure-free outcome after temporal lobe surgery in 165 patients with drug resistant temporal lobe epilepsy with mesial sclerosis. Seizure-free is defined as free of any seizures and auras for the observed follow-up (ILAE 1, Özkara et al., 2008). The study showed significant attrition of patients available for long-term follow-up, ranging from 165 patients after one year to 6 patients ten years after surgery. Thus reporting the proportion of seizure-free patients in a subgroup of patients available for review (A) provides better outcome data than reporting seizure-free outcome in relation to all 165 patients who had surgery and were followed-up for one year (B). Reporting outcome in relation to all patients undergoing treatment is preferable as it protects against reporting inflated outcome in subgroups of patients, it also provides a worst outcome scenario when all patients not available for review are considered as not proven to be seizure-free.

15 years, 53% (17/32) were class I (Jarrar *et al.*, 2002). The median proportion of seizure-free patients after resection for extratemporal lobe epilepsy was lower: 46% for occipital and parietal resections and 27% with frontal resections (Téllez-Zenteno *et al.*, 2005). In a study from the Cleveland Clinic, 6 of 22 (27%) patients available for review or 6 of all 70 patients (9%) undergoing surgery were seizure-free (Engel 1) 5 years after frontal lobe surgery (Jeha *et al.*, 2008). In summary, the studies reviewed above indicate that one in two patients undergoing temporal lobe surgery are long-term seizure-free. However, there is consistent convergent evidence that postoperative outcomes tend to decline in some studies. In a worst case scenario, where all patients not available for long-term review are considered as not being seizure-free, the documented proportion of seizure-free patients in several studies may be as low as 10% of all patients undergoing temporal lobe surgery. Long-term seizure-free outcome is approximately 30% after extratemporal lobe surgery. One further question is how many of the seizure-free surgical patients are off AEDs. This will be discussed in the next paragraph.

Seizure-free outcome off AEDs after surgery

On average, 20% (95% CI 17-23) of patients undergoing temporal lobe surgery were seizure-free and off AEDs (Téllez-Zenteno *et al.*, 2007). On average, 27% (95% CI 23-31) of children undergoing temporal lobe surgery were seizure-free and off AEDs (Téllez-Zenteno *et al.*, 2007). Children achieved better outcome than adults. During long-term evaluation, only 16% of temporal lobe surgery patients were seizure-free and off AEDs (Téllez-Zenteno *et al.*, 2007). In a report of long-term seizure outcome of 48 adult patients undergoing temporal lobe surgery from a single center, 10/48 (21%) were seizure-free on AEDs after 5 years and 14/48 (29%) seizure free off AEDs after a follow-up of 30 years, and 10 had died (Kelley & Theodore 2005). In summary, the studies reviewed above indicate that one in five patients undergoing temporal lobe surgery are long-term seizure-free and off AEDs. No data are available for the subgroups of patients seizure free on or off AEDs with extra-temporal resections only (Téllez-Zenteno *et al.*, 2007). Other types of surgery will not be covered in this chapter.

Is surgery better than medical treatment in non-operated patients with apparently drug-resistant epilepsy?

The efficacy of surgery in the management of drug-resistant epilepsy versus a change of medical regimen in non-operated patients can be determined by answering two questions. One is surgery rendering more patients seizure-free compared to drug treatment, and two, is a larger proportion of patients seizure-free off AEDs after surgery?

Comparing surgical and medical treatment is fraught with methodological issues. These include the definition of seizure freedom, nonrandomized study design (except for one randomized benchmark study to be discussed below), a possibly larger placebo effect of surgery compared to continued AED treatment, and heterogeneity patient populations and their respective treatment. Some patients with medically refractory localization-related epilepsy cannot be offered surgical resection because of inadequate localization of the epileptogenic zone, documentation of bilateral ictal onsets, or functionally important areas of cortex that prohibit resection. Other studies compared the surgical outcome with that of medical treatment in those waiting for surgery. These nonsurgical candidates have served as a medical control group. Only one controlled study of adjunctive temporal lobe surgery for epilepsy compared outcome versus continued AED treatment in those waiting for surgery (Wiebe et al., 2001). In this controlled trial patients with drug resistant temporal lobe epilepsy were randomized prior to presurgical evaluation. At one year, the cumulative proportion of patients who were free of all seizures, including auras (Engel class Ia), was 15/40 (38%) patients in the surgical group and (1/40) 3% in the medical group. The odds ratio was 23.40 in favor of surgery (95% CI: 2.91-188.36, $p < 0.001$). Using the definition of Engel Class I, 58% were free of seizures impairing awareness in the surgical group and 8% in the medical group ($p < 0.001$, Intention to treat analysis). The patients in the surgical group had fewer seizures impairing awareness and a significantly better quality of life ($p < 0.001$ for both comparisons) than the patients in the medical group. In a per protocol analysis, 23 of 36 patients (64%) who actually underwent surgery were free of seizures with impaired awareness and 15 of the 36 patients (42%) were free of all seizures.

Four patients (10%) had adverse effects of surgery. In one patient, a small thalamic infarct developed, causing sensory abnormalities in the left thigh; in one, the wound became infected; and in two, there was a decline in verbal memory that interfered with the patients' occupations at one year. Asymptomatic, superior subquadrantic visual-field defects occurred in 22 patients in the surgical group (55%), as expected. No neurologic abnormalities occurred in the patients in the medical group. Depression occurred in seven patients in the surgical group (18%) and eight patients in the medical group (20%). Transient psychosis developed in one patient in each group. One patient in the medical group died. The AEDs were switched or their doses increased in all patients in the medical group, and in 9 (22%) in the surgical group. In the medical group, the antiepileptic drug was switched once in 19 patients (48%), twice in 9 patients (22%), three times in 3 patients (8%), and four times in 1 patient (2%). All doses of anticonvulsants were increased to therapeutic levels or to the maximal tolerated dose. The trial's authors concluded that in temporal-lobe epilepsy, surgery is superior to prolonged medical therapy and that randomized trials of surgery for epilepsy are feasible and appear to yield precise estimates of treatment effects (Wiebe et al., 2001). No other controlled studies were found in which information on long-term use of resective surgery versus drug treatment in non-operated patients was found.

In a review of three nonrandomized comparative studies of surgical versus medical treatment the pooled proportion of patients free of AEDs was 0%, while 21% were on monotherapy (CI95 16-27), and 77% on several AEDs (CI95 71-83) (Téllez-Zenteno et al., 2006). In this review two of three studies reported from the same epilepsy center of Bonn and overlapping patient populations (Bien et al., 2001; Helmsteadter et al., 2003), the third study was from Norway (Guldvog et al., 2001). In preparation of a systematic review, we identified a number of nonrandomized studies comparing surgery with medical treatment. For illustration, one recent major study from the University of Bonn will be discussed here (Bien et al., 2006). Among surgical patients 68/131 (52%) were seizure-free. In contrast, 12/49 (24%) non-operated patients ineligible for surgery were seizure-free after a change of medication (Bien et al., 2006). The odds ratio of seizure freedom of surgical versus non-operated patients was 3.33 (95%CI 1.59-6.95). AEDs may have been discontinued in either group. The authors' defined being seizure free as having no seizures at the last year of follow-up. One further important finding of that study was the proportion of seizure free patients was only 5% among those awaiting presurgical assessment with a follow-up of only 0.8 years, and only 14% in those who withdrew from waiting for presurgical assessment with a follow-up of 6 years (Bien et al., 2006). This result outlines that the selection of the medical control group and the duration follow-up are confounding factors influencing the result of the medical arm of the study. The authors described surgical outcome in 131 patients with at least a 75% seizure reduction of whom 68/131 patients (52%) were seizure-free at the last year of 6.9 year follow-up. However, of all 175 surgical patients who underwent surgery, 68/175 (39%) patients undergoing surgery were reported to be seizure free. This important study underlines the efficacy of chronic AED treatment in chronic epilepsy of inherently severe epilepsy to warrant surgical evaluation (Bien et al., 2006). In addition, the authors noted that the difference between adjunctive surgical and medical treatment seems to become smaller with a longer follow-up (Bien et al., 2006). The authors interpreted their observations as follows: Patients with drug resistant epilepsies present to a surgical center at the peak severity of their disorder in terms of seizure frequency and well-being. If surgery is performed in this group, the difference to the outcome of medical treatment is greatest. Those who are not undergoing surgery and receive medical treatment, in the words of Bien and coworkers are "catching up" in their seizure outcome response over the years. The improvement in the medical group could thus be due to regression of the mean or improved medical care or both. This raises the question if the same is true for patients undergoing surgery, if this is so, regression of the mean could explain, at least in part, why the surgical outcome is lower with longer follow-up. Nevertheless, the study by Bien et al. (2006) shows that even after 6.5 years of follow-up surgery plus medical care is three times more efficacious than AED treatment alone. Finally, a caveat should be added that a systematic review of all available studies is needed to determine how much better surgery is compared to medical treatment in non-operated patients.

How many patients become seizure-free *because* of surgery?

The above analysis suggest that, after temporal lobe surgery, approximately 50% of patients will become seizure-free. However this calculation is based on no patients in similar studies becoming seizure-free without surgery, so it does not estimate the percentage of patients who become seizure-free *because* of surgery. The data given above suggest that in individual studies as many as 24% of patients may become seizure free without surgery (Bien et al., 2006). These data suggests that approximately 26% (50% seizure control with surgery minus 24% seizure control without surgery = 26%) of patients become seizure free because of surgery. Furthermore, according to a review by Téllez-Zenteno et al. (2007), 20% (95% CI 17-23) of patients undergoing temporal lobe surgery were seizure-free and off AEDs (Téllez-Zenteno et al., 2007). In summary, an estimated 20%-26% of patients (which is half of all patients seizure free after surgery) can be concluded to be seizure-free because of temporal lobe surgery. As no data seem to be available how many patients undergoing extra-temporal lobe surgery become seizure-free compared to similar patients without surgery, the extent to which patients undergoing extratemporal surgery are seizure-free *because* of surgery, if any, cannot be determined at present. The next question is then search for an explanation how surgery does achieve a better seizure outcome compared to drug treatment alone. This difficult question will be discussed in the following section.

How does surgery eliminate drug resistance and the need for AED treatment?

The intriguing and impressive ability of surgery to restore the efficacy of AEDs and thus eliminate drug-resistance, in one of two patients undergoing temporal lobe epilepsy, and the need for AEDs to remain seizure free after surgery in one of five patients undergoing temporal lobe surgery as reviewed above, raises the question of how surgery might be able to do this.

A number of challenges stand in the way of understanding how surgery eliminates drug resistance or fails to do so. The reasons for surgical failure are not completely understood, and include bitemporal, pseudotemporal and temporal plus epilepsies as well as incorrect localization or insufficient resection of mesial temporal lobe structures (Ryvlin, 2003; Gonzalez-Martin et al., 2007). One major issue to consider here is whether the cause or causes of drug resistance are only localized in the epileptogenic zone or whether changes outside of the resected epileptogenic zone are responsible for failure to eliminate drug resistance. Another major issue is how to better understand why about half of the patients becoming seizure free after surgery remain seizure free after planned discontinuation of AEDs while the other half starts to have seizures again when AEDs have been withdrawn (Schmidt et al., Schmidt & Löscher, 2005). Also, the mechanisms of drug resistance may change in the course of the epilepsy. A longitudinal study found that a proportion of patients may switch in the course of the disorder from being uncontrolled to becoming controlled and vice versa (Sillanpää & Schmidt, 2006). In addition, prognosis varies considerably in the epilepsies, even between patients with seemingly the same epilepsy syndrome, and its determinants are largely unknown (Schmidt & Löscher, 2005). Clinical features such as the epilepsy syndrome or the etiology may reasonably predict if temporal lobe epilepsy in children will turn out to be drug resistant (Spooner et al., 2006). Seizure cluster occurring during drug therapy was significantly associated with drug resistant epilepsy compared to those without clusters (42% *versus* 13%; p = 0.0102), a lower rate of entering 5-year terminal remission (p = 0.0039) and 5-year remission (p = 0.0230). In addition, the risk for death was significantly increased among patients with clustering during AED therapy compared with those without any clusters ever (42% *versus* 14%; p = 0.0299 two-sided Fisher's exact test). The risk ratio for patients with clusters was 3.49 (95% CI 1.25-9.78). In contrast, patients with seizure clustering prior to treatment versus no clustering showed no difference in seizure outcome or mortality risk (Sillanpää & Schmidt, 2008).

A *clinical/presurgical hypothesis* on how surgery eliminates drug resistance and obviated the need for AEDs to remain seizure free after surgery

Insight how surgical therapy of drug-resistant epilepsy works has benefited from new developments in structural and functional neuroimaging, improvements in diagnosis, particularly involving EEG and long-term monitoring and refinements in surgical techniques. These efforts have led to a conceptual framework how epilepsy might work as seen from a clinical and presurgical perspective *(Table I)*.

Table I. How does surgery eliminate drug resistance and need for AEDs? Conceptual framework from a clinical/surgical perspective. The concepts of an epileptogenic zone, an actual and a potential seizure onset zone led to an admittedly speculative hypothesis on the seizure outcome of epilepsy surgery

Three surgical outcome scenarios and their surgical hypotheses
• *No remission after surgery:* failure to resect the epileptogenic zone, the actual and the potential seizure onset zone.
• *Remission on AEDs:* the epileptogenic zone and the actual seizure onset zone have been affected or resected, but not the potential seizure onset zone.
• *Remission off AEDs:* the epileptogenic zone, the actual seizure onset zone have been resected, there is no evidence for a potential seizure onset zone.

Definitions: *Epileptogenic zone:* the minimum amount of cortex that must be resected (inactivated or completely disconnected) to produce seizure freedom (Lüders et al., 2006). *Actual seizure onset zone:* (the only one we can measure with direct presurgical measurements). *Potential seizure onset zone:* either cortex participating in early seizure spread or areas with potential to generate seizures once actual seizure onset zone has been resected.

A *pathophysiological hypothesis* on how surgery eliminates drug resistance and obviated the need for AEDs to remain seizure free after surgery

A conceptual framework from a pathophysiological perspective includes the concepts of limbic and extralimbic seizure generators. Such scenarios led to an admittedly speculative hypothesis on the seizure outcome of epilepsy surgery *(Table II)*.

According to the simplified concept, remission off AEDs requires not only a complete resection of the localized epileptogenic zone but also that there is no epileptogenic activity outside of the resected area. If this is the case, as in one of five patients undergoing temporal lobe surgery, the epilepsy is cured by surgery and AEDs are not needed for seizure control. In patients who entertain epileptogenic activity outside of the resected area after surgery, AEDs are required and discontinuation of AEDs leads to loss of seizure freedom. Furthermore, initially seizure-free patients may relapse on AEDs during the course of post-surgical follow-up (Schmidt *et al.*, 2005). In case of relapse, there may have been a build-up of a new epileptogenic zone.

However, a number of diagnostic challenges stand in the way of understanding how surgery eliminates drug resistance. For example, as shown in *Table II* temporal "plus" epilepsies are characterized by seizures involving a complex epileptogenic network including the temporal lobe and the closed neighboured structures such as the orbito-frontal cortex, the insula, the frontal and parietal operculum and the temporo-parieto-occipital junction

Table II. How does surgery eliminate drug resistance and need for AEDs?
Conceptual framework from a pathophysiological perspective. The concepts of limbic and extralimbic seizure generators led to an admittedly speculative hypothesis on the seizure outcome of epilepsy surgery (with data from Barba *et al.*, 2007; Löscher *et al.*, 2008; McIntyre & Gilby, 2008)

Dependent limbic seizure generators:
- Hippocampus
- Dentate gyrus
- Piriform/perirhinal cortex
- Amygdala
- Entorhinal cortex

Independent limbic seizure generators:
- Insula
- Frontal lobe

Independent non-limbic seizure generators:
- Parietal lobe
- Occipital lobe
- Multilobe
- Network

Independent limbic and non-limbic seizure generators:
- Temporal plus epilepsies

Three surgical outcome scenarios and their pathophysiological hypotheses
- *No remission after surgery:* failure to affect or resect dependent limbic seizure generators and independent limbic and non-limbic seizure generators:
- *Remission on AEDs:*
  – Dependent limbic seizure generators have been affected or resected but not independent limbic seizure generators.
  – Dependent limbic seizure generators have been incompletely affected or resected.
- *Remission off AEDs:*
  Dependent limbic seizure generators have been completely resected, no evidence for other seizure generators

(Barba et al., 2007). Temporal "plus" epilepsies are currently identified with the help of intracerebral electrodes. The study by Barba et al. (2007) assessed whether their diagnosis can be suspected non-invasively. The aim of this retrospective study was to address this issue in 80 consecutive patients who were thought to suffer from non-lesional temporal lobe seizures which finally proved, on the basis of stereotactic intracerebral EEG (SEEG) recordings, to be "purely" temporal (TL group, n = 58) or temporal "plus" (T+ group, n = 22). The results of Barba et al. (2007) showed that the two groups of patients were difficult to differentiate on the basis of general clinical features or MRI data. Even the presence of hippocampal sclerosis did not distinguish the two groups.

However, a synopsis of both ictal clinical symptoms and scalp-EEG findings significantly differentiated TL from T+ patients. Patients with TL epilepsies more frequently presented an ability to warn at seizure onset, an abdominal aura, gestural automatisms and a post-ictal amnesia. Patients suffering from T+ epilepsies more frequently had gustatory hallucinations, rotatory vertigo and auditory illusions at seizure onset; they exhibited more frequently contraversive manifestations of the eyes and/or head, piloerection and ipsilateral tonic motor signs, and they were more often dysphoric in the post-ictal phase. Cluster analysis mainly indicated that some associations of symptoms were relevant for differentiating TL cases from T+ cases. Interictal EEG of T+ patients more frequently exhibited bilateral or pre-central abnormalities, while ictal EEG more frequently pointed over the anterior frontal, temporo-parietal and pre-central regions. Neither TL interictal spikes, nor TL ictal EEG onset, allowed to definitely diagnose T+ epilepsies (Barba et al. 2007). Another conceptual frame work is to consider the current suggestions for the molecular mechanisms of drug-resistance.

Pharmacological hypothesis on which molecular mechanisms of drug-resistance, if any, are affected by surgery

Before we consider how surgery might eliminate drug-resistance, we need to consider the current suggestions for the mechanism(s) of drug resistance in non-operated patients (*Table III*). A recent example is the growing insight that target insensitivity of specific AEDs may be one reason why epilepsy is drug resistant (Remy et al., 2003, 2006). A detailed review of the numerous mechanisms of drug resistance in non-operated patients is beyond the scope of this brief chapter. Readers are referred to recent reviews of the topic (Schmidt & Löscher, 2005; and the chapter by Löscher in this volume).

Table III. Possible mechanisms of drug resistance (for review see Schmidt & Löscher, 2005)

Disease-related mechanisms
- etiology of disease;
- progression of disease;
- structural brain alterations and/or network changes;
- alterations in drug target(s);
- alterations in drug uptake into the brain;
- genetics, *e.g.*, nodular hyperplasia.

Drug-related mechanisms
- ineffective mechanism of drug action;
- insufficient drug penetration into the brain;
- loss of efficacy (tolerance);
- genetics, *e.g.*, gene polymorphisms in drug target or transporter genes.

For our discussion it is worthwhile to note that several mechanisms outlined in *Table III* may act together and possibly even interact. It is probably naïve to think that only one mechanism explains drug resistance in an individual patient. Also, the mechanisms of drug resistance may change in the course of the epilepsy. A longitudinal study found that a proportion of patients may switch in the course of the disorder from being uncontrolled to becoming controlled and vice versa (Sillanpää & Schmidt, 2006). In addition, prognosis varies considerably in the epilepsies, even between patients with seemingly the same epilepsy syndrome, and its determinants are largely unknown (Schmidt & Löscher, 2005). Clinical features such as the epilepsy syndrome or the etiology may reasonably predict if temporal lobe epilepsy in children will turn out to be drug resistant (Spooner et al., 2006). Seizure cluster occurring during drug therapy was significantly associated with drug resistant epilepsy compared to those without clusters (42% *versus* 13%; $p = 0.0102$), a lower rate of entering 5-year terminal remission ($p = 0.0039$) and 5-year remission ($p = 0.0230$). In addition, the risk for death was significantly increased among patients with clustering during AED therapy compared with those without any clusters ever (42% *versus* 14%; $p = 0.0299$ two-sided Fisher's exact test). The risk ratio for patients with clusters was 3.49 (95%CI 1.25-9.78). In contrast, patients with seizure clustering prior to treatment versus no clustering showed no difference in seizure outcome or mortality risk (Sillanpää & Schmidt, 2008).

Basic research conducted on the human brain in epilepsy surgery centers has led to a better understanding of the pathophysiology of the epileptic disorders that are amenable to surgery, and has also been instrumental to detect underlying mechanisms of drug-resistance. Theoretically, a number of pharmacological and disease related mechanisms may be affected by resection of epileptogenic brain tissue. The considerations are listed in *Table IV*.

A number of additional challenges need to be considered that stand in the way of understanding how surgery eliminates drug resistance. One major issue is whether the cause or causes of drug resistance are localized in the epileptogenic zone or whether changes outside of the resected epileptogenic zone are responsible for failure to eliminate drug resistance. Another major issue is how to better understand why about half of the patients becoming seizure free after surgery remain seizure free after planned discontinuation of AEDs while the other half starts to have seizures again when AEDs have been withdrawn (Schmidt *et al.*, 2003, Schmidt & Löscher, 2005; Schmidt, 2006).

Table IV. Overview on possible mechanisms of the effect of temporal lobe surgery on drug resistance (adapted from Schmidt & Löscher, 2005; Regesta & Tanganelli, 1995)

Genetic variation
- The prion story (Waltz *et al.*, 2003, retracted)*.

Disease-related mechanisms
- Surgery eliminates the etiology of disease, *e.g.*, removal of tumors.
- Surgery reverses drug resistance by removal of epileptogenic tissue**.
- Surgery eliminates structural brain alterations, that may contribute to drug resistance *e.g.*, cortical dysplasia.
- Surgery indirectly affects pathological network outside of the resected epileptogenic zone.

* no evidence, ** suggestive evidence.

Two more working hypotheses on how surgery eliminates drug-resistance and obviated the need for AEDs

Two further considerations are raised for further discussion:

- Surgery restores the ability of AEDs or of mechanism(s) of natural remission to control seizures. This hypothesis is supported by the clinical observation that seizure outcome after temporal lobe surgery appears to be similar to that of AEDs in drug-naïve temporal lobe epilepsy.

- Restoring the AED response involves mechanisms of plasticity that were blocked or inactivated by the structural or functional substrate(s) of drug resistance. The critical question remains: What are the functional and structural substrates of drug resistance?

■ Conclusions

Epilepsy surgery has the inexplicable and incontrovertible ability to restore the efficacy of AEDs in patients with chronic drug-resistant temporal lobe epilepsy. Reliable long-term data indicate that surgery leads to seizure freedom, as defined by the study authors, in one of two patients with apparently drug resistant temporal lobe epilepsy, including a subgroup of one in five who become free of seizures and free of AEDs. In addition to those being rendered free of any seizures and auras, a number of patients have a reduction of seizure frequency after surgery. Two major methodological issues may lead to reporting inflated surgical seizure outcome and make it difficult to compare outcome of AED treatment versus surgical treatment. One issue is that in many reports seizure outcome is inflated because it is expressed as proportion of patients available for review not as percent of all patients who have undergone treatment. Furthermore, many surgical studies do not provide the proportion of patients free of any seizures including auras for a defined duration but consider patients who continue to have auras or simple partial seizures or "non-disabling" seizures as seizure free and thus also provide an inflated seizure outcome after surgery. According to several reports temporal lobe surgery is rendering 50% of patients seizure-free, by any definition, compared to up to 24% following medical treatment in non-operated patients. However, the determination of long term prognosis of surgery versus continued AED treatment in non-operated patients requires more work as does the question of how exactly surgery is able to reverse drug resistance and to render patients seizure free off AEDs.

■ Summary

This analysis suggests that one in two drug-resistant patients undergoing temporal lobe surgery are long-term seizure-free. In these patients surgery has eliminated drug resistance. However this calculation is based on the premise that no patients in similar studies are becoming seizure-free without surgery, so it does not estimate the percentage of patients who become seizure-free *because* of surgery. In individual studies as many as 24% of patients ineligible for surgery have become seizure free without surgery. These preliminary data suggest that approximately 26% (50% seizure control with surgery minus 24% seizure control without surgery = 26%) of patients become seizure free *because* of surgery. The above calculation is supported by a number of long-term observations indicating that 20-25% of patients undergoing temporal lobe surgery are long-term seizure-free and off

AEDs. No data are available for extratemporal surgery. A definitive systematic review is needed to address this issue. In patients who need AEDs after surgery to become or remain seizure-free, AEDs are thought to be needed to lower epileptogenic activity in areas that could not be resected. Becoming seizure-free because of surgery (without the help of AEDs) requires not only a complete resection of the localized epileptogenic zone but also that there is no clinically relevant network of epileptogenic activity outside of the resected area.

References

Barba C, Barbati G, Minotti L, Hoffmann D, Kahane P. Ictal clinical and scalp-EEG findings differentiating temporal lobe epilepsies from temporal "plus" epilepsies. *Brain* 2007; 130: 1957-67.

Bien CG, Kurthen M, Baron K, *et al*. Long-term seizure outcome and antiepileptic drug treatment in surgically treated temporal lobe epilepsy patients: a controlled study. *Epilepsia* 2001; 42 (11): 1416-21.

Bien CG, Schulze-Bonhage A, Soeder BM, Schramm J, Elger CE, Tiemeier H. Assessment of the long-term effects of epilepsy surgery with three different reference groups. *Epilepsia* 2006; 47: 1865-9.

Callaghan BC, Anand K, Hesdorffer D, Hauser WA, French JA. Likelihood of seizure remission in an adult population with refractory epilepsy. *Ann Neurol* 2007; 62 (4): 382-9.

Engel J Jr, Wiebe S, French J, *et al.*; Quality Standards Subcommittee of the American Academy of Neurology; American Epilepsy Society; American Association of Neurological Surgeons. Practice parameter: temporal lobe and localized neocortical resections for epilepsy: report of the Quality Standards Subcommittee of the American Academy of Neurology, in association with the American Epilepsy Society and the American Association of Neurological Surgeons. *Neurology* 2003; 60 (4): 538-47.

Helmsteadter C, Kurthen M, Lux S, Reuber M, Elger CE. Chronic epilepsy and cognition: a longitudinal study in temporal lobe epilepsy. *Ann Neurol* 2003; 54: 425-32.

Jarrar RG, Buchhalter JR, Meyer FB, Sharbrough FW, Laws E. Long-term follow-up of temporal lobe epilepsy in children. *Neurology* 2002; 59: 1635-7.

Guldvog B, Loyning Y, Hauglie-Hansen E, Flood S, Björnaes H. Surgical versus medical treatment of epilepsy. I. Outcome relkated to survival seizures, and neurologic deficit. *Epilepsia* 1991; 32: 375-88.

Kelley K, Theodore WH. Prognosis 30 years after temporal lobectomy. *Neurology* 2005; 64: 1974-6.

Kwan P, Brodie MJ. Early identification of refractory epilepsy. *N Engl J Med* 2000; 342: 314-9.

Löscher W, Gernert M, Heinemann U. Cell and gene therapies in epilepsy - promising avenues or blind alleys? *Trends Neurosci* 2008; 31 (2): 62-73.

Lüders HO, Aurad I. Conceptual considerations. In: *Epilepsy Surgery*, ed. by H. Lüders. Raven Press, Ltd., New York, 1991: 51-73.

Luciano Al, Shorvon SD. Results of treatment changes in patients with apparently drug-resistant chronic epilepsy. *Ann Neurol* 2007; 62: 375-81.

McIntyre D, Gilby KL. Mapping seizure pathways in the temporal lobe. *Epilepsia* 2008; (suppl 3): 23-30.

Regesta G, Tanganelli P. Clinical aspects and biological bases of drug-resistant epilepsies. *Epilepsy Res* 1999; 34: 109-22.

Remy S, Gabriel S, Urban BW, *et al*. A novel mechanism underlying drug resistance in chronic epilepsy. *Ann Neurol* 2003; 53: 469-79.

Remy S, Beck H. Molecular and cellular mechanisms of pharmacoresistance in epilepsy. *Brain* 2006; 129: 18-35.

Schiller Y, Najjar Y. Quantifying the response to antiepileptic drugs: effect of past treatment history. *Neurology* 2008; 70 (1): 54-65.

Schmidt D, Löscher W. Drug resistance in epilepsy: putative neurobiological and clinical mechanisms. *Epilepsia* 2005; 46: 858-77.

Schmidt D, Löscher W. How effective is surgery to cure seizures in drug-resistant temporal lobe epilepsy? *Epilepsy Research* 2003; 56: 85-91.

Schmidt D, Baumgartner C, Löscher W. Seizure recurrence after planned discontinuation of antiepileptic drugs in seizure-free patients after epilepsy surgery: a review of current clinical experience. *Epilepsia* 2004; 45: 179-86.

Schmidt D. How often does surgery "cure" drug-resistant epilepsy in adults? In: Miller JF, Silbergeld DL (eds). *Epilepsy Surgery. Principles and Controversies*. New York: Taylor and Francis, 2006, Chapter XIII-41, p. 648-52.

Selwa LM, Schmidt SL, Malow BA, Beydoun A. Long-term outcome of nonsurgical candidates with medically refractory localization-related epilepsy. *Epilepsia* 2003; 44: 1568-72.

Sillanpää M, Schmidt D. Natural history of treated childhood-onset epilepsy: prospective, long-term population-based study. *Brain* 2006; 129: 617-24.

Sillanpää M, Schmidt D. Seizure clustering during drug treatment affects seizure outcome and mortality of childhood-onset epilepsy. *Brain* 2008; 131: 438-44.

Spooner CG, Berkovic SF, Mitchell LA, Wrennall JA, Harvey AS. New-onset temporal lobe epilepsy in children: lesion on MRI predicts poor seizure outcome. *Neurology* 2006; 26: 2147-53.

Téllez-Zenteno JF, Dhar R, Wiebe S. Long-term seizure outcomes following epilepsy surgery: a systematic review and meta-analysis. *Brain* 2005; 128: 1188-98.

Téllez-Zenteno JF, Dhar R, Hernandez-Ronquillo L, Wiebe S. Long-term outcomes in epilepsy surgery: antiepileptic drugs, mortality, cognitive and psychosocial aspects. *Brain* 2007; 130: 334-45.

Walz R, Castro RM, Velasco TR, *et al*.. Surgical outcome in mesial temporal sclerosis correlates with prion gen variant. *Neurology* 2003; 11: 1204-10 (retracted: Neurology 2007).

Wiebe S, Blume WT, Girvin JP, *et al*.. A randomized, controlled trial of surgery for temporal-lobe epilepsy. *N Engl J Med* 2001; 345: 311-8.

Neurostimulation for epilepsy: myth or reality?

Philippe Kahane[1,2,4], S. Saillet[1], Lorella Minotti[1,2],
Laurent Vercueil[1,2], Stephan Chabardès[2,3], Antoine Depaulis[1]

[1] *Institut des Neurosciences, INSERM U836-UJF-CEA, Grenoble, France*
[2] *Neurology Department, Grenoble University Hospital, France*
[3] *Neurosurgery Department, Grenoble University Hospital, France*
[4] *Institute for Children and adolescents with epilepsy – IDEE, Hospices Civils de Lyon, France*

About 30% of epileptic patients do not respond to antiepileptic drugs (Kwan & Brodie, 2000), of whom only a minority can benefit from resective surgery. Such a therapeutic option, indeed, is considered only in patients suffering from focal seizures, and in whom the epileptogenic zone has been clearly identified and can be safely removed. Therefore, those patients whose seizures arise from eloquent cortices, or whose seizures are multifocal, bilateral, or generalized, represent a particular challenge to "new" or "alternative" therapies, among which neurostimulation has interesting potential (Polkey et al., 2003). Different types of neurostimulation exist in epileptic patients, depending on the region which is targeted, and the way this stimulation is administered (Morrell, 2006; Oommen et al., 2005; Theodore & Fisher, 2004; Vonck et al., 2007). In general, stimulation is applied with the intention of reducing the probability of seizures and/or seizure propagation, either by manipulating remote control systems (vagus nerve stimulation, deep brain stimulation), or by interfering with the epileptogenic zone itself (repetitive transcranial magnetic stimulation, cortical stimulation). In most cases, stimulation is delivered continuously or intermittently according to a scheduled stimulation protocol (nonresponsive – or open loop – stimulation). Vast progress in biotechnology and EEG signal analysis now also allows stimulation in response to detection of electrographic seizures (closed loop stimulation). We will review here the various attempts that have been made to influence epilepsy by stimulation techniques, focusing attention on clinical aspects.

■ Vagus-nerve stimulation (VNS)

The vagus nerve, through the nucleus tractus solitarius and parabrachial nucleus, accesses the limbic, autonomic, and reticular structures of the forebrain (Henry, 2002). It projects to the noradrenergic and serotoninergic neurotransmission systems of the brain and spinal cord, to the amygdala, insula, hypothalamus, periaqueductal grey matter, and thalamus (Henry, 2002; Vonck et al., 2001). These widespread, bilateral, and multisynaptic projections account for possible multiple therapeutic mechanisms of Vagus Nerve Stimulation (VNS) therapy in epilepsy. In animals, VNS has been studied in many models of epilepsy (rat, cat, dog and monkey) and a number of effects were observed, including an acute abortive effect on seizures (McLachlan, 1993), and an acute as well as a chronic prophylactic effect on seizure frequency and severity (Lockard, 1990; Takaya et al., 1996). In humans, the first treatment with VNS was done in 1988 and preliminary results, obtained in 4 patients, demonstrated that such a therapy was safe and potentially effective (Penry & Dean, 1990). Later, 5 clinical trials were conducted (E01-E05), including 2 double-blind, randomized, controlled studies (E03, E05) (Handforth et al., 1998; The Vagus Nerve Stimulation Study Group, 1995). This provided the foundation for VNS therapy approval by the European Community (1994) and FDA (1997) for complex partial and secondarily generalized seizures in patients aged 12 years and older. To date, over 40,000 patients around the world have been treated with VNS.

The overall efficacy as evaluated from the 5 clinical trials shows a median seizure reduction of 35%, 44%, and 44% at one, two, and 3 years, respectively (Morris & Mueller, 1999). Post-marketing experience, as provided by manufacturer-supported open databases, suggests that VNS reduces seizure frequency by 50% or more in 50-60% of the cases. Efficacy has a tendency to improve over time (Handforth et al., 1998) and AEDs may be reduced in a number of cases (Labar, 2002). Children seem to respond similarly to adults (Wheless & Maggio, 2002).

Beyond seizure control, VNS also reduces daytime sleepiness and promotes alertness (Malow, 2001), it improves mood (Harden et al., 2000) and memory (Clark et al., 1999), and leads to a global improvement in quality of life (Dodrill & Morris, 2001). It is also cost-effective, as suggested by a few European studies (Ben-Menachem et al., 2002; Boon et al., 1999). Serious complications are rare (Ben-Menachem, 2001) and there has been no evidence of increased mortality and overall morbidity in patients with VNS compared with uncontrolled epilepsy (Annegers et al., 2000). Side effects, which mainly include hoarseness, cough, local paresthesia and dyspnea (Morris & Mueller, 1999) are typically stimulation-related and transient, and generally resolve over time (Boon et al., 1999). No interference with AEDs has been found and there is no evidence of impaired fertility or teratogenicity due to VNS.

Overall, VNS appears as effective as AEDs in terms of seizure control and it may bring additional benefit in terms of general health. A European multi-centric phase IV post-marketing study aiming at evaluating this aspect is in progress (PULSE study). However, no clear predictive factors for responders to VNS therapy have emerged, and the precise mechanism of action of this treatment remains to be elucidated. Neuroimaging studies, including PET (Henry et al., 1998, 1999; Ko et al., 1996), SPECT (Van Laere et al., 2000; Vonck et al., 2000) and fMRI (Liu et al., 2003; Narayanan et al., 2002) might support thalamic involvement in VNS efficacy.

■ Deep brain stimulation (DBS)

For more than two decades, stimulation of a number of deep brain targets has been shown to be feasible, safe, and effective in humans suffering from different forms of movement disorders. This has led to its development and application in an increasing number of neurological and non-neurological diseases, including epilepsy (Benabid et al., 2001). Although the cortex plays a crucial role in seizure generation, accumulating evidence has pointed to the role of subcortical structures in the clinical expression, propagation and control of epileptic seizures in humans (Semah, 2002; Vercueil & Hirsch, 2002). Based on more or less consistent findings from experimental studies, deep brain stimulation (DBS) has been applied to a number of targets, including the cerebellum, different nuclei of the thalamus, and several structures of the basal ganglia system. Although encouraging, published results do not reach a definite conclusion. Many issues remain unresolved, including patient selection criteria, optimal target, optimal stimulation parameters, and continuous versus intermittent stimulation protocols.

Cerebellum

During the 1950s and 1960s, cerebellar stimulation demonstrated antiepileptic properties on different animal models of epilepsy, mostly penicillin and cobalt foci in cats (Cooke & Snider, 1955; Dow et al., 1962; Mutani et al., 1969). Following this, and based on the assumption that cerebellar outflow is inhibitory in nearly all patients (Cooper, 1978), the first trials in epileptic patients were carried out in the early 1970s by Cooper and colleagues (Cooper et al., 1973), who showed that seizures were modified or inhibited in 10 out of their 15 patients, without any adverse events (Cooper et al., 1976). Although the procedure was not strictly DBS, it raised the issue of distant modulation of cortical epileptogenicity by electrical currents, and it demonstrated for the first time the feasibility and safety of a therapeutic stimulation technique in epileptic patients. Later, a large uncontrolled study of 115 patients reported that 31 became seizure-free and 56 were improved (Davis & Emmonds, 1992). Such promising results, however, were not confirmed in 3 controlled clinical trials involving 14 patients, of whom only 2 were improved (Krauss & Fisher, 1993; Van Buren et al., 1978; Wright et al., 1984). Additional animal studies conducted in alumina cream focus in monkeys, or in kindled cats, did not confirm previous experimental findings (Ebner et al., 1980; Lockard et al., 1979; Majkowski et al., 1980). This resulted in the discontinuation of cerebellar stimulation for many years. Recently, however, a double-blind, randomized controlled pilot study conducted in 5 patients suffering from intractable motor seizures has rekindled interest in cerebellar stimulation (Velasco et al., 2005). Stimulation was applied at 10 Hz to the upper medial surface of each cerebellar hemisphere, and parameters were adjusted to deliver a constant charge density of 2.0 microC/cm^2/phase. During the initial 3-month double-blind phase, seizures were significantly reduced in the patients who received cerebellar stimulation, compared with no change in seizure frequency in the patients who received sham stimulation. Over the subsequent 6-month open-label phase, where all the patients were stimulated, seizures were reduced by 41% (14-75%) and the difference was statistically significant for tonic and tonic-clonic seizures. Effectiveness was maintained over the study period of 2 years. One patient developed an infection of the implanted system which had to be removed, and 3 required further surgery because of lead/electrode displacement. Altogether, although cerebellar stimulation appears to possess antiepileptic effects in some patients and/or some forms of epilepsy, the rationale of such suppressive effects remains to be determined.

Thalamus

Since the 1980s, interest has been focused on the thalamus, a structure with many interactions with the cortex and with an organization and connectivity that has been deciphered in many details during the last 20 years. Several thalamic targets have been stimulated in an attempt to suppress seizures, mainly the anterior nucleus and the centromedian nucleus. There is limited proof from animal studies that stimulation of these structures can influence seizure threshold, however, continuous stimulation of the thalamus in epileptic humans has shown some effects on seizure frequency and severity in a few – mostly uncontrolled – studies.

Anterior thalamus (AN)

The anterior nucleus (AN) of the thalamus appears to be in close interaction with the circuit of Papez. It receives projections from the hippocampus via the mammillary bodies and the fornix and has outputs to the cingulate cortex and, via the cingulum, to the entorhinal cortex and back to the hippocampus. AN therefore occupies a central position in the network which underlies limbic seizures and, as such, represents an attractive target for DBS in epileptic patients. Cooper and his group, encouraged by their experience of cerebellar stimulation, were the first to direct their interest to this nucleus, based on the idea that AN was a pacemaker for the cortex. They therefore performed bilateral chronic stimulation of AN in 6 epileptic patients, of whom five showed a 60% reduction in seizure frequency, and three a decrease in EEG spikes (Cooper & Upton, 1985). These clinical findings were not really considered to be up to the standard of the more robust experimental data which had been published. It was then shown that AN and mammillary bodies actively participated in the genesis of pentylenetetrazol-induced seizures, that they were selectively activated during ethosuximide-induced suppression of these seizures (Mirski and Ferrendelli, 1986a; 1986b), and that section of the mamillo-thalamic bundle prevented seizures in epileptic guinea pigs (Mirsky & Ferrendelli, 1984). Furthermore, it was demonstrated that 100 Hz electrical stimulation of mammillary nuclei (Mirski & Fisher, 1994) and AN (Mirski *et al.*, 1997) increased the seizure threshold of pentylenetetrazol in rats, and that 100 Hz AN stimulation delayed (but did not prevent) pilocarpine-induced *status epilepticus* (Hamani *et al.*, 2004). These data gave weight to the argument for reassessing the effect of AN stimulation in epileptic patients, although recent findings have suggested that 100 Hz AN stimulation might have an aggravating effect on seizures of kainate-treated rats (Lado, 2006).

Four small open-label trials have been reported in 18 patients, showing that seizure frequency was reduced from 92% to 2%, this reduction being statistically significant in 12 of the 18 cases (Hodaie *et al.*, 2002; Kerrigan *et al.*, 2004; Lim *et al.*, 2007; Osorio *et al.*, 2007). Two patients presented a complication (small frontal hemorrhage and extension erosion over the scalp), which did not result in major or permanent neurological deficit. One study showed that insertion of AN electrodes could produce a reduction in seizures (Lim *et al.*, 2007), another that the observed benefits did not differ between stimulation-on and stimulation-off periods (Hodaie *et al.*, 2002), thus raising the issue of a lesional, placebo or carry-over effect. Therefore, although possibly effective, deep brain stimulation of the AN requires further controlled studies. In this way, a large multicenter prospective randomized trial of AN stimulation for partial and secondarily generalized seizures is now under way in the USA. Another clinical trial is required to evaluate the antiepileptic effect of DBS of other targets of the circuit of Papez, namely the mammillary bodies and mamillo-thalamic tract (Duprez et al., 2005; van Rijckevorsel et al., 2005). Whether AN stimulation could be more effective in temporal lobe epilepsy cases, as suggested by an anecdotal report of hippocampal inhibition produced by AN stimulation, remains an interesting issue (Zumsteg et al., 2006).

Centromedian thalamus (CM)

In parallel to the development of AN stimulation, attention was also directed towards an intralaminar nucleus of the thalamus, the centromedian nucleus (CM), which is part of the reticulothalamocortical system mediating cerebral cortex excitability (Jasper, 1991), and which participates in the modulation of vigilance states (Velasco et al., 1979). Although experimental findings remain serendipitous (Arduini & Lary Bounes, 1952), a first open-label bilateral CM stimulation study was conducted in 5 patients at the end of the 1980s (Velasco et al., 1987), mainly based on anatomical grounds. CM is a well-located and easily-accessible structure in the center of the thalamus, and "the reason to prefer stimulation of CM to other intralaminar and midline nuclei [was] based on general considerations of the stereotactic targets" (Velasco et al., 2001a). Preliminary results indicated improvement over baseline of seizure frequency and EEG spiking for 3 months of chronic stimulation. At the same period, an anecdotal case report showed that 50 Hz stimulation of the mesothalamic reticular formation, performed to alleviate chronic pain in one single case, also relieved absence seizures that had been present for many years (Andy & Jurko, 1986).

Later, Velasco's group accumulated experience in a large cohort of 49 patients suffering from different forms of seizures and epilepsies (Velasco et al., 2001a; 2002), including long term follow-up studies in a more restricted number of cases that varied from five to 13 (Velasco et al., 1993, 1995, 2000ab, 2006). Overall, the procedure was said to be beneficial and was generally well-tolerated, although a central nystagmus was induced at times (Taylor et al., 2000). A few patients were explanted because of repeated and multiple skin erosions (Velasco et al., 2006). Better clinical outcomes were obtained in generalized tonic-clonic seizures and atypical absences of the Lennox-Gastaut syndrome, which decreased by up to 80% on average, with a global improvement of patients in their ability scale scores (Velasco et al., 2006). No improvement was found for either complex partial seizures or focal spikes in temporal regions, although a recent animal study found that 60 Hz stimulation of the reticular nucleus of the thalamus could reduce kindled seizure severity (Nanobashvili et al., 2003). The best clinical results were seen when both electrodes contacts used for stimulation were located within the CM on both sides and when stimulation at 6-8 Hz and 60 Hz induced recruiting responses and regional DC shifts, respectively (Velasco et al., 2000a). Optimal parameters were 2 hours of daily 130 Hz stimulation sessions (1-minute on, 4 minutes off), alternating the right and left CM, that could be changed to continuous bilateral instead of intermittent unilateral stimulation to obtain faster and more obvious results (Velasco et al., 2001b). As for AN stimulation, persistent antiepileptic effects were found three months or more after discontinuation of the stimulation (the "off effect"), and the authors have suggested that this could be due to functional (and possibly plastic) changes which developed during the stimulation procedure (Velasco et al., 2001b).

Although promising, the findings emerging from Velasco's group were not replicated in a small placebo-controlled study conducted in seven patients, which failed to demonstrate a statistically significant difference from the baseline in frequency of tonic-clonic seizures when the stimulator was on (mean reduction: 30%) versus off (mean reduction: 8%) (Fisher et al., 1992). In the open-label follow-up phase, however, three of 6 patients reported at least a 50% decrease in seizure frequency.

Up to now, very few animal studies have examined the role of the CM or the parafascicular nucleus (PF) in the control of epileptic seizures. In the genetic model of absence epilepsy in the rat (GAERS), pharmacological activation of the PF was found to suppress spike-and-wave discharges (Nail-Boucherie et al., 2005). More recently, 130 Hz stimulation of this structure was reported to interrupt focal hippocampal seizures in a mouse model of mesiotemporal lobe epilepsy (Langlois et al., in preparation). Because of its unique location between cortical and limbic structures and basal ganglia structures, the CM/PF nuclei could well constitute an interesting target for DBS. However, more animal studies are required to understand the role of this structure in the modulation of epileptic seizures.

Basal ganglia

Since the beginning of the 1980s, evidence from experimental animal studies has suggested the existence of a "nigral control" of epileptic seizures (for review see Depaulis et al., 1994). Inhibition of the *Substantia Nigra pars Reticulata* (SNR) has potent antiepileptic effects in different animal models of epilepsy (Deransart & Depaulis, 2002) and the GABAergic SNR output to the superior *colliculus* appears to be a critical relay in this control (Paz et al., 2005, 2007). Importantly, local manipulations of the basal ganglia that lead to an inhibition of the SNR neurons (e.g., activation of the *striatum* or *pallidum*, inhibition of the sub-thalamic nucleus) also had significant antiepileptic effects (for review see Deransart & Depaulis, 2002), suggesting that different striato-nigral circuits are involved in the control of epileptic seizures. In humans, EEG, clinical and imaging data also support the involvement of the basal ganglia in the propagation and/or the control of epileptic discharges (Biraben et al., 2004; Bouilleret et al., 2008; Vercueil & Hirsch, 2002). Altogether, experimental and clinical data suggest a privileged role for the basal ganglia in the control of generation and/or spread of epileptic discharges in the cortex. Paradoxically, the therapeutic relevance of such findings was rarely considered until the 1990s.

Caudate nucleus (CN)

Following experimental evidence that stimulation of the caudate nucleus (CN) could have antiepileptic properties in different animal models of epilepsy (La Grutta et al., 1971, 1988; Mutani, 1969; Oakley & Ojemann, 1982; Psatta, 1983), Chkhenkeli and his group, as well as Sramka and colleagues, were the first to suggest the potential beneficial effect of striatal stimulation in epileptic patients (Chkhenkeli, 1978; Sramka et al., 1980). A decrease in focal and generalized interictal discharges was observed among 57 patients who had been stimulated thus far using low frequency (4-6 Hz) stimulation of the CN (Chkhenkeli & Chkhenkeli, 1997). The study, however, was uncontrolled and the effect on seizures was not assessed. Interestingly, epileptic activity was worsened by stimulating the CN at high frequency, a finding that was also reported in the aluminium-hydroxide monkey model of motor seizures (Oakley & Ojemann, 1982). Therefore, if we assume that low-frequency stimulation is excitatory and high-frequency stimulation is inhibitory, these data are in agreement with the concept of a basal ganglia control of epileptic seizures, since activation of the *striatum* inhibits SNR via its GABAergic projections, while its inhibition leads to the reverse effect. Although further studies are needed, these results highlight the ability of the basal ganglia system to modulate cortical epileptogenicity.

Subthalamic nucleus (STN)

In 1998, Vercueil et al. (1998) were the first to show that 130 Hz stimulation of the subthalamic nucleus (STN) could interrupt absence seizures in GAERS, a well-established genetic model of absence epilepsy (Danober et al., 1998; Marescaux et al., 1992), in agreement with the antiepileptic effects of its pharmacological inhibition (Deransart et al., 1996). This led the group of Benabid at Grenoble University Hospital to perform the first STN stimulation in a 5-year-old girl with pharmacologically resistant inoperable epilepsy caused by a focal centroparietal dysplasia (Benabid et al., 2002). Later, 11 additional patients suffering from different forms of epilepsy received high frequency STN stimulation at different institutions (Chabardès et al., 2002; Loddenkemper et al., 2001; Vesper et al., 2007). Overall, seizure frequency was reduced by at least 50% in 7/12 cases, and the stimulation was well tolerated. Good responders suffered from very different epilepsy types including focal epilepsy, Dravet syndrome, Lennox-Gastaut syndrome and progressive myoclonic epilepsy. Surgical complications occurred in two patients, including infection of the generator in one, and a postimplantation subdural hematoma in another who later underwent surgical treatment, without sequelae (Chabardès et al., 2002). Bilateral stimulation appeared more effective than unilateral stimulation, in agreement with experimental data (Depaulis et al., 1994). However, whether it should be applied continuously or intermittently remains questionable (Chabardès et al., 2002). Furthermore, whether the optimal target in epileptic patients is the STN itself or, as is suggested in some patients, the SNR, remains an important issue (Chabardès et al., 2002; Vesper et al., 2007). A recent study in the GAERS suggested that SNR stimulation was more effective but that continuous stimulation could aggravate seizures (Feddersen et al., 2007). Currently, a double-blind cross over multi-centric study is in progress in France (STIMEP) aiming at evaluating the clinical effect of 130 Hz stimulation of the STN/SNR in patients with ring chromosome 20 epilepsy. These patients, indeed, exhibit a deficit of dopaminergic activity in the *striatum* as compared with normal subjects (Biraben et al., 2004), a finding which is in accordance with the critical role of striatal dopamine in the control of seizures (Deransart et al., 2000).

■ Stimulation at seizure focus

Stimulating the epileptogenic cortex to interrupt epileptic seizures may appear paradoxical. Indeed, "stimulation" classically means "excitation", and the epilepsies are characterized by a pathological hyperexcitability and hypersynchrony of cortical neurons. The effects provoked by cortical stimulation, however, depend on the stimulation parameters used, the region which is stimulated, as well as the way that the stimulation is delivered (indirectly or directly). To date, a few studies have been conducted, including a limited number of patients, and therapeutic results are equivocal at best.

Repetitive transcranial magnetic stimulation (rTMS)

A simple and non-invasive way of indirectly stimulating the cortex is to use transcranial magnetic stimulation (TMS). TMS is widely utilized in neurophysiology for diagnostic purposes (*e.g.*, to evaluate motor cortex excitability); it has also therapeutic uses in various brain diseases when delivered in series or trains of pulses, a method known as repetitive TMS or rTMS (Kobayashi & Pascual-Leone, 2003; Tassinari et al., 2003; Wassermann & Lisanby, 2001). Low frequency (0.5 Hz) rTMS was reported to have anticonvulsive effects against pentylenetetrazol-induced seizures in rats (Akamatsu et al., 2001), while high frequency rTMS had opposite results (Jennum and Klitgaard, 1996). In humans, low frequency rTMS reduces motor cortex excitability, while high frequency stimulation can lead to seizures, even in healthy subjects (Chen et al., 1997). The first attempt at rTMS therapy in epilepsy was carried out at the end of the 1990s, using a round coil placed over the vertex in order to achieve global depression of excitability (Tergau et al., 1999). This open study showed that eight of 9 patients submitted to five consecutive days of 0.33 Hz rTMS had a mean seizure reduction of 38.6%. Later, effects on rTMS were evaluated in three placebo-controlled studies, of which two failed to demonstrate any significant effect (Cantello et al., 2007; Theodore et al., 2002). In the remaining one, however, conducted in patients with malformations of cortical development, rTMS focally targeting the malformation significantly decreased the number of seizures in the active compared with sham rTMS group (Fregni et al., 2006).

These data might support the idea that rTMS is more likely to be effective for patients with clearly identifiable foci in the cortical convexity, a finding also suggested by the Theodore et al. (2002) study which showed a nonsignificant tendency towards a greater effect in patients with neo-cortical foci than in those with mesial temporal lobe foci. Other – uncontrolled – studies (Brasil-Neto et al., 2004; Kinoshita et al., 2005a; Santiago-Rodriguez et al., 2008), as well as anecdotal case reports (Menkes & Gruenthal, 2000; Misawa et al., 2005), are also in line with this hypothesis. However, recent data have shown that rTMS did not always work on seizures, and that stimulation site and structural brain lesions did not necessarily influence the seizure outcome (Joo et al., 2007). Thus, although most studies have found a significant decrease of interictal EEG epileptiform abnormalities, which supports a detectable biologic effect, additional trials are needed to ascertain whether rTMS is an effective and convenient method for stimulation in epilepsy. In that respect, a placebo-controlled study is in progress in Strasbourg (France), aiming at evaluating the efficacy of rTMS in the specific group of patients suffering from drug-resistant seizures arising from the sensorimotor cortex.

Direct cortical stimulation

Several preclinical studies have found potential antiepileptic effects of brain stimulation in animal models. Notably, low frequency (1 Hz) stimulation applied after kindling stimulation of the amygdala was found to inhibit the development of afterdischarges, an effect named *quenching* (Weiss et al., 1995). This quenching effect seems effective in adult as well as immature rats (Velisek et al., 2002). Interestingly, when applied immediately before the kindling stimulus, preemptive 1 Hz sine wave stimulation was also effective, thus suggesting some potential benefit for seizure prevention (Goodman et al., 2005). Other regions such as the hippocampus or the central piriform cortex may also serve as potentially effective targets for 1 Hz stimulation treatment of epilepsy (Barbarosie & Avoli, 1997; Zhu-Ge et al., 2007).

In humans, both low- (around 1 Hz) and high- (around 50 Hz) frequency stimulation have proven effective to reduce interictal epileptiform discharges (Kinoshita et al., 2005b; Yamamoto et al., 2002). Therapeutic stimulation, however, was applied at high frequency in almost all studies. The first attempt of therapeutic stimulation of temporal lobe structures was reported in 1980, in three patients, without clear benefit (Sramka et al., 1980). More recently, several investigators have tried continuous scheduled stimulation of epileptic foci, including hypothalamic hamartoma (Kahane et al., 2003), neo-cortical structures

(Elisevich et al., 2006) and, mostly, mesio-temporal lobe (Tellez-Zenteno et al., 2006; Velasco et al., 2000c; 2007; Vonck et al., 2002). The first pilot study of mesio-temporal lobe stimulation, conducted in 10 patients studied by intracranial electrodes before surgery, showed that stimulation stopped seizures and decreased the number of interictal EEG spikes in the 7 patients in whom the stimulated electrode was placed within the hippocampus or hippocampal gyrus (Velasco et al., 2000c). There were no side-effects on language and memory, and no histological damage was found in the stimulated tissue. Whether such an antiepileptic effect could be observed over a more prolonged stimulation procedure was later evaluated in a small open series conducted in three patients, all of whom exhibited more than 50% of seizure reduction after a mean follow-up of 5 months, without adverse events (Vonck et al., 2002). Following this, two additional trials of hippocampal stimulation were conducted, leading to opposing results. Seizure outcome was dramatically improved in all 9 patients of the double-blind long-term follow-up study of Velasco et al. (2007), which showed more than 95% seizure reduction in the 5 patients with normal MRI, and 50-70% seizure reduction in the 4 patients who had hippocampal sclerosis. No adverse events were found but three patients were explanted after 2 years due to skin erosion in the trajectory system. It was suggested that beneficial effects of stimulation were associated with a high GABA tissue content and a low rate of cell loss (Cuellar-Herrera et al., 2004). By opposition, seizure frequency was reduced by only 15% in average in the 4 patients of the double-blind, multiple cross-over, randomized study of Tellez-Zenteno et al. (2006), and the results were not significant. Additionally, effects seemed to carry over into the off period, thus raising the issue of an implantation effect. Yet, no adverse events were found. Overall, stimulation of hippocampal foci shows beneficial trends, but whether the effect size is high or weak, and of clear clinical relevance, remains debatable.

Closed-loop stimulation

Continuous scheduled brain stimulation, whatever the target (DBS, cortical stimulation), has appeared to be safe and of potential benefit in treating medically intractable epilepsies (see above). Limited, but growing experience suggests that responsive (seizure-triggered) stimulation might also be effective (Morrel, 2006). Such a strategy is distinct from continuous scheduled stimulation in that it aims at blocking seizures acutely, rather than at decreasing cortical excitability on a chronic basis. In addition to a cranially implanted device, this requires a seizure-detection algorithm which in turn allows delivery of stimulation to interrupt seizure prior to the onset of clinical symptoms. A number of such algorithms do exist, but optimal stimulation parameters to abort seizures have not been clearly established. In humans, responsive stimulation can shorten or terminate electrically-elicited afterdischarges using brief bursts of 50 Hz electrical stimulation (Lesser et al., 1999), the effect being greater at primary sites than at adjacent electrodes (Motamedi et al., 2002). Preliminary trials of responsive stimulation, however, did not consistently use a similar paradigm (Fountas et al., 2005; Kossof et al., 2004; Osorio et al., 2005). The effects of responsive stimulation were first evaluated in 4 patients using an external neurostimulator, which proved effective at automatically detecting electrographic seizures, delivering targeted electrical stimuli, and altering or suppressing ictal discharges (Kossov et al., 2004). Another feasibility study confirmed these results using a cranially implantable device in 8 patients (Fountas et al., 2005). Detection and stimulation were performed using electrodes placed over the seizure focus, and seven of the 8 patients exhibited more than a 45% decrease in their seizure frequency, with a mean follow-up time of 9.2 months. In the third pilot study, conducted in 8 patients, stimulation was delivered either directly to the epileptogenic zone (local closed-loop, n = 4), or indirectly through the anterior thalami (remote closed-loop, n = 4), depending on whether the epileptogenic zone was single, or multiple (Osorio et al., 2005). On average, a 55.5% and 40.8% decrease of seizure frequency was observed in the local closed-loop group and in the remote closed-loop, respectively. Overall, none of the 20 patients enrolled in these three pilot studies had adverse events. Although promising, this new therapy needs further evaluation and a multi-institutional prospective clinical trial is underway in the USA. Whether, in the near future, closed-loop stimulators will be able to react using seizure-prediction algorithms represents a particularly challenging issue.

■ Conclusions

Neurostimulation in nonsurgically remediable epileptic patients represents an emerging treatment. It has the advantages of reversibility and adjustability, but it remains palliative so that surgical resection remains the gold standard treatment of drug-resistant epilepsies whenever this option is possible. VNS is the only approved stimulation therapy for epilepsy and, as such, it is licensed in many countries as an adjunctive therapy. Other stimulation techniques must be considered experimental. Notably, results of direct brain stimulation, although encouraging, are not conclusive and further investigations are required to evaluate the real benefit of this emerging therapy, in as much as the risks of haemorrhage and infection, although low (around 5%), do exist. However, pathological examination in post-mortem studies and temporal lobe resection, in Parkinson's disease or epilepsy, suggest that chronic stimulation does not induce neural injury and can be delivered safely (Haberler et al., 2000; Pilitsis et al., 2008; Velasco et al., 2000c). In any case, seizure types or epileptic syndromes which may respond to stimulation should be identified, as well as the type of stimulation that is likely to be of potential efficacy depending on the patient's characteristics. This requires to improve our knowledge on the neural circuits in which seizures start and propagate, to better understand the precise mechanisms of the supposed effect of neurostimulation, and to search for optimal stimulation parameters. The development of experimental research in this field, as well as rigorous clinical evaluation, is essential for further improvements in clinical efficacy.

References

Akamatsu N, Fueta Y, Endo Y, Matsunaga K, Uozumi T, Tsuji S. Decreased susceptibility to pentylenetetrazole-inducded seizures after low frequency transcranial magnetic stimulation in the rat. *Neurosci Lett* 2001; 310: 153-6.

Andi OJ, Jurko MF. Seizure control by mesothalamic reticular stimulation. *Clin Electroencephalography* 1986; 17: 52-60.

Arduini D, Lary Bounes GC. Action de la stimulation électrique de la formation réticulaire du bulbe et des stimulations sensorielles sur les ondes strychniques. *Electroencephalogr Clin Neurophysiol* 1952; 4: 502-12.

Annegers J, Coan SP, Hauser WA, Lesteema J. Epilepsy, vagal nerve stimulation by the NCP system, all-cause mortality, and sudden, unexpected, unexplained death. *Epilepsia* 2000; 41: 549-53.

Barbarosie M, Avoli M. CA3-driven hippocampal-entorhinal loop controls rather than sustains in vitro limbic seizures. *J Neurosci* 1997; 17: 9308-14.

Ben-Menachem E. Vagus nerve stimulation, side effects, and long-term safety. *J Clin Neurophysiol* 2001; 18: 415-8.

Ben-Menachem E, Hellström K, Verstappen D. Analysis of direct hospital costs before and 18 months after treatment with vagus nerve stimulation therapy in 43 patients. *Neurology* 2002; 59 (suppl 4): S44-S47.

Benabid AL, Koudsié A, Benazzouz A, Vercueil L, Fraix V, Chabardès S, Lebas JF, Pollak P. Deep brain stimulation of the corpus luysi (subthalamic nucleus) and other targets in Parkinson's disease. Extension to new indications such as dystonia and epilepsy. *J Neurol* 2001; 248 (suppl 3): III37-47.

Benabid AL, Minotti L, Koudsie A, de Saint Martin A, Hirsch E. Antiepileptic effect of high-frequency stimulation of the subthalamic nucleus (corpus luysi) in a case of medically intractable epilepsy caused by focal dysplasia: a 30-month follow-up: technical case report. *Neurosurgery* 2002; 50: 1385-91.

Biraben A, Semah F, Ribeiro MJ, Douaud G, Remy P, Depaulis A. PET evidence for a role of the basal ganglia in patients with ring chromosome 20 epilepsy. *Neurology* 2004; 63: 73-7.

Boon P, Vonck K, D'Have M, O'Connor S, Vandekerckhove T, De Reuck J. Cost-benefit of vagus nerve stimulation for refractory epilepsy. *Acta Neurol Belg* 1999; 99: 275-80.

Bouilleret V, Semah F, Chassoux F, Mantzaridez M, Biraben A, Trebossen R, Ribeiro MJ. Basal ganglia involvement in temporal lobe epilepsy: a functional and morphologic study. *Neurology* 2008; 70: 177-84.

Brasil-Neto JP, de Arauja DP, Teixeira WA, Araujo VP, Boechat-Barros R. *Arq Neuropsiquiatr* 2004; 62: 21-5.

Cantello R, Rossi S, Varrasi C, *et al*. Slow repetitive TMS for drug-resistant epilepsy: clinical and EEG findings of a placebo-controlled trial. *Epilepsia* 2007; 48: 366-74.

Chabardès S, Kahane P, Minotti L, Koudsie A, Hirsch E, Benabid A-L. Deep brain stimulation in epilepsy with particular reference to the subthalamic nucleus. *Epileptic disord* 2002; 4 (suppl 3): 83-93.

Chen R, Classen J, Gerloff C, *et al*. Depression of motor cortex excitability by low-frequency transcranial magnetic stimulation. *Neurology* 1997; 48: 1398-403.

Chkhenkeli SA. The inhibitory influence of the nucleus caudatus electrostimulation on the human's amygdalar and hippocampal activity at temporal lobe epilepsy. *Bull Georgian Acad Sci* 1978; 4/6: 406-11.

Chkhenkeli SA, Chkhenkeli IS. Effects of therapeutic stimulation of nucleus caudatus on epileptic electrical activity of brain in patients with intractable epilepsy. *Stereotact Funct Neurosurg* 1997; 69: 221-4.

Clark KB, Naritoku DK, Smith DC, Browning RA, Jensen RA. Enhanced recognition memory following vagus nerve stimulation in human subjects. *Nat Neurosci* 1999; 2: 94-8.

Cooke PM, Snider RS. Some cerebellar influences on electrically-induced cerebral seizures. *Epilepsia* 1955; 4: 19-28.

Cooper I. *Cerebellar stimulation in man*. New York: Raven Press, 1978: 1-212.

Cooper IS, Amin I, Riklan M, Waltz JM, Poon TP. Chronic cerebellar stimulation in epilepsy. Clinical and anatomical studies. *Arch Neurol* 1976; 33: 559-70.

Cooper IS, Upton ARM. The effect of chronic stimulation of cerebellum and thalamus upon neurophysiology and neurochemistry of cerebral cortex. In: Lazorthes Y, Upton ARM (eds). *Neurostimulation: an overview*. New York: Futura, 1985: 207-11.

Cooper IS, Amin I, Gilman S. The effect of chronic cerebellar stimulation upon epilepsy in man. *Trans Am Neurol Assoc* 1973; 98: 192-6.

Cuellar-Herrera M, Velasco M, Velasco F, Velasco AL, Jimenez F, Orozco S, Briones M, Rocha L. Evaluation of GABA system and cell damage in parahippocampus of patients with temporal lobe epilepsy showing antiepileptic effects after subacute electrical stimulation. *Epilepsia* 2004; 45: 459-66.

Danober L, Deransart C, Depaulis A, Vergnes M, Marescaux C. Pathophysiological mechanisms of genetic absence, epilepsy in rat. *Progr Neuronal* 1998; 55: 27-57.

Davis R, Emmonds SE. Cerebellar stimulation for seizure control: 17-year study. *Stereotact Funct Neurosurg* 1992; 58: 200-8.

Depaulis A, Vergnes M, Depaulis A. Endogenous control of epilepsy: the nigral inhibitory system. *Prog Neurobiol* 1994; 42: 33-52.

Deransart C, Depaulis A. The control of seizures by the basal ganglia? A review of experimental data. *Epileptic Disord* 2002; 4 (suppl 3): S61-S72.

Deransart C, Marescaux C, Depaulis A. Involvement of nigral glutamatergic inputs in the control of seizures in a genetic model of absence epilepsy in the rat. *Neuroscience* 1996; 71: 721-8.

Deransart C, Riban V, Lê BT, Marescaux C, Depaulis A. Dopamine in the nucleus accumbens modulates seizures in a genetic model of absence epilepsy in the rat. *Neuroscience* 2000; 100: 335-44.

Dodrill CB, Morris GL. Effects of Vagal Nerve Stimulation on Cognition and Quality of Life in Epilepsy. *Epilepsy Behav* 2001; 2: 46-53.

Dow RS, Ferandez-Guardiola A, Manni E. The influence of the cerebellum on experimental epilepsy. Electroencephalogr *Clin Neurophysiol* 1962; 14: 383-98.

Duprez TP, Serieh BA, Raftopoulos C. Absence of memory dysfunction after bilateral mammillary body and mammillothalamic tract electrode implantation: preliminary experience in three patients. *AJNR Am J Neuroradiol* 2005; 26: 195-7.

Ebner TJ, Bantli H, Bloedel JR. Effects of cerebellar stimulation on unitary activity within a chronic epileptic focus in a primate. *Electroencephalogr Clin Neurophysiol* 1980; 49: 585-99.

Elisevich K, Jenrow K, Schuh L, Smith B. Long-term electrical stimulation-induced inhibition of partial epilepsy. Case report. *J Neurosurg* 2006; 105: 894-7.

Feddersen B, Vercueil L, Noachtar S, David O, Depaulis A, Deransart C. Controlling seizures is not controlling epilepsy: a parametric study of deep brain stimulation for epilepsy. *Neurobiol Dis* 2007; 27: 292-300.

Fisher RS, Uematsu S, Krauss GL, *et al.* Placebo-controlled pilot study of centromedian thalamic stimulation in treatment of intractable seizures. *Epilepsia* 1992; 33: 841-51.

Fountas KN, Smith JR, Murro AM, Politsky J, Park YD, Jenkins PD. Implantation of a closed-loop stimulation in the management of medically refractory focal epilepsy: a technical note. *Stereotact Funct Neurosurg* 2005; 83: 153-8.

Fregni F, Otachi PT, Do Valle A, *et al.* A randomized clinical trial of repetitive transcranial magnetic stimulation in patients with refractory epilepsy. *Ann Neurol* 2006; 60: 447-55.

Goodman JH, Berger RE, Tcheng TK. Preemptive low-frequency stimulation decreases the incidence of amygdala-kindled seizures. *Epilepsia* 2005; 46: 1-7.

Haberler C, *et al.* No tissue damage by chronic deep brain stimulation in Parkinson's disease. *Ann Neurol* 2000; 42: 372-6.

Harden CL, Pulver MC, Ravdin LD, Nikolov B, Halper JP, Labar DR. A Pilot Study of Mood in Epilepsy Patients Treated with Vagus Nerve Stimulation. *Epilepsy Behav* 2000; 1: 93-9.

Hamani C, Ewerton FI, Bonilha SM, Ballester G, Mello LE, Lozano AM. Bilateral anterior thalamic nucleus lesions and high-frequency stimulation are protective against pilocarpine-induced seizures and status epilepticus. *Neurosurgery* 2004; 54: 191-5.

Handforth A, DeGiorgio CM, Schachter SC. Vagus nerve stimulation therapy for partial-onset seizures: a randomized active-control trial. *Neurology* 1998; 51: 48-55.

Henry TR, Bakay RA, Votaw JR, *et al*. Brain blood flow alterations induced by therapeutic vagus nerve stimulation in partial epilepsy, I: acute effects at high and low levels of stimulation. *Epilepsia* 1998; 39: 983-90.

Henry TR, Votaw JR, Pennell PB, *et al*. Acute blood flow changes and efficacy of vagus nerve stimulation in partial epilepsy. *Neurology* 1999; 52: 1166-73.

Henry TR. Therapeutic mechanisms of vagus nerve stimulation. *Neurology* 2002; 59 (suppl 4): S3-S14.

Hodaie M, Wennberg RA, Dostrovsky JO, Lozano AM. Chronic anterior thalamus stimulation for intractable epilepsy. *Epilepsia* 2002; 43: 603-8.

Jasper H. Current evaluation of the concepts of centrencephalic and cortico-reticular seizures. *Electroencephalogr Clin Neurophysiol* 1991; 78: 2-11.

Jennum P, Klitgaard H. Repetitive transcranial magnetic stimulations of the rat. Effect of acute and chronic stimulations on pentylenetetrazole-induced clonic seizures. *Epilepsy Res* 1996; 23: 115-22.

Joo EY, Han SJ, Chung S-H, Cho J-W, Seo DW, Hong SB. Antiepileptic effects of low frequency repetitive transcranial magnetic stimulation by different stimulation durations and locations. *Clinical Neurophysiology* 2007; 118: 702-8.

Kahane P, Ryvlin P, Hoffmann D, Minotti L, Benabid AL. From hypothalamic hamartoma to cortex: what can be learnt from depth recordings and stimulation? *Epileptic Disord* 2003; 5: 205-17.

Kerrigan JF, Litt B, Fisher RS, *et al*. Electrical stimulation of the anterior nucleus of the thalamus for the treatment of intractable epilepsy. *Epilepsia* 2004; 45: 346-54.

Kinoshita M, Ikeda A, Begum T, Yamamoto J, Hitomi T, Shibasaki H. Low-frequency repetitive transcranial magnetic stimulation for seizure suppression in patients with extratemporal lobe epilepsy – a pilot study. *Seizure* 2005a; 14: 387-92.

Kinoshita M, Ikeda A, Matsuhashi M, *et al*. Electric cortical stimulation suppresses epileptic and background activities in neo-cortical epilepsy and mesial temporal lobe epilepsy. *Clin Neurophysiol* 2005b; 116: 1291-9.

Ko D, Heck C, Grafton S, *et al*. Vagus nerve stimulation activates central nervous system structures in epileptic patients during PET H2(15)O blood flow imaging. *Neurosurgery* 1996; 39: 426-30.

Kobayashi M, Pascual-Leone A. Transcranial magnetic stimulation in neurology. *Lancet Neurol* 2003; 2: 145-56.

Kossoff EH, Ritzl EK, Politsky JM, *et al*. Effect of an external responsive neurostimulator on seizures and electrographic discharges during subdural electrode monitoring. *Epilepsia* 2004; 45: 1560-7.

Krauss GL, Fisher RS. Cerebellar and thalamic stimulation for epilepsy. *Adv Neurol* 1993; 63: 231-45.

Kwan P, Brodie M. Early identification of refractory epilepsy. *N Engl J Med* 2000; 342: 314-9.

Labar DR. Antiepileptic drug use during the first 12 months of vagus nerve stimulation therapy: a registry study. *Neurology* 2002; 59 (suppl 4): S38-S43.

Lado FA. Chronic bilateral stimulation of the anterior thalamus of kainate-treated rats increases seizure frequency. *Epilepsia* 2006; 47: 27-32.

La Grutta V, Amato G, Zagami MT. The importance of the caudate nucleus in the control of convulsive activity in the amygdaloid complex and the temporal cortex of the cat. *Electroencephalogr Clin Neurophysiol* 1971; 31: 57-69.

La Grutta V, Sabatino M, Gravante G, Morici G, Ferraro G, La Grutta G. A study of caudate inhibition on an epileptic focus in the cat hippocampus. *Arch Int Physiol Biochim* 1988; 96: 113-20.

Lesser RP, Kim SH, Beyderman L, *et al*. Brief bursts of pulse stimulation terminate afterdischarges caused by cortical stimulation. *Neurology* 1999; 53: 2073-81.

Lim SN, Lee ST, Tsai YT, *et al*. Electrical stimulation of the anterior nucleus of the thalamus for intractable epilepsy: a long term follow-up study. *Epilepsia* 2007; 48: 342-7.

Liu WC, Mosier K, Kalnin AJ, Marks D. BOLD fMRI activation induced by vagus nerve stimulation in seizure patients. *J Neurol Neurosurg Psychiatry* 2003; 74: 811-3.

Lockard JS, Ojemann GA, Congdon WC, DuCharme LL. Cerebellar stimulation in alumina-gel monkey model: inverse relationship between clinical seizures and EEG interictal bursts. *Epilepsia* 1979; 20: 223-34.

Lockard JS, Congdon WC, DuCharme LL. Feasibility and safety of vagal stimulation in monkey model. *Epilepsia* 1990; 31 (suppl 2): S20-S26.

Loddenkemper T, Pan A, Neme S, *et al.* Deep brain stimulation in epilepsy. *J Clin Neurophysiol* 2001; 18: 514-32.

Majkowski J, Karlinski A, Klimowicz-Mlodzik I. Effect of cerebellar stimulation of hippocampal epileptic discharges in kindling preparation. *Monogr Neural Sci* 1980; 5: 40-5.

Malow BA, Edwards J, Marzec M, Sagher O, Ross D, Fromes G. Vagus nerve stimulation reduces daytime sleepiness in epilepsy patients. *Neurology* 2001; 57: 879-84.

Marescaux C, Vergnes M, Depaulis A. Genetic absence epilepsy in rats from Strasbourg. *J Neurol Trans Suppl* 1992; 35: 37-69.

McLachlan RS. Suppression of interictal spikes and seizures by stimulation of the vagus nerve. *Epilepsia* 1993; 34: 918-23.

Menkes DL, Gruenthal M. Slow-frequency repetitive transcranial magnetic stimulation in a patient with focal cortical dysplasia. *Epilepsia* 2000; 4: 240-2.

Mirski MA, Ferrendelli JA. Interruption of the mammillothalamic tract prevents seizures in guinea pigs. *Science* 1984; 226: 72-4.

Mirski MA, Ferrendelli JA. Anterior thalamic mediation of generalized pentylenetetrazol seizures. *Brain Res* 1986a; 399: 212-23.

Mirski MA, Ferrendelli JA. Selective metabolic activation of the mammillary bodies and their connections during ethosuximide-induced suppression of pentylenetetrazol seizures. *Epilepsia* 1986b; 27: 194-203.

Mirski MA, Fisher RS. Electrical stimulation of the mammillary nuclei increases seizure threshold to pentylenetetrazol in rats. *Epilepsia* 1994; 35: 1309-16.

Mirski MA, Rossell LA, Terry JB, Fisher RS. Anticonvulsant effect of anterior thalamic high frequency electrical stimulation in the rat. *Epilepsy Res* 1997; 28: 89-100.

Misawa S, Kuwabara S, Shibuya K, Mamada K, Hattori T. Low-frequency transcranial magnetic stimulation for epilepsia partialis continua due to cortical dysplasia. *J Neurol Sci* 2005; 234: 37-9.

Morrell M. Brain stimulation for epilepsy: can scheduled or responsive neurostimulation stop seizures? *Curr Opin Neurol* 2006; 19: 164-8.

Morris GL 3rd, Mueller WM. Long-term treatment with vagus nerve stimulation in patients with refractory epilepsy. The Vagus Nerve Stimulation Study Group E01-E05. *Neurology* 1999; 53: 1731-5.

Motamedi GK, Lesser RP, Miglioretti DL, *et al.* Optimizing parameters for terminating cortical afterdischarges with pulse stimulation. *Epilepsia* 2002; 43: 836-46.

Mutani R. Experimental evidence for the existence of an extrarhinencephalic control of the activity of the cobalt rhinencephalic epileptogenic focus, part 1: the role played by the caudate nucleus. *Epilepsia* 1969; 10: 337-50.

Mutani R, Bergamini L, Doriguzzi T. Experimental evidence for the existence of an extrarhinencephalic control of the activity of the cobalt rhinencephalic epileptogenic focus. Part 2. Effects of the paleocerebellar stimulation. *Epilepsia* 1969; 10: 351-62.

Nail-Boucherie K, Lê-Pham BT, Gobaille S, Maitre M, Aunis D, Depaulis A. Evidence for a role of the parafascicular nucleus of the thalamus in the control of epileptic seizures by the superior colliculus. *Epilepsia* 2005; 46: 141-5.

Nanobashvili Z, Chachua T, Nanobashvili A, Bilanishvili I, Lindvall O, Kokaia Z. Suppression of limbic motor seizures by electrical stimulation in thalamic reticular nucleus. *Exp Neurol* 2003; 181: 224-30.

Narayanan JT, Watts R, Haddad N, Labar DR, LiPM, Filippi CG. Cerebral activation during vagus nerve stimulation: a functional MR study. *Epilepsia* 2002; 43: 1509-14.

Oakley JC, Ojemann GA. Effects of chronic stimulation of the caudate nucleus on a preexisting alumina seizure focus. *Exp Neurol* 1982; 75: 360-7.

Oommen J, Morrell M, Fisher RS. Experimental electrical stimulation for epilepsy. *Curr Treat Options Neurol* 2005; 7: 261-71.

Osorio I, Frein MG, Sunderam S, *et al*. Automated seizure abatement in humans using electrical stimulation. *Ann Neurol* 2005; 57: 258-68.

Osorio I, Overman J, Giftakis J, Wilkinson SB. High frequency thalamic stimulation for inoperable mesial temporal epilepsy. *Epilepsia* 2007; 48: 1561-71.

Paz JT, Deniau JM, Charpier S. Rhythmic Bursting in the Cortico-Subthalamo-Pallidal Network during Spontaneous Genetically Determined Spike and Wave Discharges. *J Neurosci* 2005; 25: 2092-101.

Paz JT, Chavez M, Saillet S, Deniau JM, Charpier S. Activity of ventral medial thalamic neurons during absence seizures and modulation of cortical paroxysms by the nigrothalamic pathway. *J Neurosci* 2007; 27: 929-41.

Penry JK, Dean JC. Prevention of intractable partial seizures by intermittent vagal stimulation in humans: preliminary results. *Epilepsia* 1990; 31 (suppl 2): S40-S43.

Pilitis JG, *et al*. Postmortem study of deep brain stimulation in the anterior thalamus: case report. *Neurosurgery* 2008; 62: 530-2.

Polkey CE. Alternative surgical procedures ti help drug-resistant epilepsy – a review. *Epileptic Disord* 2003; 5: 63-75.

Psatta DM. Control of chronic experimental focal epilepsy by feedback caudatum stimulations. *Epilepsia* 1983; 24: 444-54.

Santiago-Rodriguez E, Cardenas-Morales L, Harmony T, Fernandez-Bouzas A, Porras-Kattz E, Hernandez A. Repetitive transcranial magnetic stimulation decreases the number of seizures in patients with focal neo-cortical epilepsy. *Seizure* 2008; May 19.

Semah F. PET imaging in epilepsy: basal ganglia and thalamic involvement. *Epileptic Disord* 2002; 4 (suppl 3): S55-S60.

Sranka M, Fritz G, Gajdosova D, Nadvomik P. Central stimulation treatment of epilepsy. *Acta Neurochir* Suppl 1980; 30: 183-7.

Tassinari CA, Cincotta M, Zaccara G, Michelucci R. Transcranial magnetic stimulation and epilepsy. *Clin Neurophysiol* 2003; 114: 777-98.

Taylor RB, Wennberg RA, Lozano AM, Sharpe JA. Central nystagmus induced by deep-brain stimulation for epilepsy. *Epilepsia* 2000; 41: 1637-41.

Takaya M, Terry WJ, Naritoku DK. Vagus nerve stimulation induces a sustained anticonvulsant effect. *Epilepsia* 1996; 37: 1111-6.

Tellez-Zenteno JF, McLachlan RS, Parrent A, Kubu CS, Wiebe S. Hippocampal electrical stimulation in mesial temporal lobe epilepsy. *Neurology* 2006; 66: 1490-4.

Tergau F, Naumann U, Paulus W, Steinhoff BJ. Low-frequency repetitive transcranial magnetic stimulation improves intractable epilepsy. *Lancet* 1999; 353: 2209.

Theodore WH, Fisher RS. Brain stimulation for epilepsy. *Lancet Neurol* 2004; 3: 111-8.

Theodore WH, Hunter K, Chen R, *et al*. Transcranial magnetic stimulation for the treatment of seizures: a controlled study. *Neurology* 2002; 59: 560-2.

The Vagus Nerve Stimulation Study Group. A randomized controlled trial of chronic vagus nerve stimulation for treatment of medically intractable seizures. *Neurology* 1995; 45: 224-30.

Van Buren JM, Wood JH, Oakley J, Hambrecht F. Preliminary evaluation of cerebellar stimulation by double blind stimulation and biological criteria in the treatment of epilepsy. *J Neurosurg* 1978; 48: 407-16.

Van Laere K, Vonck K, Boon P, Brans B, Vandekerckhove T, Dierckx R. Vagus nerve stimulation in refractory epilepsy: SPECT activation study. *J Nucl Med* 2000; 41: 1145-54.

van Rijckevorsel K, Abu Serieh B, de Tourtchaninoff M, Raftopoulos C. Deep EEG recordings of the mammillary body in epilepsy patients. *Epilepsia* 2005; 46: 781-5.

Velasco F, Velasco M, Cepeda C, Munoz H. Wakefulness-sleep modulation of thalamic multiple unit activity and EEG in man. *Electroencephalogr Clin Neurophysiol* 1979; 47: 597-606.

Velasco F, Velasco M, Ogarrio C, Fanghanel G. Electrical stimulation of the centromedian thalamic nucleus in the treatment of convulsive seizures: a preliminary report. *Epilepsia* 1987; 28: 421-30.

Velasco F, Velasco M, Velasco AL, Jimenez F. Effect of chronic electrical stimulation of the centromedian thalamic nuclei on various intractable seizure patterns, I: clinical seizures and paroxysmal EEG activity. *Epilepsia* 1993; 34: 1052-64.

Velasco F, Velasco M, Velasco AL, Jimenez F, Marquez I, Rise M. Electrical stimulation of the centromedian thalamic nucleus in control of seizures: long term studies. *Epilepsia* 1995; 36: 63-71.

Velasco F, Velasco M, Jimenez F, et al. Predictors in the treatment of difficult to control seizures by electrical stimulation of the centromedian thalamic nucleus. *Neurosurgery* 2000a; 47: 295-305.

Velasco M, Velasco F, Velasco AL, Jimenez F, Brito F, Marquez I. Acute and chronic electrical stimulation of the centromedian thalamic nucleus: modulation of reticulo-cortical systems and predictor factors for generalized seizure control. *Arch Med Res* 2000b; 31: 304-15.

Velasco M, Velasco F, Velasco AL, et al. Subacute electrical stimulation of the hippocampus blocks intractable temporal lobe seizures and paroxysmal EEG activities. *Epilepsia* 2000c; 41: 158-69.

Velasco F, Velasco M, Jimenez F, Velasco AL, Marquez I. Stimulation of the central median thalamic nucleus for epilepsy. *Stereotact Funct Neurosurg* 2001a; 77: 228-32.

Velasco M, Velasco F, Velasco AL. Centromedian-thalamic and hippocampal electrical stimulation for the control of intractable epileptic seizures. *J Clin Neurophysiol* 2001b; 18: 495-513.

Velasco F, Velasco M, Jimenez F, Velasco AL, Rojas B. Centromedian nucleus stimulation for epilepsy. Clinical, electroencephalographic, and behavioral observations. *Thalamus & Related systems* 2002; 1: 387-98.

Velasco F, Carrillo-Ruiz JD, Brto F, et al. double-blind, randomized controlled pilot study of bilateral cerebellar stimulation for treatment of intractable motor seizures. *Epilepsia* 2005; 46: 1071-81.

Velasco AL, Velasco F, Jimenez F, et al. Neuromodulation of the centromedian thalamic nuclei in the treatment of generalized seizures and the improvement of the quality of life in patients with Lennox-Gastaut syndrome. *Epilepsia* 2006; 47: 1203-12.

Velasco AL, Velasco F, Velasco M, Trejo D, Castro G, Carrillo-Ruiz JD. Electrical stimulation of the hippocampal epileptic foci for seizure control: a double-blind, long-term follow-up study. *Epilepsia* 2007; 48: 1895-903.

Velisek L, Velsikova J, Stanton PK. Low-frequency stimulation of the kindling focus delays basolateral amygdala kindling in immature rats. *Neurosci Lett* 2002; 326: 61-3.

Vercueil L, Hirsch E. Seizures and the basal ganglia: a review of the clinical data. *Epileptic Disord* 2002; 4 (suppl 3): S47-S54.

Vercueil L, Benazzouz A, Deransart C, et al. High-frequency stimulation of the sub-thalamic nucleus suppresses absence seizures in the rat: comparison with neurotoxic lesions. *Epilepsy Res* 1998; 31: 39-46.

Vesper J, Steinhoff B, Rona S, et al. Chronic high-frequency deep brain stimulation of the STN/SNr for progressive myoclonic epilepsy. *Epilepsia* 2007; 48: 1984-9.

Vonck K, Boon P, Van Laere K, et al. Acute single photon emission computed tomographic study of vagus nerve stimulation in refractory epilepsy. *Epilepsia* 2000; 41: 601-9.

Vonck K, Van Laere K, Dedeurwaerdere S, Caemaert J, De Reuck J, Boon P. The mechanism of action of vagus nerve stimulation for refractory epilepsy. *J Clin Neurophysiol* 2001; 18: 394-401.

Vonck K, Boon P, Achten E, De Reuck J, Caemaert J. Long-term amygdalohippocampal stimulation for refractory temporal lobe epilepsy. *Ann Neurol* 2002; 52: 556-65.

Vonck K, Boon P, Van Roost D. Anatomical and physiological basis and mechanism of action of neurostimulation for epilepsy. *Acta Neurochir* 2007; 97 (suppl): 321-8.

Wassermann EM, Lisanby SH. Therapeutic application of repetitive transcranial magnetic stimulation: a review. *Clin Neurophysiol* 2001; 112: 1367-77.

Weiss SRB, Li XL, Rosen JB, Li H, Heynen T, Post RM. Quenching: inhibition of the development and expression of amygdala kindled seizures with low frequency stimulation. *Neuroreport* 1995; 4: 2171-6.

Wheless JW, Maggio V. Vagus nerve stimulation therapy in patients younger than 18 years. *Neurology* 2002; 59 (suppl 4): S21-S25.

Wright GD, Mc Lellan DL, Brice JG. A double-blind trial of chronic cerebellar stimulation in twelve patients with severe epilepsy. *J Neurol Neurosurg Psychiatry* 1984; 47: 769-74.

Yamamoto J, Ikeda A, Satow T, *et al*. Low-frequency electric cortical stimulation has an inhibitory effect on cortical focus in mesial temporal lobe epilepsy. *Epilepsia* 2002; 43: 491-5.

Zhu-Ge ZB, Zhu YY, Wu DC, *et al*. Unilateral low-frequency stimulation of central piriform cortex inhibits amygdaloid-kindled seizures in Sprague-Dawley rats. *Neuroscience* 2007; 146: 901-6.

Zumsteg D, Lozano AM, Wennberg RA. Mesial temporal inhibition in a patient with deep brain stimulation of the anterior thalamus for epilepsy. *Epilepsia* 2006; 47: 1958-62.

Beyond seizure reduction

Frank G. Gilliam and Piero Perucca

Department of Neurology, Columbia University, New York, USA

This chapter is written on the 10th anniversary of the publication of the final report of the Commission on Outcome Measurement in Epilepsy (COME) (Baker *et al.*, 1998), a remarkable document that elucidated the need for more complete, patient-oriented assessments of the results of epilepsy interventions. Interestingly, a major portion of the paper focused on the interictal state:

"Although by definition, epilepsy is a condition characterized by brief paroxysmal disturbances of brain function, the supposition that between seizures every person with epilepsy reverts to a condition without epilepsy is obviously too optimistic. The mere need for uninterrupted AED therapy implies a risk of treatment-emergent adverse events (AE). Symptomatic epilepsies are a co-morbidity, with disorders affecting the brain and, as indicated by the label cryptogenic, probably many more epilepsies than those diagnosed as symptomatic fall into that category. The primary brain disorder itself may determine to a great extent the condition of the person with epilepsy in the interictal period. Accurate recording of the effects of co-morbidity should not be limited to routine neurological, psychological, and psychiatric examination, but should include a measure of quantification" (Baker *et al.*, 1998).

The reader is encouraged to review the COME final report, and carefully consider its clear and insightful recommendations regarding outcomes research in epilepsy. The current chapter will summarize and review some of the advances in patient-oriented research during the past decade.

Epilepsy is a disorder defined by the tendency toward recurrent seizures. In the large majority of persons with epilepsy, the occurrence of the next seizure is unpredictable, and appears as a stochastic event. The results of patient-oriented outcomes research have made evident that complete cessation of seizures allows the greatest improvement in a person's health-related quality of life (HRQOL) (Devinsky, 1995). The impact of a partial reduction of a previously determined seizure rate remains less well defined. Some authors have even suggested that the emphasis of a reduction in seizures (*e.g.*, > 50% reduction from baseline) as a positive result could be misleading (Walker & Sander, 1997).

From a broader social and psychological perspective, epilepsy is a more complex disorder than might be assumed based on a medical definition. Although quality of life in persons with complete seizure control appears to be similar to those without a history of epilepsy, some studies have showed decreased rates of success and achievement in multiple areas of function in adults with a history of epilepsy limited to childhood (Sillanpaa et al., 2004). Such data suggest that even a few seizures can have highly consequential and long lasting effects. On the other hand, the quality of life of persons with recurrent seizures despite optimal treatment may be strongly influenced by non-seizure factors (Baker et al., 1998). Accumulating evidence indicates that multiple influences, such as adverse medication effects, depression, and learning disabilities, may affect overall health status independent of seizure rate (Gilliam, 2002; Boylan et al., 2004; Gilliam et al., 2004; Gilliam et al., 2006; Johnson et al., 2004).

The following sections review and examine the results of studies of health-outcomes in epilepsy that support the contention that quality of life in epilepsy can often be substantially improved, even when recurrent seizures cannot be completely controlled. Although research on the psychosocial effects of epilepsy has an elaborate and extensive history, we will focus on more recent studies that use reliable and valid assessments of health in order to quantify the relative influences on overall health in epilepsy.

Patient-oriented assessments

Prior position statements by groups advocating for health outcomes research, such as the World Health Organization (WHO, 1947), the Agency for Health Policy and Research (Clancy & Eisenberg, 1998), and the International League Against Epilepsy (Baker et al., 1998) have summarized the importance of overall functioning in addition to physiological aspects of illness. A relevant study of persons with recurrent seizures allowed the subjects to rank their concerns; driving, independence, work, education, mood, medication issues, and safety were listed in this rank order of importance by the patients (Figure 1) (Gilliam et al., 1997). The protocol designated termination of the study when 30 consecutive participants provided no new concerns, and so the prospective study ended after the 81st subject. These findings indicate that persons with epilepsy are readily able to designate a well circumscribed set of problems that affect their daily lives.

Driving limitations in epilepsy have been investigated from multiple perspectives, and their importance is unequivocal Driving in the most common and important concern of adults with epilepsy regardless of age (Gilliam et al., 1997; Martin et al., 2005). A history of pharmacoresistance is associated with increased risk of motor vehicle accidents, occurring in one-third of patients (Berg et al., 2000). Additionally, lack of a license to drive may be influenced by demographic and cultural factors, such as sex (Berg et al., 2000; Sillanpaa & Shinnar, 2005). Driving status appears to be associated with quality of life, independent of seizure rate or other epilepsy-related factors (Gilliam et al., 1999). The need to protect driving privileges may influence some patients to underreport seizure occurrences to their physicians, which is a critically important consideration for clinical care and research (Dalrymple & Appleby, 2000).

Employment, education, and cognition also are major concerns of persons with recurrent seizures. Several studies indicate that even pediatric epilepsy that does not continue into adulthood can have long lasting negative effects (Sillanpaa et al., 1998). For example, a prospective cohort study of children diagnosed with epilepsy found that rates of educational achievement, employment, and child-bearing were lower in persons with a prior history of epilepsy compared to non-epilepsy controls (Sillanpaa et al., 2004). Similarly, studies of pediatric epilepsy surgery suggest that parental worry continues at a considerable level even after seizures have abated (Gilliam et al., 1997).

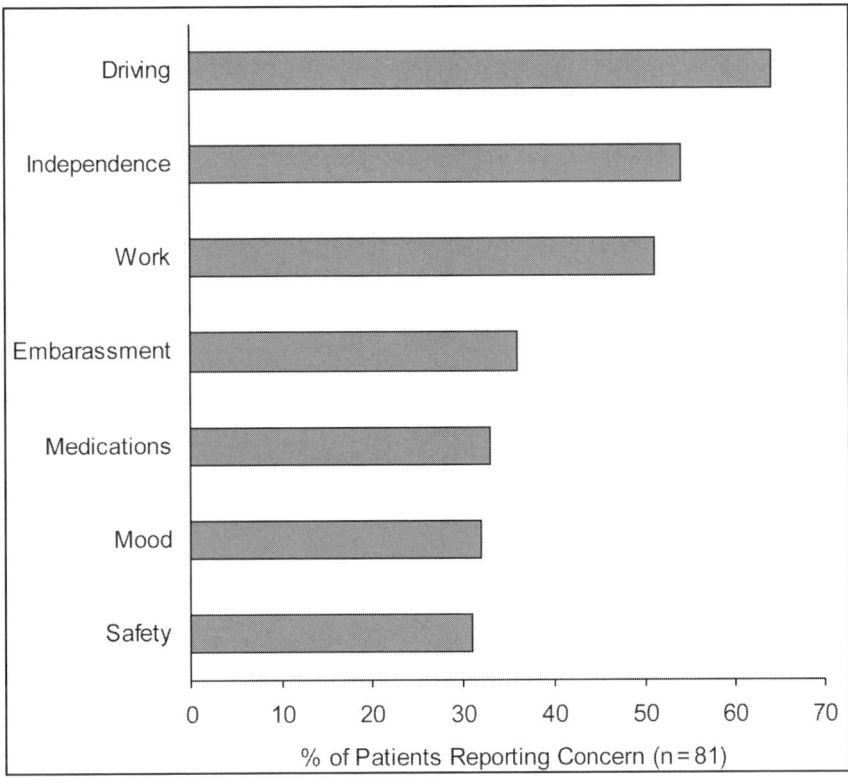

Figure 1. Concerns listed by one-third or more of 81 patients with moderately severe epilepsy (Gilliam et al., 1997).

■ Reliable and valid measures of subjective health status

Health Outcomes researchers in the past 15 years have made substantial advances in methodologies to quantify patient-oriented end-point of epilepsy studies (Devinsky, 1995; Vickrey, 1993; Ware, 1987). The development of the Epilepsy Surgery Inventory (ESI)-55 (Vickrey, 1993) and subsequent Quality of Life in Epilepsy (QOLIE)-89 (Devinsky et al., 1995; Hermann, 1993; Perrine, 1993; Meador, 1993; Leidy et al., 1999) was supported through US samples, while researchers in Europe completed parallel initiatives using other batteries (Baker et al., 1993; Baker, 1998; O'Donoghue et al., 1998). These instruments with established reliability and validity have provided the opportunity to use an external standard to determine the value of traditional clinical variables, such as seizure rate and medication number, from the patients' perspective (Leidy et al., 1999). For example, Vickrey et al. (1994) compared the Short Form-36 postsurgical scores in patients with no seizures, only simple partial seizures, or continued complex partial and/or generalized tonic-clonic seizures to patients with hypertension, diabetes mellitus, heart disease, or depression. Most domains of quality of life were significantly better in the seizure-free group than all other groups, whereas patients with recurrent simple partial seizures had a quality of life in many areas similar to hypertension and diabetes. Recurrent complex partial or generalized tonic-clonic seizures were associated with worse or similar quality of life to heart disease in most areas other than pain and physical function. O'Donoghue et al. (1998, 1999) found similar results in a community-based study using the Subjective Handicap of Epilepsy Scale (SHE).

Table I. Subscales of the quality of life in epilepsy inventory (Devinsky et al., 1995)

Seizure worry	Role limitations-emotional
Medication effect	Social isolation
Health discouragement	Social support
Work/Driving/Social function	Energy/fatigue
Language	Health perceptions
Attention/concentration	Physical function
Memory	Role limitations-physical
Overall quality of life	Pain
Emotional well-being	Overall score

The QOLIE-89 is a representative instrument that was designed to measure HRQOL in epilepsy (Devinsky et al., 1995). It uses the SF-36 (Jacoby et al., 1999; Ware & Kosinski, 2001) as the generic core, and includes an additional 53 items that are more specific to epilepsy. Seventeen subscales are used to evaluate areas of function and wellbeing ranging from cognition and mental health to work, driving, and socialization, as listed in *Table I*. The questions are generally framed in a specific time period, such as "during the past four weeks, how have you had difficulty with your ability to...?". Most items are scored on a Likert-like scale, which provides an adequate range to allow the scales to be correlated with other continuous or ordinal variables. The QOLIE-89, and the shorter 31 and 10 item instruments, have been used in dozens of clinical studies during the past decade, which have provided a more complete and patient-oriented understanding of the multifaceted effects of epilepsy.

■ Adverse antiepileptic medication effects

Toxic effects of pharmacological treatment of epilepsy have been well documented since the initial experiences with bromides, but few studies have attempted to quantify the severity or frequency of adverse events using reliable and valid measures. The VA Cooperative Studies (Mattson et al., 1985; 1992) used a combination of subjective self-report with clinicians physical examination findings to create a composite score in combination with seizure control. At the final 36 month outcome assessment in the VA Cooperative I trial, the composite scores were closer to the poor than the good outcome category for each of the study drugs (Mattson et al., 1985). The authors concluded that "the outcome of this project underscores the unsatisfactory status of antiepileptic therapy with the medications currently available. Most patients whose epilepsy is reasonably controlled must tolerate some side effects. These observations emphasize the need for new AEDs and other approaches to treatment" (Mattson et al., 1985). A multi-center Italian survey (Beghi et al., 1986) reported that 31% of epilepsy patients described an adverse drug reaction. The rates per center varied from 6% to 79%, suggesting that differences between centers in the organization of the clinical interviews may have affected the ability of the patients to report their adverse experiences. Also of note was the observation that only 53% of the adverse reactions resulted in a decision to change treatment. Furthermore, most studies that have included medication use in the predictors of HRQOL have found an association of poorer QOL with seizure-free patients taking AEDs compared to seizure-free patients not taking AEDs (Sillanpaa et al., 1998; O'Donoghue et al., 1999). The large prospective study of immediate versus delayed treatment for epilepsy (MESS Trial) found that medication toxicity was significantly worse in the group with recurrent seizures while taking AEDs, compared to all other groups (Jacoby et al., 2007).

Based on the evident importance of adverse events from AEDs for overall clinical outcome in epilepsy, researchers from the UK (Baker et al., 1994; 1997; 1998), Holland (Aldenkamp & Baker, 1997), and the US (Salinsky & Storzbach, 2005) developed specific self-report instruments to assist and supplement clinical evaluation. The items in the Adverse Events Profile were selected based on the results of small group interviews of patients taking AEDs. It contains 19 items that are brief descriptions of a subjective experience of a toxic medication effect. The instructions ask the person to rank the frequency of each adverse effect on a 1 to 4 Likert-like scale during the past four weeks. The psychometric properties of reliability and validity of the AEP are robust (Baker et al., 1994). In a European studies including 15 countries and over 5,000 participants, the AEP demonstrated that 40% to 50% of patients on the most common AEDs reported excessive tiredness, poor concentration, sleepiness and/or memory problems (Baker et al., 1997). In another study, the AEP strongly correlated with HRQOL (partial r = 0.61; p < 0.001), independent of seizure rate (Gilliam, 2002). This observation was replicated in a multi-center study (partial r = 0.60; p < 0.0001), after controlling for depression symptoms *(Figure 2)* (Gilliam et al., 2006).

In order to demonstrate the clinical utility of the AEP to improve outcomes in the outpatient treatment of epilepsy, a randomized trial compared the use of the AEP by clinicians to usual care without the AEP (Gilliam et al., 2004). In this four month trial, the group for which the treating neurologists had access to the AEP at each visit had a 24% reduction in AEP scores *(Figure 3)* and were nearly three fold more likely to have a medication change or dosage adjustment. Improvement in the AEP was significantly associated with improvement in QOLIE-89 scores. This study demonstrated the importance of systematic screening in clinical epilepsy care, and also the value of quantification of medication toxicity in health outcomes research in epilepsy (Gilliam et al., 2004).

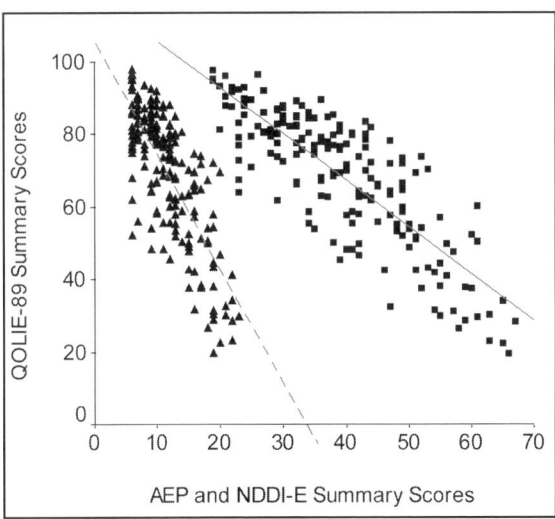

Figure 2. Scatterplot of the comparison of Quality of Life in Epilepsy Inventory-89 (QOLIE-89) summary scores with Neurological Disorders Depression Inventory for Epilepsy (AEP ■; partial r = -0.60, *p* < 0.0001) and Adverse Events Profile (NDDI-E ▲; partial r = -0.39, *p* < 0.0001). Adjusted R^2 was 0.72 (*p* < 0.0001) for regression model with QOLIE-89 as the dependent variable (Gilliam et al., 2006).

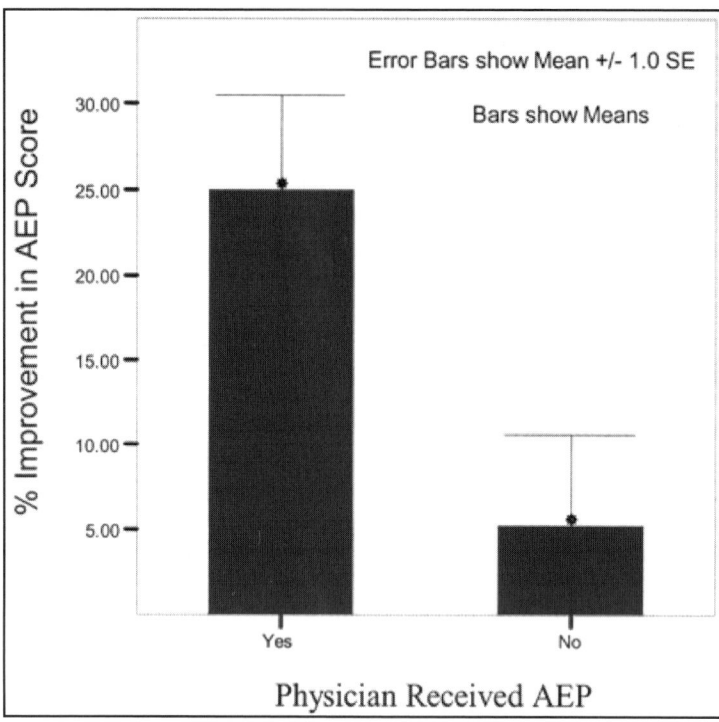

Figure 3. Improvement in Adverse Event Profile (AEP) total scores during the 4-month study for the AEP-provided and AEP-inaccessible (usual care) groups; t-test p value = 0.01 (Gilliam et al., 2004).

■ Co-morbid disorders: depression and anxiety

Similar to epilepsy, depression is a term used for a variety of medical disorders with multiple etiologies and complex interactions with social, vocational, and neuropsychological functioning (Santos et al., 2006). Depression has long been recognized as a common co-morbid condition in persons with epilepsy, especially in tertiary care samples (Robertson & Trimble, 1993; Lambert & Robertson, 1999; Beghi et al., 2002) and more recently in population (Tellez-Zenteno et al., 2007; Gaitatzis et al., 2004) and community-based studies (Ettinger et al., 2004). Although interpretation of the literature on depression in epilepsy is complicated by varying ascertainment methods, definitions of depression, and sample characteristics, current estimates suggest that the prevalence of clinically relevant depression is 30-50% in persons with refractory epilepsy and 10-30% in controlled epilepsy. Further support for the significance of depression in epilepsy is the observation that suicide rates are significantly higher than the general population (Christensen et al., 2007; Jones et al., 2003).

The etiology of depression in epilepsy is not fully understood and is very likely multifactorial, even on an individual level (Kanner, 2003; Hecimoric et al., 2003). However, specific psychological and neurological factors have been associated with depression in epilepsy. Hermann et al. performed a study based on the learned helplessness theory and found that a pessimistic attributional style was significantly associated with increased self-reported depression and remained significant when the effects of several confounding variables were controlled [age, age at epilepsy onset, laterality of TLE, sex, and method variance] (Hermann, 1996). Other investigators have found association of depression with brain abnormalities based on structural and functional imaging (Gilliam et al., 2007; Bromfield et al., 1992; Quiske et al., 2000; Savic et al., 2004; Giovacchini et al., 2005; Hasler et al., 2007; Theodore et al., 2007; Salzberg et al., 2006; Richardson et al., 2007; Briellmann et al., 2007). For example, extent of abnormal creatine/NAA MR spectroscopic maps in the hippocampi of a sample of patients with refractory temporal lobe epilepsy strongly correlated with severity of depression symptoms (Gilliam et al., 2007). Less information is available regarding the neurobiology of anxiety symptoms and epilepsy (Minter & Lopez, 2002; Satishchandra et al., 2003).

The importance of depression and anxiety in epilepsy is supported by their strong and consistent correlation with HRQOL, independent of seizure-rates, in multiple clinical studies (Gilliam, 2002; Gilliam et al., 2006; Boylan et al., 2004; Johnson et al., 2004). A recent study of 200 epilepsy patients from five academic centers in the US found that 72% of the variance in HRQOL was explained by reliable and valid measures of depression and adverse medication effects, shown in *Figure 2* (Gilliam, 2006). Furthermore, depression is associated with increased health-care utilization and costs in persons with epilepsy (Cramer et al., 2004).

The best approach to treatment of depression and anxiety in epilepsy has received relatively little attention compared to its impact on the epilepsy community. Multiple important issues must be considered, such as efficacy of antidepressant medications in the setting of epileptic brain dysfunction, additional adverse effects of antidepressants, and the unique social and vocational disabilities in epilepsy that may make cognitive and behavioural therapies particularly valuable (Gilliam et al., 2004). In 1985, Robertson and Trimble described the results of a randomized, double-blind comparison of amitriptyline, nomifesine, and placebo in 42 patients with depression and epilepsy (Robertson & Trimble, 1985). Although the mean scores of the Hamilton Depression Rating Scale and the Beck Depression Inventory scores improved by 50% after treatment, similar improvement in the placebo group resulted in no significant difference in outcome between any groups at 6 weeks. A second 6-week treatment phase without placebo control compared higher doses of each drug (150 mg), and found that the nomifesine group had significantly better Hamilton Depression Rating Scale but not Beck Depression Inventory scores. The authors concluded "our results suggest that, in patients with depression and epilepsy, immediate prescription with antidepressants may not be indicated" (Robertson & Trimble, 1985). A more recent study compared the efficacy of citalopram, mirtazapine, and roboxetine in 75 subjects with temporal lobe epilepsy and major depression (Kühn et al., 2003). Although each of the drugs was associated with significant reduction in depression symptoms at the 24-30 week assessment, mirtazapine had a higher dropout rate due to unacceptable side effects. Although the results indicate efficacy and differential tolerability of the antidepressants in temporal lobe epilepsy, only a small minority of the minority of the subjects achieved an improvement consistent with complete remission of depression. Similar to another study using sertraline (Kanner et al., 2000), no significant increase in seizure was observed (Kühn et al., 2003). Non-pharmacological treatments for depression have not received adequate systematic evaluations to make conclusions about efficacy in persons with epilepsy. Additional research is needed to provide the necessary evidence to guide optimal care of persons with epilepsy and co-morbid depression and anxiety.

Cognition

Although the majority of individuals with epilepsy have normal intelligence, overall, they are more prone to suffer from impaired cognitive performance when compared to age- and education-matched healthy controls (Motamedi, 2003; Kwan & Brodie, 2001; Hermann et al., 2008).

Table II. Factors affecting cognition in individuals with epilepsy (Meador, 2006)

Etiology of seizures
Cerebral lesions acquired prior to onset of seizures
Seizure type
Age at onset of epilepsy
Seizure frequency, duration and severity
Intarictal, interictal, or postictal physiologic dysfunction from seizures
Structural cerebral damage due to repetitive or prolonged seizures
Hereditary factors
Psychosocial factors (*e.g.* depression)
Sequelae of epilepsy surgery
Untoward effects of antiepileptic drugs

A wide spectrum of different variables underlies cognitive impairment in people with epilepsy, including biological, psychosocial and treatment-related factors, as summarized in *Table II* (Meador, 2006). In this respect, the effects of epilepsy *per se* may be particularly deleterious (Helmstaedter et al., 1996; Hermann et al., 2002, 2003; Jokeit et al., 1999). In a prospective controlled study, 46 subjects with chronic temporal lobe epilepsy and 65 age- and sex- matched healthy controls underwent extensive neuropsychological assessment at baseline and reevaluation 4 years later (Hermann et al., 2006). Significant worsening of cognitive performances was observed exclusively among epilepsy patients, in particular in those subjects characterized by longer duration of epilepsy, older age, lower intellectual ability, and more baseline abnormalities in quantitative magnetic resonance volumetrics.

Epilepsy treatment is also a potential cause of cognitive impairment (Gilliam et al., 2006; Kwan & Brodie, 2001; Bourgeois, 2004). Although several AEDs have no apparent effect on cognitive function, other agents such as phenytoin, carbamazepine, valproic acid and topiramate moderately affect cognitive performance and phenobarbital has the greatest potential for adverse cognitive effects (Meador et al., 1991, 1995; Aldenkamp et al., 2000; Lee et al., 2003). Epilepsy surgery is also associated with impairment of cognitive performances in a significant proportion of cases, but such effects can often be minimized or avoided (Rausch et al., 2003; Blanchette et al., 2002; Trevathan & Gilliam, 2003). Vagal nerve stimulation appears not to be associated with cognitive disturbance (Hoppe et al., 2001; Aldenkamp et al., 2002).

■ Sleep disturbances

The interaction between epilepsy and sleep has been recognized for centuries, but only in recent years it has received appropriate attention (Bazil, 2004; Malow, 2007; Rodriguez & Kuzniecky, 2008). Sleep state influences seizures and epileptic discharges (Sammaritano et al., 1991; Bazil & Walczak, 1997; Hermann et al., 2001). On the other hand, epilepsy and its treatment may cause decreased sleep efficiency, increased sleep fragmentation, and excessive daytime sleepiness (Malow, 2007). In addition, a variety of sleep disorders may coexist with epilepsy, such as obstructive sleep apnea, restless legs syndrome, narcolepsy, insufficient sleep, and REM behaviour disorder (Malow et al., 2000; Manni & Terzaghi, 2005). Although sleep disturbance is known to be associated with impairment of quality of life in people with chronic illnesses (Manocchia et al., 2001), only few studies have attempted to elucidate the impact of sleep disturbance on subjective health status in individuals with epilepsy (de Weerd et al., 2005; Piperidov et al., 2008). A large study of 486 adult epilepsy patients and 492 controls, which included a number of reliable and valid health assessments, found that respondents with partial epilepsy had a twofold higher prevalence of sleep disturbance compared with controls (38.6 vs. 18.0%; p < 0.0001) (de Weerd et al., 2004). Subjects with epilepsy displayed a higher number of abnormalities in the sleep-disorder subscales compared to controls. The presence of sleep disturbance in individuals with epilepsy was associated with the greatest impact on subjective health status. These findings were replicated recently in different epilepsy samples (Alanis-Guevara et al., 2005; Piperidov et al., 2008).

Migraine and headache

Despite over 100 years of investigations, the association between epilepsy and migraine has not been fully understood (Winawer, 2007). Both conditions are characterized by transient, paroxysmal alterations of neurologic function, and it often occurs that one disorder is mistaken for the other (Gilliam et al., 2005). Abundant evidence supports the association of migraine and epilepsy (Andermann, 1987). The risk of migraine has been found to more than twice as great in adults with epilepsy compared to those without epilepsy (Ottman & Lipton, 1994). In children, an association between migraine and specific epilepsy syndromes, such as benign childhood epilepsy with centro-temporal spikes (BECTS) and childhood epilepsy with occipital paroxysms (CEOP), has been demonstrated (Giroud et al., 1990; Andermann & Zifkin, 1998). Moreover, a recent population-based case-control study in Iceland showed that migraine with aura is associated with a fourfold increased risk for developing epilepsy (Ludvigsson et al., 2006). Although common pathopysiological mechanisms may exist (Terwindt et al., 1998; Aurora et al., 1998), the nature of this association remains complex and largely obscure. Obscure is also the reason for the complete absence of studies on the effects of such common co-morbidity on quality of life. As in epilepsy and other chronic illnesses, overall quality of life has been found to be significantly reduced in patients with uncontrolled migraine headaches (Terwindt et al., 2000; Lipton et al., 2003; Bussone et al., 2004). In a large population-based cross-sectional study, subjective health status, as measured by the SF-36, was found to be inversely correlated to migraine attack frequency (p < 0.0002) (Terwindt et al., 2000). These findings were confirmed by subsequent studies (Lipton et al., 2003).

Motor function and coordination

Several studies have recently found that people with epilepsy are at increased risk for progressive deterioration in motor function, independent of epilepsy syndrome and treatment (Hermann et al., 2006; Ciumas et al., 2008). These findings seem to have a neurobiological correlate in specific anatomic structures (Sandok et al., 2000; Szabo et al., 2006; Hermann et al., 2004). A recent study utilized magnetic resonance imaging (MRI) to measure volumes of cerebellar hemispheres in 185 surgical candidates with temporal lobe epilepsy (TLE) and 80 healthy controls (Sandok et al., 2000). Cerebellar volumes were found to be significantly reduced among TLE patients, in particular in those with an early age at onset and longer duration of epilepsy. Similar findings have been reported by other investigators (Szabo et al., 20006; Hermann et al., 2004), and suggest that motor dysfunction arising from cerebral disturbance may be a clinically relevant concern in epilepsy management and outcomes.

■ Conclusions

Although complete seizure control is an indisputable goal of epilepsy treatment, other factors also have strong influence on overall health outcome. For patients who cannot achieve seizure cessation, appropriate management of adverse antiepileptic drug effects and mood disorders can lead to significant improvements in quality of life. Addressing other common co-morbid conditions such as cognitive disturbances, sleep disorders, migraine, and motor problems may also improve function and well being, although less research has specifically addressed these areas. Epilepsy can be a complex disorder with multiple types of psychological, neurological, social, and vocational disabilities, but systematic screening with reliable and valid instruments to efficiently identify common co-morbidities can facilitate and improve the results of clinical care. Optimal management of epilepsy remains a major challenge to the neurological community, and advances in basic, translational, and health outcomes research should support continued improvement in the delivery and results of epilepsy treatment.

References

Alanis-Guevara I, Pena E, Corona T, Lopez-Ayala T, Lopez-Meza E, Lopez-Gomez M. Sleep disturbances, socioeconomic status, and seizure control as main predictors of quality of life in epilepsy. *Epilepsy Behav* 2005; 7: 481-5.

Aldenkamp AP, Baker GA. The Neurotoxicity Scale--II. Results of a patient-based scale assessing neurotoxicity in patients with epilepsy. *Epilepsy Res* 1997; 27: 165-73.

Aldenkamp AP, van Bronswijk K, Braken M, Diepman LA, Verwey LE, van den Wittenboer G. A clinical comparative study evaluating the effect of epilepsy versus ADHD on timed cognitive tasks in children. *Neuropsychol Dev Cogn Sect C Child Neuropsychol* 2000; 6: 209-17.

Aldenkamp AP, Majoie HJ, Berfelo MW, *et al.* Long-term effects of 24-month treatment with vagus nerve stimulation on behaviour in children with Lennox-Gastaut syndrome. *Epilepsy Behav* 2002; 3: 475-9.

Andermann E, Andermann F. Migraine-Epilepsy Relationships: Epidemiological and Genetic Aspects. In: Andermann F, Lugaresi E (eds). *Migraine and Epilepsy*. Boston: Butterworth Publishers, 1987: 281-91.

Andermann F, Zifkin B. The benign occipital epilepsies of childhood: an overview of the idiopathic syndromes and of the relationship to migraine. *Epilepsia* 1998; 39 (suppl 4): S9-23.

Aurora SK, Ahmad BK, Welch KM, Bhardhwaj P, Ramadan NM. Transcranial magnetic stimulation confirms hyperexcitability of occipital cortex in migraine. *Neurology* 1998; 50: 1111-4.

Baker GA, Smith DF, Dewey M, Jacoby A, Chadwick DW. The initial development of a health-related quality of life model as an outcome measure in epilepsy. *Epilepsy Res* 1993; 16: 65-81.

Baker GA, Frances P, Middleton E. Initial development, reliability, and validity of a patient-based adverse events scale. *Epilepsia* 1994; 35 (suppl 7): 80.

Baker GA, Jacoby A, Buck D, Stalgis C, Monnet D. Quality of life of people with epilepsy: a European study. *Epilepsia* 1997; 38: 353-62.

Baker GA, Camfield C, Camfield P, *et al.* Commission on Outcome Measurement in Epilepsy, 1994-1997: final report. *Epilepsia* 1998; 39: 213-31.

Baker GA. Quality of life and epilepsy: the Liverpool experience. *Clin Ther* 1998; 20 (suppl A): A2-12.

Bazil CW. Sleep, Sleep Apnea, and Epilepsy. *Curr Treat Options Neurol* 2004; 6: 339-45.

Bazil CW, Walczak TS. Effects of sleep and sleep stage on epileptic and nonepileptic seizures. *Epilepsia* 1997; 38: 56-62.

Beghi E, Mascio R-cD, Sasanelli F. Adverse Reactions to Antiepileptic Drugs: A Multicenter Survey of Clinical Practice. *Epilepsia* 1986; 27: 323-30.

Beghi E, Spagnoli P, Airoldi L, *et al*. Emotional and affective disturbances in patients with epilepsy. *Epilepsy & Behavior* 2002; 3: 255-61.

Berg AT, Vickrey BG, Sperling MR, *et al*. Driving in adults with refractory localization-related epilepsy. Multi-Center Study of Epilepsy Surgery. *Neurology* 2000; 54: 625-30.

Blanchette N, Smith ML. Language after temporal or frontal lobe surgery in children with epilepsy. *Brain Cogn* 2002; 48: 280-4.

Boylan LS, Flint LA, Labovitz DL, Jackson SC, Starner K, Devinsky O. Depression but not seizure frequency predicts quality of life in treatment-resistant epilepsy. *Neurology* 2004; 62: 258-61.

Bourgeois BF. Determining the effects of antiepileptic drugs on cognitive function in pediatric patients with epilepsy. *J Child Neurol* 2004; 19 (suppl 1): S15-24.

Boylan LS, Flint LA, Labovitz DL, Jackson SC, Starner K, Devinsky O. Depression but not seizure frequency predicts quality of life in treatment-resistant epilepsy. *Neurology* 2004; 62: 258-61.

Briellmann RS, Hopwood MJ, Jackson GD. Major depression in temporal lobe epilepsy with hippocampal sclerosis: clinical and imaging correlates. *J Neurol Neurosurg Psychiatry* 2007; 78: 1226-30.

Bromfield EB, Altshuler L, Leiderman DB, *et al*. Cerebral metabolism and depression in patients with complex partial seizures [published erratum appears in Arch Neurol 1992 Sep; 49 (9): 976]. *Arch Neurol* 1992; 49: 617-23.

Bussone G, Usai S, Grazzi L, Rigamonti A, Solari A, D'Amico D. Disability and quality of life in different primary headaches: results from Italian studies. *Neurol Sci* 2004; 25 (suppl 3): S105-107.

Christensen J, Vestergaard M, Mortensen PB, Sidenius P, Agerbo E. Epilepsy and risk of suicide: a population-based case-control study. *The Lancet Neurology* 2007; 6: 693-8.

Ciumas C, Robins Wahlin TB, Jucaite A, Lindstrom P, Halldin C, Savic I. Reduced dopamine transporter binding in patients with juvenile myoclonic epilepsy. *Neurology* 2008; [epub].

Clancy CM, Eisenberg JM. Outcomes research: measuring the end results of health care. *Science* 1998; 282: 245-6.

Cramer JA. A clinimetric approach to assessing quality of life in epilepsy. *Epilepsia* 1993; 34 (suppl 4): S8-13.

Cramer JA, Blum D, Fanning K, Reed M. The impact of co-morbid depression on health resource utilization in a community sample of people with epilepsy. *Epilepsy & Behavior* 2004; 5: 337-42.

Dalrymple J, Appleby J. Cross sectional study of reporting of epileptic seizures to general practitioners. *BMJ* 2000; 320: 94-7.

de Weerd A, de Haas S, Otte A, *et al*. Subjective sleep disturbance in patients with partial epilepsy: a questionnaire-based study on prevalence and impact on quality of life. *Epilepsia* 2004; 45: 1397-404.

Devinsky O, Vickrey BG, Cramer J, *et al*. Development of the quality of life in epilepsy inventory. *Epilepsia* 1995; 36: 1089-104.

Devinsky O. Outcome research in neurology: incorporating health-related quality of life. *Ann Neurol* 1995; 37: 141-2.

Ettinger A, Reed M, Cramer J. Depression and co-morbidity in community-based patients with epilepsy or asthma. *Neurology* 2004; 63: 1008-14.

Gaitatzis A, Carroll K, Majeed A, Sander JW. The Epidemiology of the Comorbidity of Epilepsy in the General Population. *Epilepsia* 2004; 45: 1613-22.

Gilliam F, Kuzniecky R, Faught E, Black L, Carpenter G, Schrodt R. Patient-validated content of epilepsy-specific quality-of-life measurement. *Epilepsia* 1997; 38: 233-6.

Gilliam F, Wyllie E, Kashden J, *et al*. Epilepsy surgery outcome: comprehensive assessment in children. *Neurology* 1997; 48: 1368-74.

Gilliam F, Kuzniecky R, Meador K, et al. Patient-oriented outcome assessment after temporal lobectomy for refractory epilepsy [see comments]. *Neurology* 1999; 53: 687-94.

Gilliam F. Optimizing Health Outcomes in Active Epilepsy. *Neurology* 2002; 58 (suppl 5): S9-S19.

Gilliam F, Carter J, Vahle V. Tolerability of antiseizure medications: Implications for health outcomes. *Neurology* 2004; 63 (suppl 4): S9-12.

Gilliam FG, Fessler AJ, Baker G, Vahle V, Carter J, Attarian H. Systematic screening allows reduction of adverse antiepileptic drug effects: A randomized trial. *Neurology* 2004; 62: 23-7.

Gilliam FG, Santos J, Vahle V, Carter J, Brown K, Hecimovic H. Depression in Epilepsy: Ignoring Clinical Expression of Neuronal Network Dysfunction? *Epilepsia* 2004; 45: 28-33.

Gilliam FG, Mendiratta A, Pack AM, Bazil CW. Epilepsy and common comorbidities: improving the outpatient epilepsy encounter. *Epileptic Disord* 2005; 7 (suppl 1): S27-33.

Gilliam FG, Barry JJ, Hermann BP, Meador KJ, Vahle V, Kanner AM. Rapid detection of major depression in epilepsy: a multicentre study. *The Lancet Neurology* 2006; 5: 399-405.

Gilliam FG, Maton BM, Martin RC, et al. Hippocampal 1H-MRSI correlates with severity of depression symptoms in temporal lobe epilepsy. *Neurology* 2007; 68: 364-8.

Giovacchini G, Toczek MT, Bonwetsch R, et al. 5-HT1A Receptors Are Reduced in Temporal Lobe Epilepsy After Partial-Volume Correction. *J Nucl Med* 2005; 46: 1128-35.

Giroud M, Bernard P, Guignier F, Gras P, Bonaiti C, Dumas R. Lack of genetic link between the HLA system and idiopathic generalized epilepsy (letter). *Presse Med* 1990; 19: 1904.

Hasler G, Bonwetsch R, Giovacchini G, et al. 5-HT1A Receptor Binding in Temporal Lobe Epilepsy Patients With and Without Major Depression. *Biological Psychiatry* 2007; 62: 1258-64.

Hecimovic H, Goldstein JD, Sheline YI, Gilliam FG. Mechanisms of depression in epilepsy from a clinical perspective. *Epilepsy & Behavior* 2003; 4: 25-30.

Helmstaedter C, Kemper B, Elger CE. Neuropsychological aspects of frontal lobe epilepsy. *Neuropsychologia* 1996; 34: 399-406.

Hermann BP. Developing a model of quality of life in epilepsy: the contribution of neuropsychology. *Epilepsia* 1993; 34 (suppl 4): S14-21.

Hermann BP. The evolution of health-related quality of life assessment in epilepsy. *Qual Life Res* 1995; 4: 87-100.

Hermann BP, Seidenberg M, Bell B, et al. The neurodevelopmental impact of childhood-onset temporal lobe epilepsy on brain structure and function. *Epilepsia* 2002; 43: 1062-71.

Hermann BP, Seidenberg M, Bell B, et al. Extratemporal quantitative MR volumetrics and neuropsychological status in temporal lobe epilepsy. *J Int Neuropsychol Soc* 2003; 9: 353-62.

Hermann BP, Seidenberg M, Sears L, et al. Cerebellar atrophy in temporal lobe epilepsy affects procedural memory. *Neurology* 2004; 63: 2129-31.

Hermann B, Jones J, Sheth R, Dow C, Koehn M, Seidenberg M. Children with new-onset epilepsy: neuropsychological status and brain structure. *Brain* 2006; 129: 2609-19.

Hermann BP, Seidenberg M, Dow D, et al. Cognitive prognosis in chronic temporal lobe epilepsy. *Annals of Neurology* 2006; 60: 80-7.

Hermann BP, Seidenberg M, Jones J. The neurobehavioural comorbidities of epilepsy: can a natural history be developed. *The Lancet Neurology* 2008; 7: 151-60.

Hermann BP, Trenerry MR, Colligan RC. Learned helplessness, attributional style, and depression in epilepsy. Bozeman Epilepsy Surgery Consortium. *Epilepsia* 1996; 37: 680-6.

Herman ST, Walczak TS, Bazil CW. Distribution of partial seizures during the sleep-wake cycle: differences by seizure onset site. *Neurology* 2001; 56: 1453-9.

Hoppe C, Helmstaedter C, Scherrmann J, Elger CE. No Evidence for Cognitive Side Effects after 6 Months of Vagus Nerve Stimulation in Epilepsy Patients. *Epilepsy Behav* 2001; 2: 351-6.

Jacoby A. Epilepsy and the quality of everyday life. Findings from a study of people with well-controlled epilepsy. *Soc Sci Med* 1992; 34: 657-66.

Jacoby A, Baker GA, Steen N, Buck D. The SF-36 as a health status measure for epilepsy: a psychometric assessment. *Qual Life Res* 1999; 8: 351-64.

Jacoby A, Gamble C, Doughty J, Marson A, Chadwick D, on behalf of the Medical Research Council MSG. Quality of life outcomes of immediate or delayed treatment of early epilepsy and single seizures. *Neurology* 2007; 68: 1188-96.

Johnson EK, Jones JE, Seidenberg M, Hermann BP. The Relative Impact of Anxiety, Depression, and Clinical Seizure Features on Health-related Quality of Life in Epilepsy. *Epilepsia* 2004; 45: 544-50.

Jokeit H, Ebner A. Long term effects of refractory temporal lobe epilepsy on cognitive abilities: a cross sectional study. *J Neurol Neurosurg Psychiatry* 1999; 67: 44-50.

Jones JE, Hermann BP, Barry JJ, Gilliam FG, Kanner AM, Meador KJ. Rates and risk factors for suicide, suicidal ideation, and suicide attempts in chronic epilepsy. *Epilepsy & Behavior* 2003; 4: 31-8.

Kanner AM, Kozak AM, Frey M. The use of sertraline in patients with epilepsy: Is it safe? *Epilepsy Behav* 2000; 1: 100-5.

Kanner AM. Depression in epilepsy: prevalence, clinical semiology, pathogenic mechanisms, and treatment. *Biological Psychiatry* 2003; 54: 388-98.

Kühn K-U, Quednow BB, Thiel M, Falkai P, Maier W, Elger CE. Antidepressive treatment in patients with temporal lobe epilepsy and major depression: a prospective study with three different antidepressants. *Epilepsy & Behavior* 2003; 4: 674-9.

Kwan P, Brodie MJ. Neuropsychological effects of epilepsy and antiepileptic drugs. *The Lancet* 2001; 357: 216-22.

Lambert MV, Robertson MM. Depression in epilepsy: etiology, phenomenology, and treatment. *Epilepsia* 1999; 40 (suppl 10): S21-47.

Lee S, Sziklas V, Andermann F, *et al*. The effects of adjunctive topiramate on cognitive function in patients with epilepsy. *Epilepsia* 2003; 44: 339-47.

Leidy NK, Elixhauser A, Rentz AM, *et al*. Telephone validation of the Quality of Life in Epilepsy Inventory-89 (QOLIE-89). *Epilepsia* 1999; 40: 97-106.

Leidy NK, Elixhauser A, Vickrey B, Means E, Willian MK. Seizure frequency and the health-related quality of life of adults with epilepsy. *Neurology* 1999; 53: 162-6.

Lipton RB, Liberman JN, Kolodner KB, Bigal ME, Dowson A, Stewart WF. Migraine headache disability and health-related quality-of-life: a population-based case-control study from England. *Cephalalgia* 2003; 23: 441-50.

Ludvigsson P, Hesdorffer D, Olafsson E, Kjartansson O, Hauser WA. Migraine with aura is a risk factor for unprovoked seizures in children. *Ann Neurol* 2006; 59: 210-3.

Malow BA, Levy K, Maturen K, Bowes R. Obstructive sleep apnea is common in medically refractory epilepsy patients. *Neurology* 2000; 55: 1002-7.

Malow BA. The interaction between sleep and epilepsy. *Epilepsia* 2007; 48 (suppl 9): 36-8.

Manni R, Terzaghi M. REM behavior disorder associated with epileptic seizures. *Neurology* 2005; 64: 883-4.

Manocchia M, Keller S, Ware JE. Sleep problems, health-related quality of life, work functioning and health care utilization among the chronically ill. *Qual Life Res* 2001; 10: 331-45.

Martin R, Vogtle L, Gilliam F, Faught E. What are the concerns of older adults living with epilepsy? *Epilepsy & Behavior* 2005; 7: 297-300.

Mattson RH, Cramer JA, Collins JF, *et al*. Comparison of carbamazepine, phenobarbital, phenytoin, and primidone in partial and secondarily generalized tonic-clonic seizures. *N Engl J Med* 1985; 313: 145-51.

Mattson RH, Cramer JA, Collins JF. A comparison of valproate with carbamazepine for the treatment of complex partial seizures and secondarily generalized tonic-clonic seizures in adults. The Department of Veterans Affairs Epilepsy Cooperative Study No. 264 Group. *N Engl J Med* 1992; 327: 765-71.

Meador KJ, Loring DW, Allen ME, et al. Comparative cognitive effects of carbamazepine and phenytoin in healthy adults. *Neurology* 1991; 41: 1537-40.

Meador KJ. Research use of the new quality-of-life in epilepsy inventory. *Epilepsia* 1993; 34 (suppl 4): S34-38.

Meador KJ, Loring DW, Moore EE, et al. Comparative cognitive effects of phenobarbital, phenytoin, and valproate in healthy adults. *Neurology* 1995; 45: 1494-9.

Meador KJ. Cognitive and memory effects of the new antiepileptic drugs. *Epilepsy Research* 2006; 68: 63-7.

Mintzer S, Lopez F. Comorbidity of ictal fear and panic disorder. *Epilepsy & Behavior* 2002; 3: 330-7.

Motamedi G, Meador K. Epilepsy and cognition. *Epilepsy & Behavior* 2003; 4: 25-38.

O'Donoghue MF, Duncan JS, Sander JW. The subjective handicap of epilepsy. A new approach to measuring treatment outcome. *Brain* 1998; 121: 317-43.

O'Donoghue MF, Goodridge DM, Redhead K, Sander JW, Duncan JS. Assessing the psychosocial consequences of epilepsy: a community-based study. *Br J Gen Pract* 1999; 49: 211-4.

Ottman R, Lipton RB. Comorbidity of migraine and epilepsy. *Neurology* 1994; 44: 2105-10.

Perrine KR. A new quality-of-life inventory for epilepsy patients: interim results. *Epilepsia* 1993; 34 (suppl 4): S28-33.

Piperidou C, Karlovasitou A, Triantafyllou N, et al. Influence of sleep disturbance on quality of life of patients with epilepsy. *Seizure* 2008; [epub].

Quiske A, Helmstaedter C, Lux S, Elger CE. Depression in patients with temporal lobe epilepsy is related to mesial temporal sclerosis. *Epilepsy Res* 2000; 39: 121-5.

Rausch R, Kraemer S, Pietras CJ, Le M, Vickrey BG, Passaro EA. Early and late cognitive changes following temporal lobe surgery for epilepsy. *Neurology* 2003; 60: 951-9.

Richardson EJ, Griffith HR, Martin RC, et al. Structural and functional neuroimaging correlates of depression in temporal lobe epilepsy. *Epilepsy & Behavior* 2007; 10: 242-9.

Robertson MM, Trimble MR. Depressive illness in patients with epilepsy: a review. *Epilepsia* 1983; 24 (suppl 2): S109-116.

Robertson MM, Trimble MR. The treatment of depression in patients with epilepsy. A double-blind trial. *J Affect Disord* 1985; 9: 127-36.

Rodriguez AJ, Kuzniecky RI. The interactions between sleep and epilepsy. *Rev Neurol Dis* 2008; 5: 1-7.

Salinsky MC, Storzbach D. The Portland Neurotoxicity Scale: Validation of a Brief Self-Report Measure of Antiepileptic-Drug-Related Neurotoxicity. *Assessment* 2005; 12: 107-17.

Salzberg M, Taher T, Davie M, et al. Depression in Temporal Lobe Epilepsy Surgery Patients: An FDG-PET Study. *Epilepsia* 2006; 47: 2125-30.

Sammaritano M, Gigli GL, Gotman J. Interictal spiking during wakefulness and sleep and the localization of foci in temporal lobe epilepsy. *Neurology* 1991; 41: 290-7.

Sandok EK, O'Brien TJ, Jack CR, So EL. Significance of Cerebellar Atrophy in Intractable Temporal Lobe Epilepsy: A Quantitative MRI Study. *Epilepsia* 2000; 41: 1315-20.

Santos JM, Chen LS, de Erausquin GA. Phenomenology of depression: towards a neuroscientific perspective. In: Gilliam FG, Kanner AM, Sheline YI (eds). *Depression and Brain Dysfunction*. New York: Taylor and Francis, 2006: 1-49.

Satishchandra P, Krishnamoorthy ES, Elst LTv, et al. Mesial Temporal Structures and Co-morbid Anxiety in Refractory Partial Epilepsy. *J Neuropsychiatry Clin Neurosci* 2003; 15: 450-2.

Savic I, Lindstrom P, Gulyas B, Halldin C, Andree B, Farde L. Limbic reductions of 5-HT1A receptor binding in human temporal lobe epilepsy. *Neurology* 2004; 62: 1343-51.

Sillanpaa M, Jalava M, Kaleva O, Shinnar S. Long-term prognosis of seizures with onset in childhood. *N Engl J Med* 1998; 338: 1715-22.

Sillanpaa M, Haataja L, Shinnar S. Perceived Impact of Childhood-onset Epilepsy on Quality of Life as an Adult. *Epilepsia* 2004; 45: 971-7.

Sillanpaa M, Shinnar S. Obtaining a driver's license and seizure relapse in patients with childhood-onset epilepsy. *Neurology* 2005; 64: 680-6.

Szabo CA, Lancaster JL, Lee S, et al. MR Imaging Volumetry of Subcortical Structures and Cerebellar Hemispheres in Temporal Lobe Epilepsy. *AJNR Am J Neuroradiol* 2006; 27: 2155-60.

Tellez-Zenteno JF, Patten SB, Jette N, Williams J, Wiebe S. Psychiatric Comorbidity in Epilepsy: A Population-Based Analysis. *Epilepsia* 2007; 48: 2336-44.

Terwindt GM, Ophoff RA, Haan J, Sandkuijl LA, Frants RR, Ferrari MD. Migraine, ataxia and epilepsy: a challenging spectrum of genetically determined calcium channelopathies. Dutch Migraine Genetics Research Group. *Eur J Hum Genet* 1998; 6: 297-307.

Terwindt GM, Ferrari MD, Tijhuis M, Groenen SM, Picavet HS, Launer LJ. The impact of migraine on quality of life in the general population: the GEM study. *Neurology* 2000; 55: 624-9.

Theodore WH, Hasler G, Giovacchini G, et al. Reduced Hippocampal 5HT1A PET Receptor Binding and Depression in Temporal Lobe Epilepsy. *Epilepsia* 2007; 48: 1526-30.

Trevathan E, Gilliam F. Lost years: delayed referral for surgically treatable epilepsy. *Neurology* 2003; 61: 432-33.

Vickrey BG. A procedure for developing a quality-of-life measure for epilepsy surgery patients. *Epilepsia* 1993; 34 (suppl 4): S22-27.

Vickrey BG, Hays RD, Rausch R, Sutherling WW, Engel J Jr., Brook RH. Quality of life of *epilepsy surgery patients as compared with outpatients with hypertension, diabetes, heart disease, and/or depressive symptoms*. *Epilepsia* 1994; 35: 597-607.

Victoroff JI, Benson F, Grafton ST, Engel J Jr., Mazziotta JC. Depression in complex partial seizures. Electroencephalography and cerebral metabolic correlates. *Arch Neurol* 1994; 51: 155-63.

Walker MC, Sander JW. Difficulties in extrapolating from clinical trial data to clinical practice: the case of antiepileptic drugs. *Neurology* 1997; 49: 333-7.

Ware JE, Jr. Standards for validating health measures: definition and content. *J Chronic Dis* 1987; 40: 473-80.

Ware JE, Kosinski M. Interpreting SF-36 summary health measures: a response. *Qual Life Res* 2001; 10: 405-13; discussion 415-20.

WHO. The constitution of the World Health Organization. *WHO Chron* 1947; 1: 29.

Winawer M. New evidence for a genetic link between epilepsy and migraine. *Neurology* 2007; 68: 1969-70.

Early identification of drug-resistant patients

Douglas R. Nordli, Jr.

Children's Memorial Hospital, Feinberg School of Medicine, Northwestern University, Chicago, USA

Estimates of medical intractability amongst patients with epilepsy vary, but generally are between 10 and 22% (Kwong et al., 2003; Berg et al., 2001). These discrepancies may be explained, at least in part, by the precise definition of intractability for there is no agreed-upon standard. Authors use the following variables, alone or in combination: frequency of seizures, duration of active epilepsy, and number of medications used (with or without documentation of therapeutic drug levels). Other causes for discrepancy may relate to differences in study designs and the source of the subjects for the studies.

Some argue that intractable epilepsy can be determined early on, but others indicate that it may take some time before the second drug failure announces intractability (Sillanpaa, 1993; Berg, 2003). It appears that the only way to firmly establish intractability is to wait and see how the patient fares with medication trials. If there were infallible biomarkers for intractability we could conceivably spare some patients and their families the agony of this whole process by intervening more aggressively with surgery, medications, special diets, or combinations of these treatments. To date, no such marker exists so the next best alternative is to identify patients with intractable epilepsy as soon as possible so that they do not languish with refractory seizures. Medical systems could be designed that incorporate the latest knowledge regarding determinants of intractability so that patients with high probabilities of developing drug-resistant epilepsy could be prioritized to receive urgent specialist care and close follow-up. This article will review the existing information on risk factors for intractable epilepsy with a primary focus on children. It will conclude with specific recommendations for evaluation and follow-up.

▪ Epidemiology of intractability

Most studies have revealed clear risk factors for development of intractability that can be identified at the first meeting of the patient, or within a month of follow-up. Kwong and colleagues examined a cohort of 309 children with epilepsy living in northwestern Hong Kong and compared 44 children with poorly controlled seizures (at least one per month for at least two years) with 211 who were seizure-free for two years (Dlugos et al., 2001). Forty of the 44 children (91%) with intractable epilepsy had remote symptomatic etiology. The first EEG was abnormal in 85.4% of cases, with focal abnormalities in half (51%). Imaging abnormalities were detected in 64.9% of those who had imaging. Independent predictors of intractability after multiple regression analysis were abnormal neurodevelopmental status, symptomatic etiology, and more than three seizures in the second six months after treatment. The odds ratio for abnormal neurodevelopmental status was 18.16 (CI 5.19-63.61), for symptomatic etiology was 16.58 (CI 4.2-65.43) and for greater than three seizures in the first six months was 21.86 (CI 7.35-65.01). The p value for all of these was < 0.001.

In perhaps the most definitive paper on prediction of intractability in children Berg et al. studied the development of intractable epilepsy (IE) in a prospective group of 613 children from Connecticut (Kwan & Brodie, 1993) Children with newly diagnosed epilepsy were identified from child neurology practices and tracked for the occurrence of IE which was defined as failure of more than two drugs and more than one seizure a month for at least 18 months. The median follow-up of this group was 4.8 years. Sixty children (10%) met the criteria for intractability. Children with cryptogenic/symptomatic forms of epilepsy were more likely to become intractable. After adjusting for epilepsy syndrome with multivariable analysis initial seizure frequency (p < 0.001), focal EEG slowing (p = 0.02), and acute symptomatic or neonatal status epilepticus (p = 0.001) were associated with an increased risk for IE.

Sillanpää reported on an incident cohort of 178 patients. On logistic regression analyses, poor short-term response to AEDs, occurrence of status epilepticus, high initial seizure frequency and remote symptomatic etiology were independent predictors of intractability (Berg et al., 2001).

Camfield et al. examined predictors of remission in a population-based study in Nova Scotia. This sample was collected from 1977 through 1985. The follow-up was an average of seven years. Multivariate analysis found that factors predicting remission- not simply the inverse of intractability-were absence of neonatal seizures, age greater than one year but less than 12 years, normal intelligence and less than 20 seizure before initiation of treatment (Camfield et al., 1993).

Oskoui and colleagues (2005) reviewed the chars of children presenting to a single neurology practice in Montreal. There were 169 children with onset between 2 and 17 years. On half had idiopathic epilepsy, 32.1% had cryptogenic, and 17.9% had remote symptomatic cause. Overall, 52.6% achieved remission. Multiple seizure types predicted a poor outcome, intractability and a lower probability of remission. As the authors note, multiple seizure types may be disproportionately seen in children with epilepsy syndromes that are associated with worse prognoses. Syndrome specific studies are probably more valuable, but larger numbers are needed to reach statistically significant results.

Geelhoed et al. reported on the accuracy of outcome predication models for children with epilepsy, combining data from the Dutch study and the study performed in Nova Scotia. While a combined model was incorrect in about one of every three patients, similar factors found to predict poor outcome were symptomatic generalized epilepsy and number of seizures before treatment (Nova Scotia study), and etiology (Dutch study) (Geelhoed et al., 2005).

In summary, children with symptomatic forms of epilepsy, antecedent neurological abnormalities, high initial seizure frequency, focal slowing on EEG, and prior neonatal or acute symptomatic status epilepticus can be predicted to be at a high risk for intractable epilepsy.

Table I. Factors that predict outcome in new onset of epilepsy in children.

Author	Year	Design	# cases	# controls	Neuro. Abnor.	Symptomatic Epilepsy	Seizure Type	Age of Onset	Prior acute status or Neonatal Seizures	Initial Seizure Frequency	Seizure Frequency after First Treatment	EEG Focal Slow	MRI Abnl.
Annegers	1979	Retrospective (Adults and Children)	457	-	YES	YES	YES	YES					
Berg	1996	Retrospective Case-control	76	96	-	YES	YES (IS)	YES					
Berg	2001	Prospective	613	-	YES	YES			YES	YES		YES	
Brorson	1987	Retrospective	195	-	YES		YES (mult. versus single)	YES					
Camfield	1993	Prospective (Predictive of Remission)	504	-	YES	YES		YES	YES	YES			
Geelhoed		Combined data from Nova Scotia and Dutch	-	-	YES	YES				YES			
Kwong	2006	Prospective	309	-	YES						YES		
Sillanpää	1993	Prospective	40	138	YES				YES	YES	YES		
Dlugos	2001	Retrospective Localization-Related	120	-							YES		
Kim	1999	Retrospective (MTS on MRI)	104	-				YES	YES (febrile seizures)				
Ohtsuka	2001	Retrospective Localization-Related Epilepsies	113	-			YES		YES	YES			
Spooner	2006	Prospective Temporal Lobe Epilepsy	77	-								YES	YES

In some cases failure of the first drug may predict intractability, but it is also possible that the failure of the first drug may not become fully apparent for many years. These epidemiological data help us to focus on the at-risk child and are combined in *Table I* in order to provide a quick overview. Data from prediction models show that these findings may not be sensitive, but may be relatively specific (Arts *et al.*, 1999).

■ Early recognition of refractory symptomatic epilepsy syndromes (Childhood epileptogenic encephalopathies)

Taking together, the data from the available studies *(Table I)* strongly supports that very young age, neurological or developmental impairment, and frequent initial seizures- either before or shortly after initiation of treatment- are robust predictors of intractable epilepsy. Many of these same factors are captured by the precise delineation of the epilepsy syndrome. It is not surprising therefore, that Berg *et al.* found epilepsy syndrome to be the best prognostic indicator of intractability (Kwan *et al.*, 2000). Key clinical components of the epilepsy syndrome are the age of presentation, the types of seizures, the presence or absence of antecedent neurological conditions, and the frequency of seizures. One unifying category combines many although not all, of the factors shown to predict intractability: symptomatic epileptogenic encephalopathies. These epilepsies are quite distinctive and notoriously intractable. They could be viewed as related conditions lying along an age-related spectrum *(Figure 1)*.

These pediatric epileptogenic encephalopathies can be identified at onset by considering the salient clinical features and the interictal EEG findings. For example, a young infant with encephalopathy, tonic seizures and an invariant burst-suppression pattern may be promptly diagnosed with Ohtahara syndrome. Having established this, one immediately knows that seizures are very unlikely to completely respond to medication and that the prognosis for long-term development or even survival is very guarded. Other refractory epileptogenic encephalopathies and their associated interictal EEG features are so distinctive that they too can be promptly diagnosed including: EME (variable burst-suppression), symptomatic infantile spasms or West syndrome (hypsarhythmia), and Lennox-Gastaut syndrome (slow generalized spike-wave discharges). All have clear and unambiguous interictal epileptiform EEG correlates that should allow for diagnosis if not immediately, within a very short time of presentation.

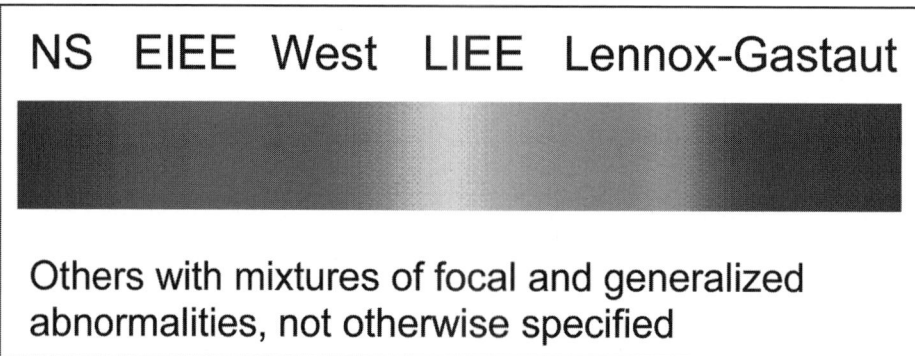

Figure 1. Pediatrics epileptogenic encephalopathies.
NS = neonatal seizures, EIEE = early infantile epileptogenic encephalopathy, LIEE = late infantile epileptogenic encephalopathy (used to describe patients with characteristics in between West and Lennox-Gastaut Syndrome).

Other epilepsy syndromes with a high rate of intractability

Epilepsies undetermined whether focal or generalized

Other young children or infants may present with a confusing clinical presentation, not easily categorized into one of the known epilepsy syndromes. These patients may present with multifocal pleomorphic epileptiform discharges against a slowed or poorly organized background. They may have tonic seizures, spasms, or mixtures of other seizures. At our institution we often use the category of "uncertain whether focal or generalized epilepsy" for this group of patients. That is because there is often a mixture of focal and some more diffuse findings that do not allow separation into either a pure generalized epilepsy or a focal process. These patients often show developmental delay or other neurological abnormalities and in our experience are difficult to control (Korff et al., 2006). We suspect that these patients may harbor genetic or metabolic abnormalities that have yet to be determined.

Other epilepsy syndromes with high rates of intractability are malignant migrating partial seizures of infancy (MMPSI) as described by Coppola et al. and Dravet syndrome (Veneselli et al., 2001; Dravet et al., 2005). Dravet syndrome has been associated with SCN1A mutations, especially those resulting in truncation of the protein, or missense mutations involving the pore region of the channel. To date, no clear cause has been found for malignant migrating partial seizures of infancy. Early recognition of MMPSI is not terribly difficult: children will have almost continuous multifocal seizures on routine EEG, and the ictal discharges appear to involve either hemisphere with little regard for the other independent ictal discharges. Dravet syndrome may be challenging to detect early since it often begins with prolonged febrile seizures, but we have noticed peculiar small amplitude spike and repetitive spikes discharges in the occipital regions with some of our patients early in their course (Korff et al., 2007).

Predicting intractable symptomatic localization-related epilepsy

In contrast to the aforementioned patients with epilepsies whose refractory nature can be anticipated almost from the onset of the disease, it may be much more challenging to accurately predict which patients with focal seizures will go on to have refractory seizures. As summarized in *Table I* several studies have examined this issue.

Spooner et al. studied a community-based cohort of 77 children from the start of their temporal lobe epilepsy (Spooner et al., 2006). The median follow-up was 13.7 years and 95% were followed for more than ten years. Lesions were found in 28, and all of these children were not seizure-free. Focal slowing on EEG was associated with persistent seizures, but this also correlated with the presence of a lesion on MRI.

Dlugos et al. performed a retrospective study on patients seen at Children's Hospital of Philadelphia. There were 120 patients who were followed for at least two years. Logistic regression analysis showed that failure of the first AED trial was the only variable to predict refractory temporal lobe epilepsy.

Ohtsuka and colleagues evaluated 113 children with symptomatic and cryptogenic localization-related epilepsy and found that there were 40 children with intractable epilepsy (Ohtsuka et al., 2001). This was defined as one or more seizure per month during the six months before the last follow-up. Multivariate analyses showed that seizure type at first visit, seizure frequency, status epilepticus before the first visit, and underlying causes were predictive factors. The rate of intractability was highest in children with multilobar epilepsy, followed by those with frontal lobe epilepsy. The intractable group had nine patients with encephalitis of unknown origin and three each with localized cortical malformation and mesial temporal sclerosis. EEG epileptiform discharges were analyzed but slowing was apparently not examined in this project.

Kim and colleagues performed a study of 104 patients with MRI evidence of mesial temporal sclerosis followed up at the Yonsei Epilepsy Clinic in Seoul (Kim et al., 1999). Of their 104 patients 75% were intractable or poorly responsive to "aggressive anticonvulsant polytherapy". Poor seizure control was related to an early age of onset of seizure, a history of febrile convulsions and epileptiform discharges on the EEG.

Older studies done before modern imaging techniques stressed different factors. Roger et al. reported on 119 patients with focal epilepsy with onset before age 12 years and found that factors predicting a poor outcome were early onset of seizures, history of prolonged febrile seizures, presence of mental retardation or a neurological abnormality, and a history of multiple seizures types (Roger et al., 1981, 1991). Scarpa and Carassini studied 261 children with non-idiopathic focal epilepsy between the ages of one month and 13 years (Gambardella et al., 2008). They found that full seizure control was possible in 72% but factors predictive of poor outcome were early onset, symptomatic cause and a high seizure frequency. More recent studies using MRI strongly argue that an imaging abnormality bodes very poorly for medication responsiveness (Spooner et al., 2006; Roger et al., 1981).

Rasmussen syndrome might be considered the prototypic intractable localization-related epilepsy syndrome. Early features might be focal signal abnormalities in the frontal regions, or early shrinkage of the caudate nucleus. A recent report, however, reinforced the notion that some cases might either stabilize, or not ever develop a relentlessly progressive course (Gambardella et al., 2008). Still, the rate of intractability remains high in this disorder.

Overall, the identification of refractory localization-related epilepsy appears to have increased slightly. Ohtsuka et al. studied the characteristic of refractory childhood epilepsy in two time periods, separated by about 15 years and published the findings in 2000 (Otsuka et al., 2000). They found that the proportion of localization-related epilepsies in the refractory group had increased over time, and of these patients were frontal lobe epilepsies were more common. The prevalence of Lennox-Gastaut syndrome amongst all children with refractory epilepsy dropped in half and overall the percentage of children with generalized epilepsies was reduced in the more recent series.

One intriguing factor that appears to predict intractability in at least two studies is the presence of focal slowing on the EEG (Kwan et al., 2000; Spooner et al., 2006). In the Spooner et al study this correlated with imaging findings and therefore was not an independent factor predicting intractability. In the Berg et al. series, however, focal slowing was a significant risk factor for intractability. It is not surprising that focal slowing correlated with the presence of an MRI abnormality since one well-established cause of focal slowing is the presence of a focal structural lesion interfering with the thalamo-cortical relations, most often in the centrum semiovale. But, experience has also shown that focal slowing is not always accompanied by a focal structural lesion, at least not one visible on standard MRI sequences. What then is the cause of this focal slowing? Could it be a physiological alteration that in some manner is associated with the epileptogenic process, and in particular the development of refractory epilepsies?

■ The special role of prolonged febrile convulsions

The role of febrile convulsions and particularly febrile status epilepticus is particularly interesting in this regard. This is currently the subject of a prospective multi-institutional study funded by the NIH examining the long term consequences of febrile status epilepticus (FEBSTAT). Children with febrile status are enrolled immediately after the status. Structured history, clinical examination, developmental assessment, MRI, EEG, viral studies and genetic studies are being performed and these same studies are being repeated one year later, with the exception of the virology and genetic studies. All patients are being followed prospectively so that they may be carefully tracked for development of epilepsy. The study is on-going and definitive results are not yet available, however a careful review of the preceding literature provides us with some intriguing hypotheses that should be answerable.

Camfield et al. examined their Nova Scotia cohort for evidence of preceding febrile seizures (Camfield et al., 1994). They described prolonged febrile seizures as those with convulsive activity lasting more than twenty minutes. There were 39 of 482 patients with intractable epilepsy. In addition there were 17 children with prolonged febrile seizures. Seven of these 17 were intractable versus 32 of the 433 without prolonged febrile seizures (p = 0.0002). These seven patients had been followed for an average of 94 months from the onset of their epilepsy. Of these 39 children, 16 had complex partial seizures. Two developed intractable complex partial seizures after prolonged febrile seizures. One of these children had a temporal lobectomy and this showed mesial temporal sclerosis. Based upon a population of 150,000, the authors estimated that the chance of finding someone with a prolonged febrile seizure who later developed intractable complex partial seizures was 1 in 75,000. However, the fact that 2/17 children with prolonged febrile seizures (12%) developed intractable epilepsy with complex partial seizures indicates that large, but not unreasonable numbers of patients, with prolonged febrile seizures would need to be studied and followed for 5-10 years to detect development of intractable focal epilepsy. The numbers in the FEBSTAT cohort (projected enrollment of 200) should be sufficient to address this issue.

A very intriguing story starts nearly 60 years ago in a study published by Margaret A. Lennox (Lennox, 1949). She examined the EEG results of 240 children with febrile seizures and correlated the findings with various features of the illness and seizure. She also contacted the patients for follow-up. Since most of these children all had EEGs, they were undoubtedly more severe than children with typical febrile seizures, and 40% of the group had severe convulsions. A severe convulsion was defined as one in which it or the following coma lasted an hour or more, or if it started in or involved chiefly on limb or one side of the body. Of these 34% had an extremely slow or focal EEG abnormality. These children were almost always under three years of age and had their EEG within seven days of the EEG convulsion. In contrast, paroxysmal abnormalities were observed in 6.7% of the group and were seen in nearly all cases in children who were over three years of age, and the majority were over 5 years of age. One third of this group had three or more febrile convulsions and there was a higher incidence of a family history of isolated convulsions, strongly suggesting a genetic component. Her EEG examples depict typical generalized spike-wave discharges. Overall, the maximum follow-up time on the patients was only three years, and Dr. Lennox conceded that this was too short to allow any broad-reaching conclusions about the development of epilepsy. Nevertheless she noted that somewhere (depending upon the groups used for analysis) between 5 and 12% of the children had afebrile seizures within the three years of follow-up. Of the 11 patients who developed afebrile seizures, two had an extremely slow or focal EEG pattern. She found that 33% of children with focal slowing on their EEG developed afebrile seizures. One of her primary conclusions was that an abnormal EEG record increases the likelihood of epilepsy.

Millichap and colleagues studied the EEG records and clinical features of unselected patients with febrile seizures (Millichap et al., 1960). This study was performed at Albert Einstein College of Medicine in the Bronx and reported in 1960, 12 years after Dr. Lennox'work. He also reported EEG abnormalities in 36% of patients whose seizures lasted more than 20 minutes, in comparison to just 10% abnormalities in those children whose seizures were less than 20 minutes ($p < 0.05$). In the short time of follow-up (an average of one year) spontaneous seizures developed in 38% of children with prolonged febrile seizures. Interstingly, 4/18 (22%) patients with later afebrile seizures had focal slowing on their initial EEGs, whereas only 3/58 (5%) had focal slowing without later development of afebrile seizures.

Lerique-Koechlin and colleagues examined the EEG and clinical features of children with febrile seizures in Paris (Lerique-Koechlin et al., 1958). There were a total of 228 cases with detailed information rgarding the initial EEG and the subsequent course. There were 105 of these children who had either a focal convulsion, a subsequent hemiparesis, or both. There were focal slow waves in 36 (34%) and overall 32% of the children in this group develop epilepsy.

Frantzen et al. studied the longitudinal EEG and clinical features of children with febrile convulsions in Denmark (Frantzen et al., 1968). They examined 200 consecutive children with febrile seizure who were admitted to hospital. Most had an EEG within one week of the seizure. In about one third, the initial EEG showed marked slowing, most marked or confied to the occipital leas and usually asymmetrical. When seven days or more had passed only one of thirteen show marked slowing. They noted that when the convluson lasted 30 minutes or more, had a focal onset or ws unilateral or followed by transient hemipareiss that nearly half of the acute EEGs showed marked slowing (47%), corresponding ot he most involved hemisphere, as indicated b the clinical localization in all cases but one. They also noted that the incidenceo f slowing was greater when the tempraature was high, and he children had been sick for 36 hours of more. Gastroenteritis seemed to be the most likely cause associated with slowing. The slowing did not predict development of later febrile convulsions. However, children who subsequently developed a spike focus more often had EEG slowing (11/19 or 58%) than children who never developed a spike focus (26/77 or 34%) and the side of the spike focus corresponded to the site of maximum EEG slowing. Most often the location of the spike focus was occipital or temporal and it did not shift from one side to the other between examinations. The p value for this was < 0.1, and the authors state that the numbers were too small to draw any definitive conclusions. Frantzen et al. observed that these findings were nearly identical to those of Lennox and Lerique-Koeclin, but there was no agreement as to the significance of the findings. In their relatively short period of follow-up and with a rather small number of patients with prolonged febrile convulsions they did not clearly demonstrate a significant association with later development of epilepsy. They did however, quote other authors who found the identical development of spike foci supplanting areas of prior slowing including Doose et al. and Prichard and McGreal (Doose et al., 1966; Prichard & McGreal, 1958).

In summary, the acute EEG features after prolonged febrile seizures are abnormal in at least one third of cases across a number of series, most of these dating back 40-60 years ago. These findings are most marked in the posterior derivations and appear to increase the chance of development of a spike focus in the same region. In at least three studies, these same children appear to have a higher incidence of afebrile seizures. A reasonable hypothesis would be that focal slowing on the acute EEG after febrile status epilepticus might predict later development of focal epilepsy. If correlated with mesial temporal sclerosis it could be further hypothesized that this finding will predict development of intractability. This hypothesis can be tested in a large prospective series such as FEBSTAT.

Another hypothesis that will be tested with FEBSTAT is that acute MRI findings will predict development of mesial temporal sclerosis. VanLandingham and colleagues showed acute MRI changes after prolonged febrile seizures in children (VanLandingham et al., 1998). These findings consisted of increased T2 signal and volume of the hippocampus. This was followed by shrinkage of the hippocampus at later scans. These initial observations raised the possibility that the acute MRI findings might predict development of epilepsy with mesial temporal sclerosis and this appears to have been confirmed, at least in some cases in a recent publication (Provenzale et al., 2008).

A third area of interest to be addressed in FEBSTAT relates to the possible role of HHV-6B infection in causing intractable epilepsy. Acute MRI changes with intractable partial seizures were observed in patients after transplantation and commensurate immunosuppression (Wainwright et al., 2001). Pathological examination revealed the presence of HHV-6 infection. Presence of HHV-6B was also detected in surgical specimens from patients who underwent temporal lobectomy for intractable seizures, but not in controls (Fotheringham et al., 2007). The hypothesis is that acute infection with HHV-6B might predispose to development of mesial temporal sclerosis and later development of epilepsy.

How long does it take to establish intractability?

Some patients with symptomatic epilepsies have catastrophic onsets, and almost from the start the medical staff can be assured of intractability. This is the case for the aforementioned early onset epileptogenic encephalopathies. Others patients, including those with partial epilepsy that ultimately undergo surgical treatment can take many years to establish intractability. Berg and colleagues examined this in a prospective multicenter study of resective epilepsy surgery (Berg et al., 2003). In 333 patients the latency between onset of epilepsy and failure of the second medication was 9.1 years. Younger age of onset was associated with a longer latency and also a high probability of a temporary remission. Children less than five years were the group reporting the longest lateccies and this was also the group that was most likely to have hasd febrile seizures and hippocampal atrphy. These findings also highlight the need for an extended follow-up period after prolonged febrile seizures to capture those patients with refractory epilepsy.

Conclusions and recommendations

There is no certain way at the current time to establish intractability without medication trials. However, certain clinical factors appear to be highly associated with the development of intractable epilepsy. Many of these features are seen in children with early onset epileptogenic encephalopathies. Other epilepsies with intractable courses are Migrating

Partial Seizures of Infancy, Dravet syndrome, and some cases of Myoclonic Astatic Epilepsy. The course of patients with non-idiopathic focal epilepsy are somewhat harder to predict and the data do not allow very firm conclusions. Even Rasmussen syndrome has recently been suggested to have a more stable course in some patients. Still, and as a general rule those with focal structural lesions, early age of onset, and poor response to medication are likely to have unfavorable courses.

Given the limited resources of neurological services in many parts of the world it is helpful to prioritize the need for urgent evaluations and close follow-up. Considering all of the foregoing, the following recommendations would seem appropriate:

1. Children with onset of epilepsy before one year of age should be urgenty referred for specialty consultation. Some of these children will undoubtedly benefit from immediate hospitalization to accelerate their evaluation and initiate treatment. The risk of refractory epilepsy is quite high in this group.

2. Among these infants, those with clearly symptomatic forms of epilepsy, particularly those following prolonged acute symptomatic seizures or neonatal seizures, should receive the highest priority. Their follow-up should be sooner and more frequent than the average patient with newly-diagnosed epilepsy.

3. Children with high initial seizure rates should also be prioritized for specialty referral and should be followed more closely than the average patient.

4. Children with notoriously refractory epilepsy syndromes should be referred promptly to specialty centers upon diagnosis. Some examples include: Early Myoclonic Encephalopathy, Early Infantile Epileptogenic Encephalopathy, West, Migrating Partial Seizures of Infancy, Lennox-Gastuat, Dravet Syndrome, and epilepsies associated with focal structural lesions. The latter may be candidates for early surgical intervention.

5. A careful analysis of the EEG background, the presence or absence of focal slowing, and type of interictal epileptiform activity may be very useful in predicting intractability. Therefore, it is recommended that the EEGs of children with new onset epilepsy be examined by personnel with experience in the special interpretation of pediatric EEGs and particularly with a intimate knowledge of the clinical and EEG features of pediatric epilepsy syndromes.

References

Annegers JF, Hauser WA, Elveback LR. Remission of seizures and relapse in patients with epilepsy. *Epilepsia* 1979; 20: 729-37.

Arts WF, Geerts AT, Brouwer OF, Boudewyn Peters AC, Stroink H, van Donselaar CA. The early prognosis of epilepsy in childhood: the prediction of a poor outcome. The Dutch study of epilepsy in childhood. *Epilepsia* 1999; 40: 726-34.

Berg AT, Levy SR, Novotny EJ, Shinnar S. Predictors of intractable epielpsy in childhood: a case-control study. *Epilepsia* 1996; 37: 24-30.

Berg AT, Shinnar S, Levy SR, Testa FM, Smith-Rapaport S, Beckerman B. Early development of intractable epilepsy in children: a prospective study. *Neurology* 2001; 56: 1445-52.

Berg AT, Langfitt J, Shinnar S, *et al.* How long does it take for partial epilepsy to become intractable? *Neurology* 2003; 60: 186-90.

Brorson LO, Wranne L. Long-term prognosis in childhood epilepsy: survival and seizure prognosis. *Epilepsia* 1987; 28: 324-30.

Camfield C, Camfield P, Gordon K, Smith B, Dooley J. Outcome of childhood epilepsy: a population-based study with a simple predictive scoring system for those treated with medication. *J Pediatr* 1993; 122: 861-8.

Camfield P, Camfield C, Gordon K, Dooley J. What types of epilepsy are preceded by febrile seizures? A population-based study of children. *Dev Med Child Neurol* 1994; 36: 887-92.

Dlugos DJ, Sammel MD, Strom BL, Farrar JT. Response to first drug trial predicts outcome in childhood temporal lobe epilepsy. *Neurology* 2001; 57: 2259-64.

Doose H, Völzke E, Petersen CE, Herzeberger E. Fieberkrämpfe und Epilepsie. II. Elektroencephalographische Verlaufsuntersuchungen bei sogenannten Fieber- order Infektkrämpfen. *Arch Psychiatr Nervenkr Z Gesamte Neurol Psychiatr* 1966; 208: 413-32.

Dravet C, Bureau M, Oguni H, Fukuyama Y, Cokar O. Severe myoclonic epilepsy in infancy: Dravet syndrome. *Adv Neurol* 2005; 95: 71-102.

Fotheringham J, Donati D, Akhyani N, *et al*. Association of human herpesvirus-6B with mesial temporal lobe epilepsy. *PLoS Med* 2007; 4: e180.

Frantzen E, Lennox-Buchthal M, Nygaard A. Longitudinal EEG and clinical study of children with febrile convulsions. *Electroencephalogr Clin Neurophysiol* 1968; 24: 197-212.

Gambardella A, Andermann F, Shorvon S, Le Piane E, Aguglia U. Limited chronic focal encephalitis: another variant of Rasmussen syndrome? *Neurology* 2008; 70: 374-7.

Geelhoed M, Boerrigter AO, Camfield P, *et al*. The accuracy of outcome prediction models for childhood-onset epilepsy. *Epilepsia* 2005; 46: 1526-32.

Kim WJ, Park SC, Lee SJ, *et al*. The prognosis for control of seizures with medications in patients with MRI evidence for mesial temporal sclerosis. *Epilepsia* 1999; 40: 290-3.

Korff CM, Nordli DR, Jr. Epilepsy syndromes undetermined whether focal or generalized in infants. *Epilepsy Res* 2006; 70 (suppl 1): S105-109.

Korff CM, Laux L, Kelley K, Goldstein J, Koh S, Nordli D, Jr. Dravet syndrome (severe myoclonic epilepsy in infancy): a retrospective study of 16 patients. *J Child Neurol* 2007; 22: 185-94.

Kwan P, Brodie MJ. Early identification of refractory epilepsy. *N Engl J Med* 2000; 342: 314-9.

Kwong KL, Sung WY, Wong SN, So KT. Early predictors of medical intractability in childhood epilepsy. *Pediatr Neurol* 2003; 29: 46-52.

Lennox MA. Febrile convulsions in childhood, a clinial and electroencephalographic study. *Am J Dis Child* 1949; 78: 868-82.

Lerique-Koechlin A, Misès J, Teyssonière de Gramont M, Losky-Nekhorocheff I. L'EEG dans les convulsions fébriles. *Rev Neurol* 1958; 99: 11-25.

Millichap JG, Madsen JA, Aledort LM. Studies in febrile seizures. V. Clinical and electroencephalographic study in unselected patients. *Neurology* 1960; 10: 643-53.

Ohtsuka Y, Yoshinaga H, Kobayashi K. Refractory childhood epilepsy and factors related to refractoriness. *Epilepsia* 2000; 41 (suppl 9): 14-7.

Ohtsuka Y, Yoshinaga H, Kobayashi K, *et al*. Predictors and underlying causes of medically intractable localization-related epilepsy in childhood. *Pediatr Neurol* 2001; 24: 209-13.

Oskoui M, Webster RI, Zhang X, Shevell MI. Factors predictive of outcome in childhood epilepsy. *J Child Neurol* 2005; 20: 898-904.

Prichard JS, McGreal DA. Febrile convulsions. *Med Clin N Amer* 1958; 42: 379-87.

Provenzale JM, Barboriak DP, VanLandingham K, MacFall J, Delong D, Lewis DV. Hippocampal MRI signal hyperintensity after febrile status epilepticus is predictive of subsequent mesial temporal sclerosis. *AJR Am J Roentgenol* 2008; 190: 976-83.

Roger J, Dravet C, Menendez P, Bureau M. Les épilepsies partielles de l'enfant: evolution et facteurs de pronostic. *Rev Electroencephalogr Neurophysiol Clin* 1981; 11: 431-7.

Roger J, Bureau M, Gobbi G, Tassinari CA, Dravet C. Les épilepsies partielles sévères de l'enfant. *Epilepsies* 1991; 213: 191-8.

Scarpa P, Carassini B. Partial epilepsy in childhood: clinical and electroencephalographic study of 261 cases. *Epilepsia* 1982; 23: 333-41.

Sillanpää M. Remission of seizures and predictors of intractability in long-term follow-up. *Epilepsia* 1993; 34: 930-6.

Spooner CG, Berkovic SF, Mitchell LA, Wrennall JA, Harvey AS. New-onset temporal lobe epilepsy in children: lesion on MRI predicts poor seizure outcome. *Neurology* 2006; 67: 2147-53.

VanLandingham KE, Heinz ER, Cavazos JE, Lewis DV. Magnetic resonance imaging evidence of hippocampal injury after prolonged focal febrile convulsions. *Ann Neurol* 1998; 43: 413-26.

Veneselli E, Perrone MV, Di Rocco M, Gaggero R, Biancheri R. Malignant migrating partial seizures in infancy. *Epilepsy Res* 2001; 46: 27-32.

Wainwright MS, Martin PL, Morse RP, *et al*. Human herpesvirus 6 limbic encephalitis after stem cell transplantation. *Ann Neurol* 2001; 50: 612-9.

Epileptic encephalopathies versus "garden variety focal epilepsies": can they be considered together?

J. Helen Cross, C. Eltze

UCL-Institute of Child Health & Great Ormond Street Hospital for Children NHS Trust, London, UK

The focal epilepsies by definition have an origin from a single area of the brain according to the proposed ILAE classification (Engel Jr., 2001). They present as the most common intractable epilepsies in adulthood (Semah *et al.*, 1998; Elwes *et al.*, 1984). By contrast, in childhood, several focal epilepsy syndromes have been delineated which follow a predictable course and which often have specific implications for treatment choice. These are categorised under idiopathic, symptomatic and presumed symptomatic (cryptogenic) focal epilepsies (ILAE, 1989, 2001). However in clinical practice classifying patients into these groups can be difficult especially at the initial diagnosis. (Kahane *et al.*, 2005).

The term "epileptic encephalopathy", has been recently introduced as a new concept and several syndromes have been listed under this category in the 2001 ILAE proposal (*Table I*) (Engel Jr., 2001). The concept involves the presumption that cognitive impairment is related to ongoing epileptic activity. In certain epileptic encephalopathy syndromes such as Landau-Kleffner syndrome (LKS) or epilepsy with continuous spike waves during slow sleep (CSWS), epileptiform activity does not predominantly manifest as seizure activity (Neville & Cross, 2006). Thus, we must consider that intractability may extend beyond the seizures themselves and its manifestations to include the cognitive effects of the epileptic activity in the brain. Fluctuation of cognitive function with clinically manifest or subclinical

Table I. Epilepsies currently classed as Epileptic Encephalopathies (ILAE 2001) (Engel Jr., 2001e)

Early myoclonic encephalopahy (EME)
Ohtahara Syndrome
West Syndrome
Dravet Syndrome (Severe Myoclonic Epilepsy of Infancy) (SMEI)
Lennox Gastaut Syndrome (LGS)
Myoclonic status in nonprogressive encephalopathies
Landau Kleffner Syndrome (LKS)
Epilepsy with continuous spike waves during slow sleep (CSWS)

epileptiform activity may also be encountered in the context of other childhood epilepsy syndromes (including some idiopathic syndromes) currently not contained in the "epileptic encephalopathies" category.

Within these contexts we will discuss the impact of therapeutic interventions on clinical course and ultimately on outcome.

▪ Idiopathic vs symptomatic: how sure can we be?

The current classification defines idiopathic epilepsy as a syndrome that is only epilepsy, presumed to be genetic and usually age dependent. Individuals have no underlying structural brain lesion or other neurological signs or symptoms (Engel Jr., 2001). Some well delineated syndromes can be recognised by a characteristic clinical picture and associated EEG, *e.g.* Benign Epilepsy with Centrotemporal Spikes (BECTS). In typical presentations of such syndromes age dependent remission is part of the natural evolution. The debate may often be whether to treat rather than when to treat, and response to treatment is typically excellent. Other idiopathic syndromes with good prognosis have also been described. They may however, be diagnosed retrospectively when a benign course becomes obvious in the absence of a diagnostic marker available at initial presentation particularly in the very young (Watanabe *et al.*, 1993). The idiopathic partial epilepsies in infancy are such an example, where normal developmental outcome is one of the criteria for diagnosis recognising subtle structural abnormalities may not be apparent on early brain imaging.

Children with symptomatic focal epilepsy can usually be identified based upon the presence of a structural lesion, the determination of which is greatly enhanced by magnetic resonance imaging. There remains a dilemma however in those children with negative neuroimaging and focal epilepsy. A cryptogenic or presumed symptomatic epilepsy is only recognised where criteria fail to fulfil those of a recognised idiopathic epilepsy syndrome, there is no precise aetiology detectable and radiological abnormalities are absent (Kahane *et al.*, 2005).Therefore the question remains as to whether there is an aetiology that is yet to be recognised or whether such epilepsies can more clearly be defined as idiopathic? Certainly surgical series do show that histopathologically confirmed abnormalities can be present where imaging is negative although the numbers of children undergoing surgery with negative imaging remains low (Harvey *et al.*, 2008). This is perhaps of more relevance in the paediatric rather than the adult population.

Another way that a distinction between symptomatic or idiopathic (although not relatively) could be made would be by response to treatment. This distinction may prove useful in terms of prognosis. (Semah *et al.*, 1998; Kwan & Brodie, 2000). Further the question arises in the young as to whether we should use associated neurological impairment as a marker of symptomatic rather than idiopathic. Where the impairment is the result of the underlying epileptic activity (*i.e.* epileptic encephalopathy), this may not be appropriate.

▪ What is an epileptic encephalopathy?

The concept of epileptic encephalopathy has developed following the observation that certain children present with developmental difficulties after the onset of epilepsy. By definition the condition is one where the epileptiform abnormalities themselves are believed to contribute to the progressive disturbance in cerebral function (Engel Jr., 2001). The developmental compromise seen in some of the more catastrophic epilepsies therefore has been presumed to be the result of continued epileptic activity particularly where the children have had normal developmental progress prior to the epilepsy. By this presumption, one would have to consider such neurodevelopmental compromise to be reversible. However it is unknown whether the cognitive losses are totally reversible. Furthermore, we do not understand why, in idiopathic or symptomatic focal epilepsies, it appears to develop in some children and not in others with similar underlying aetiologies, and to what extent focal pathology contributes to this phenomenon.

The premise is that such epilepsies should be treated aggressively. But what evidence do we have that reversal of the epilepsy will lead to cognitive improvement, and what treatments can be effective? By definition, this is more likely to be determined by the inherent treatability of the disorder, but we have no predictive markers of this.

The current concept of epileptic encephalopathy within the classification only recognizes certain severe syndromes as epileptic encephalopthies. The concept of epileptic encephalopthy, especially if viewed as a spectrum of severity of disturbance, could, however, be applicable to a wide variety of syndromes. We will consider evidence regarding this for idiopathic and nonidiopathic epilepsies separately, despite the concern of the degree of possible overlap.

■ Idiopathic focal epilepsies

The most common syndrome within this group is benign epilepsy with centrotemporal spikes. It is characterised by onset typically between the ages of 7 and 10 years, seizures of a specific semiology (motor partial), characteristic centrotemporal spikes on EEG, absence of neurological deficits and spontaneous remission of seizures in adolescence (Dalla Bernardina *et al.*, 2005). There is increasing literature now on the issue of the true benign nature of centrotemporal spikes (Staden *et al.*, 1998; Metz Lutz & Filippini, 2006). In particular, there is concern over whether cognition may be impaired in some individuals, and whether there may be a spectrum of severity with typical BECTS representing the mild end and Landau-Kleffner Syndrome in association with electrical status epilepticus of slow sleep (ESES) at the most severe end.

To this end, it would be especially useful to have markers that identify the subpopulation that may act in an atypical fashion, either electrically or clinically, or who are already on an evolutionary trajectory toward ESES (Saltik *et al.*, 2005). Saltik *et al.* examined clinical and EEG parameters in 16 individuals with idiopathic partial epilepsy (IPE) who subsequently developed epilepsy with ESES and compare them to those of 25 who had a course "typical" of idiopathic partial epilepsy. They determined children in the ESES group were more likely to have a higher seizure frequency, variability in seizure types and resistance to a single AED (75% in ESES group in early stage, 16% control group). Focal slowing on EEG at the site of the predominant epileptogenic foci was seen early in the course of 25% of those later to develop ESES compared to none of the controls.

Despite the relative belief of the "benign" nature of BECTS some authors have reported specific neuropsychological deficits when children with an apparent typical course are studied in detail. Staden *et al.* conducted standardised neuropsychological assessment in children to review specifically aspects of language processing (Staden *et al.*, 1998). They examined 20 children and showed patients with BECTS to fail five of twelve standardized language tests significantly more often than the normative population. Thirteen of the 20 children showed language dysfunction with difficulties in two or more of the twelve standardized language tests. Other studies have also shown cognitive deficits to be associated with the prevalence of seizures and degree of EEG abnormality (Metz-Lutz et al., 1999); however, the relevance of this to long term outcome has been unclear. How do these deficits relate to the centrotemporal spike activity and are they reversible when children grow out of the disorder? In a further study of 55 children comparing performance on the different subtests of the Wechsler Intelligence Scale for Children, significant decreases were seen in four subtests for children tested 18-32 months after the onset of epilepsy. In the group with frequent spike wave discharges on waking EEG these cognitive deficits correlated with frequency and lateralisation of discharges to the right hemisphere (Metz-Lutz, et al.. Massa et al.). were able to determine interictal EEG patterns that distinguished between BECTS patients with complications and without complications (Massa et al., 2001). Groups were a priory separated according to presence of significant behavioural and schooling difficulties. Patients with complications (atypical group) had significantly lower verbal IQ (VIQ) and full scale IQ (FSIQ) at onset and recovery compared with the group of patients without complications (typical group).

Metz-Lutz et al. used the electro-clinical criteria established by Massa et al. to compare children with typical and atypical BECTS longitudinally at three points:
– two months following seizure onset;
– the active period when there was greatest amount of spike wave discharges;
– recovery set after one year with normal waking and sleep EEG following withdrawal of antiepileptic medication (Metz-Lutz & Filippini, 2006).

Similarly they found that the atypical group had significantly lower FSIQ and VIQ's at onset until recovery. Performance IQ's were lower only at onset and during the active phase. Performance subtests that required executive functions such as attention and behavioural regulation showed impairment in both groups in the active phase and improvement at recovery. After recovery from epilepsy a significant improvement in performance in all cognitive domains was seen except verbal short term memory in the atypical group. Certain EEG features were associated with poorer overall cognitive function from onset to recovery. These results suggest that the groups are different prior to onset of the disorder and that another pathophysiological mechanism other than epileptiform activity in the active phase is likely to be responsible for the deficits. The duration of the possible subclinical EEG abnormalities in the atypical group however remains unknown and may be of clinical significance. Thus there is little evidence to show that treatment in the active phase would make a difference to the overall cognitive outcome.

There is limited information in the literature to suggest that other idiopathic epilepsies can present us with the same dilemma. Some studies suggest a degree of dysfunction on detailed assessment in select children with other idiopathic epilepsies, but provide no detail on correlation with EEG abnormality or severity (Gulgonen et al., 2000; Chilosi et al., 2006) However in theory there may be no lesser reason why idiopathic occipital epilepsy cannot be associated with intellectual deficits, perhaps secondary to medication. Would this raise doubts about the diagnosis of idiopathic epilepsy? In the absence of a visible lesion and typical semiology, can we be so sure?

▪ What influence may we have with treatment?

The general principle to the treatment of epilepsy is that we consider treatment after two epileptic seizures; we treat frequency and occurrence of seizures not the presence of epileptiform activity on EEG. The exception to the rule of course is ESES; the exact difference in spike wave index between wake and sleep required to treat may lead to further discussion. However, if we are suspecting spikes to be related to cognitive deficit in these idiopathic epilepsies do we have evidence that treatment with the aim of suppressing interictal discharges leads to benefit? Studies reveal in fact that carbamazepine although quoted as effective in the treatment of seizures, is not effective at suppressing epileptiform discharges *(Table II)*. Furthermore, evidence suggests that such medication may lead to aggravation of discharges, and seizures in selected children with BECTS (Fejerman *et al.*, 2000; de Saint-Martin *et al.*, 2000; Corda *et al.*, 2001). Others have demonstrated development of negative myoclonus, and suggest spike wave rather than sharp waves on EEG at presentation may be a marker of an abnormal response to carbamazepine (Parmeggiani *et al.*, 2004). A similar deterioration has been demonstrated with lamotrigine (Cerminara *et al.*, 2004; Catania *et al.*, 1999). Such deterioration may also be seen in symptomatic focal epilepsies *(Figure 1)*.

Sulthiame has been demonstrated in a randomised controlled study to be effective in the treatment of seizures (Rating *et al.*, 2000), but also shown to be effective in abolishing centrotemporal spikes (Bast *et al.*, 2003). This aside, there is only limited and contradictory evidence that effective suppression of spikes may improve cognition in the long-term (Baglietto *et al.*, 2001; Wirrell *et al.*, 2008).

What evidence is there that symptomatic focal epilepsies may develop an epileptic encephalopathy? There is no question that children presenting to epilepsy surgery for focal epilepsy have a high rate of learning disability, and this is more likely in children with early onset of seizures (Vasconcellos *et al.*, 2001; Cormack *et al.*, 2007). Neuropsychological data from children with congenital hemiplegia also show us that children with

Table II. Effect of medication on centrotemporal discharges in children with BECTS: percentge of children showing complete suppression of electroencephalographic interictal discharges (Nicolai *et al.*, 2006)

Study	Study design	Carbamazepine	Valproate	Sulthiame	Clonazepam	Placebo
Gross-Selbeck, 1995 N = 42	Retrospective	0/16 (0%)	–	7/17 (41%)	–	–
Mitsudome *et al.*, 1997 N = 40	Prospective	0/10	1/10 (10%)	–	15/20 (75%)	–
Kramer *et al.*, 2002 N = 111	Retrospective	8/19 (42%)	–	5/7 (71%)	–	–
Bast *et al.* 2003 N = 66	RCT	–	–	4 wks 20/29 (29%) 6 m 10/26 (38%)		4/5 (16%) 1/10 (10%)
Engler *et al.*, 2003 N = 16	Prospective			3-6 m 3/13 (23%) > 6 m 6/16 (38%)		–

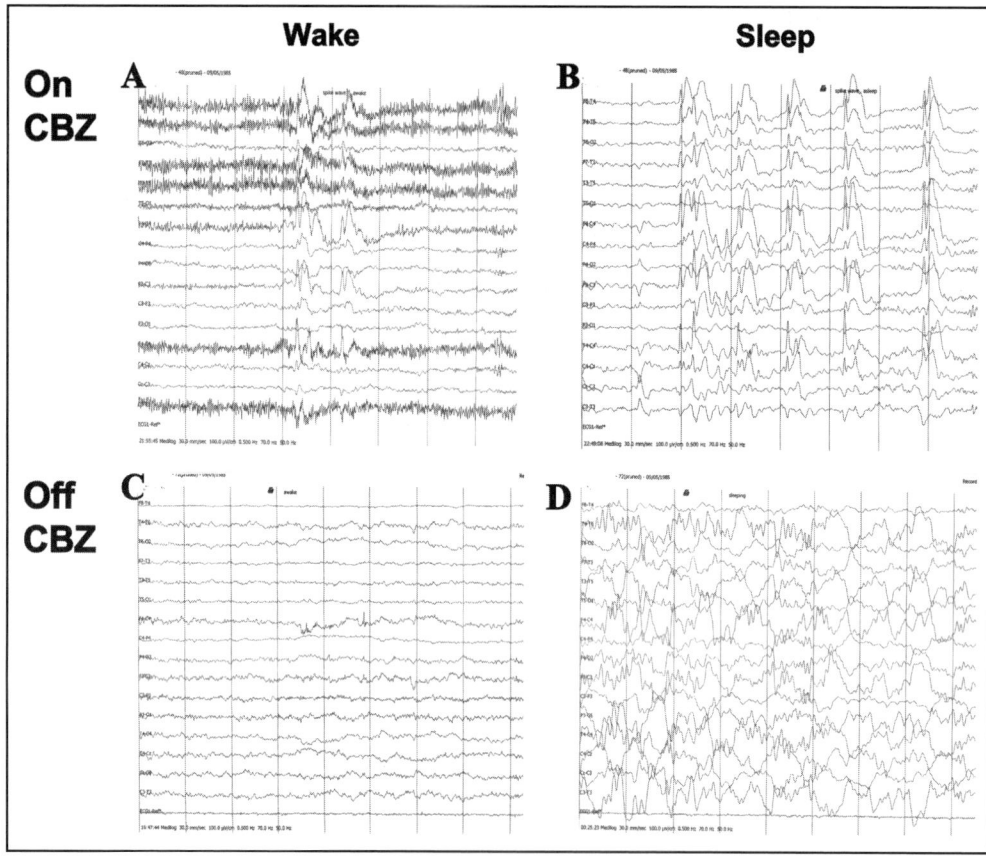

Figure 1. EEG in wake and sleep state in a five year old girl who presented with temporal lobe seizures, the result of a temporal DNET. Carbamazepine was initiated but she developed poor concentration at school and regression in abilities. Wake (A) and Sleep (B) EEG demonstrate her to have developed ESES. Weaning from the carbamazepine led to resolution of this (D).
Courtesy of Mary O'Regan, Yorkhill Childrens Hospital, Glasgow.

early onset of epilepsy have a lower cognitive performance at 6 years than those that do not develop epilepsy (Vargha-Khadem et al., 1992) Furthermore, children with pervasive developmental disorder in association with epilepsy and temporal lobe lesions also have a significantly lower age of onset than others presenting for temporal lobe surgery (McLellan et al., 2005). There is other evidence that duration of epilepsy may also influence ultimate cognitive outcome following surgery (Jonas et al., 2005).This has led to the premise that early onset of symptomatic focal epilepsy has a high risk of epileptic encephalopathy and those failing to respond to medical management should be aggressively considered for resective surgery early in their clinical course.

One then has to review the evidence that we make a difference to outcome with such treatment. Recognising children with early onset epilepsy are at high risk of cognitive impairment, there is evidence that those with castastrophic early onset of symptomatic focal epilepsy are at a particular risk, many of whom have epilepsy the result of multilobar or hemispheric structural abnormalities. Pulsifer et al. reported on neuropsychological outcome following hemispherectomy 71 children, split into three groups dependent on aetiology – cortical dysplasia, Rasmussens and vascular abnormalities including stroke (Pulsifer et al., 2004). Little change was seen as a group between pre and postoperative scores in any of the three groups. This study also showed that children with developmental pathology had a significantly lower IQ presurgery, with no significant gain post surgery. However, it was also evident that the group of children undergoing surgery for developmental malformations had a significantly lower age of onset of epilepsy (< 12 m) than the other groups, which is likely as suggested from other studies to have had a significant impact on outcome. In our own study of 33 patients undergoing hemidisconnection (the majority undergoing functional hemispherectomy), similar results were found (Devlin et al., 2003). Most studies report little longitudinal change in IQ following hemidisconnection procedures. When IQ is considered as a measure of ability relative to peers, this implies any decline or arrest of intellectual function took place prior to surgery, and cessation of seizures may have led to a maintained trajectory (and therefore longitudinal progress relative to peers) as opposed to a decline. Review of EEG data from these children suggest an impact on the contralateral hemisphere with spike and wave activity as well as generalised slow activity, does not necessarily influence the likelihood of seizure free outcome, (Doring et al., 1999; Wyllie et al., 2007).

With regard to children undergoing focal resection data are less clear. A recent study of children coming to surgery between the ages of 3 and 7 years (16 temporal, 9 frontal, 18 multilobar and 7 hemispherectomy) showed that, at 12 months postoperatively, 82% were functioning at a similar level to their preoperative level (Freitag & Tuxhorn, 2005). Notably development was delayed in 84% coming to surgery. Two to three years post surgery 29/40 (72%) performed at their preoperative levels, and eight children showed significant gains of > 15 IQ points from preoperative levels. This suggests that developmental gains may accumulate over a longer period and do not necessarily become evident in early postoperative months. Duration of epilepsy prior to surgery was the only predictor of long term cognitive change; children with shorter intervals between onset of epilepsy and surgery had greater gains in developmental quotient. However in this study seizure outcome did not significantly contribute to the prediction of postoperative cognitive change.

One problem with surgical series is that cognitive outcome is assessed on the analysis of group data. Therefore it could be presumed that children with any degree of epileptic encephalopathy may be hidden within such an analysis amongst those without evidence of such, particularly if the latter form a greater proportion. Who specifically is at risk is unclear. Conversely, this may presume that all children presenting with early onset seizures may have some degree of epileptic encephalopathy. Data from a population based study with 12 months review of all children presenting under the age of two years, suggest at present that the underlying pathology is the greater predictor of outcome rather than control of seizures (Whitney et al., 2008). To what degree is epileptic encephalopathy accountable for ultimate outcome and how much is therefore reversible? There is no question that in isolated cases gains can be made (Figure 2); however, a demonstration of group effect is more difficult. The clinical data to date are not able to answer the question as to whether the ongoing epileptic activity is of relevance, or whether permanent change to developmental pathways takes place if seizures occur at a critical age, and therefore by early intervention we are eliminating the occurrence of further compromise rather than reading is further improvement.

Children with late onset of epilepsy do not appear to be at the same risk, but data may be clearer on the degree of reversibility possible.

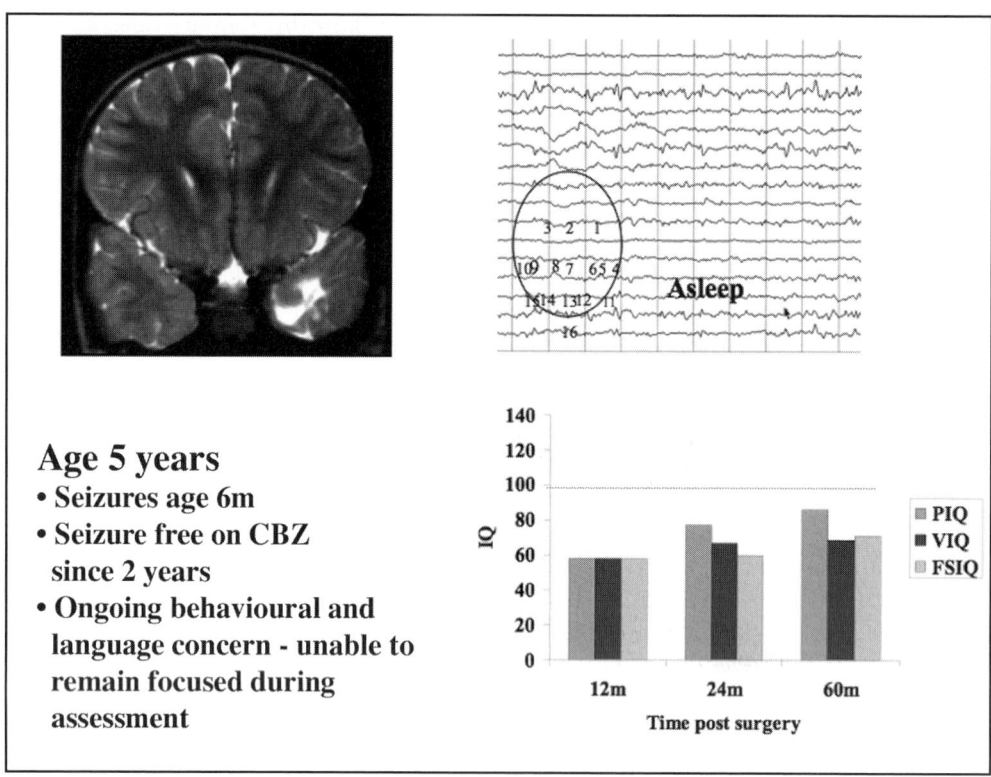

Figure 2. Clinical and developmental progress in a girl who underwent a temporal lobe resection for dysembryoplastic neuroepithelial tumour at 5 years, despite seizure freedom on medication since 2 years. Developmental progress had been slow and the EEG continued to show continuous epileptiform activity over this region.

There is clear evidence from certain studies that children with focal brain malformations may develop a more widespread epilepsy process associated with cognitive regression and therefore by definition an epileptic encephalopathy. Longitudinal studies in children with hemipolymicrogyria have shown that although epilepsy may start with focal seizures, with time drop attacks appear and their EEG demonstrates evidence of ESES (Figure 3). Although the limited, temporal course of spike wave discharges has been demonstrated, as well as the cognitive ability limited the degree to which these cognitive deficits recover on resolution of the EEG abnormality is unclear. Furthermore it is also unclear whether effective aggressive early treatment might have resulted in better cognitive outcomes (Guerrini et al. 1998). There are children in whom there is no question that surgical intervention resulting in removal of clinically manifest or subclinical epileptiform activity leads to dramatically increased awareness, but others where medical treatment improves the EEG with little change in cognitive function and behaviour (Figure 4). What factors are responsible for the observed differences in outcome? Is resistance to medication a marker of the likely cognitive impact from epileptic activity, or the results of differences in the underlying pathology? The association between subclinical epileptiform activity and cognitive/behavioural function is complex. Other factors such a side effects of pharmacological treatment may play an important role in this context.

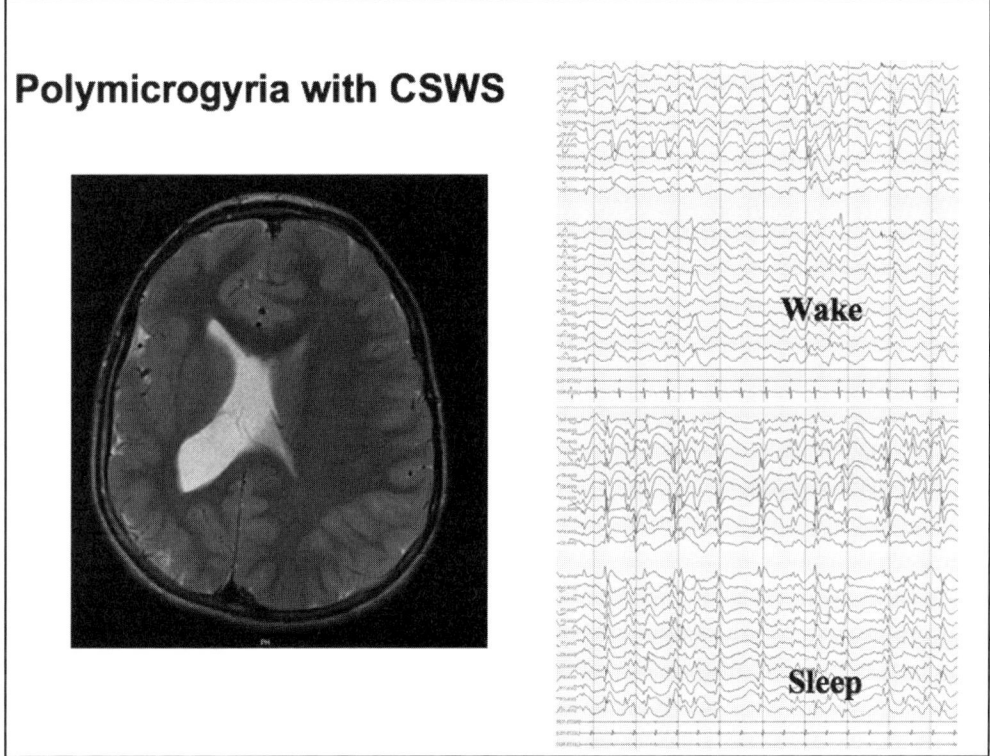

Figure 3. EEG in wake and sleep in a boy presenting with drug resistant epilepsy in association with right hemipolymicrogyria. "Drop" attacks ad become almost continuous. Sleep EEG shows the development of ESES.

■ What is the evidence that epileptic encephalopathy may have a focal onset

To answer this question, much evidence is anecdotal rather than substantially evidence based. Certain syndromes are linked to the concept of epileptic encephalopathy (Lennox Gastaut Syndrome, Dravet), and these traditionally do not appear to have a focal onset. A clinical phenotype with some charactertistics of Lennox-Gastaut Syndrome may however develop from focal brain malformations. ESES, may also develop from a structural brain malformation, and even where one is not shown, a localised prominence to the EEG may be demonstrated. Some correlation has been shown between frontal prominence on EEG and children with global cognitive deficit, and temporal prominence on EEG in children with language regression, so called Landau Kleffner syndrome (Rouselle & Revol, 1995). On the one hand, such an EEG abnormality may be seen to be a developmental disorder, as with those associated with structural malformations described above. There is a good prognosis with regard to resolution of the seizures and EEG abnormalities in these disorders. However the prognosis for the cognitive and language deficit is typically poor. The reason for aggressive treatment would be to minimise long-term cognitive and language morbidity.

The premise that such EEG abnormalities in some cases may be focal in origin has led to the question of surgical treatment in selected cases of those associated with language regression (Landau Kleffner Syndrome). Morrell first described the possible use of multiple

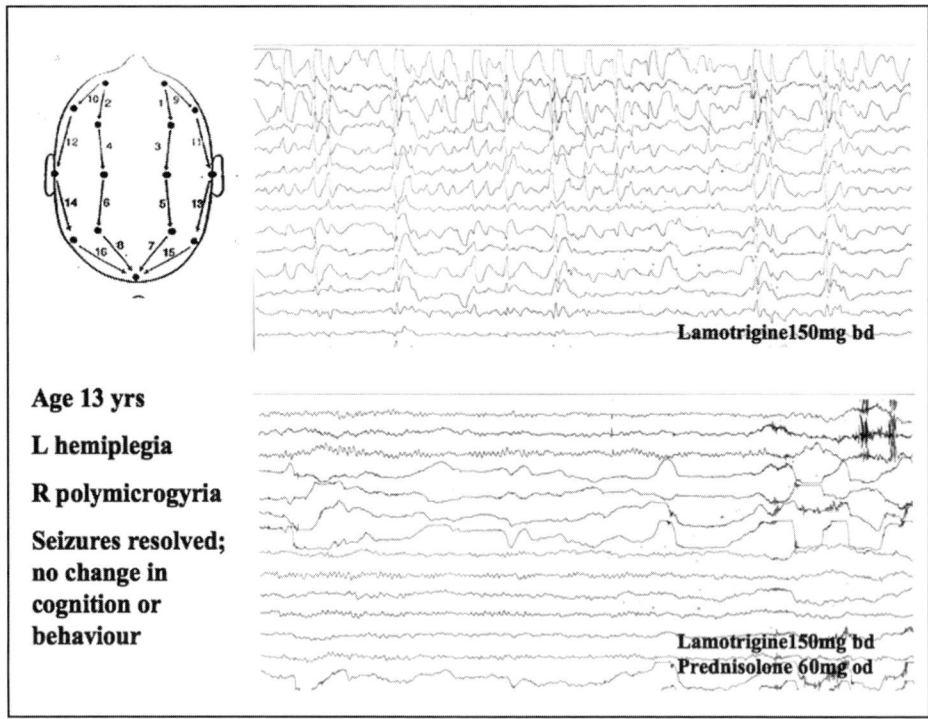

Figure 4. EEG before and after treatment in a 13 year old boy who demonstrated ESES with a right lateralisation in association with right polymicrogyria. Neuropsychological assessment before and after treatment showed no change.

sub-pial transections over Wernickes area deep into the sylvian fissure under corticographic control (until abolition of ESES) (Morrell et al., 1995; Grote et al., 1999) with good outcome, although followup data suggest the longer duration following surgery the better outcome. Repeat literature has been scant resulting in difficulty assessing whether the natural course is in fact altered by such intervention (Irwin et al., 2001).

■ The future: where from here?

In the treatment of focal epilepsy, from the data we have available it is apparent that a single treatment is unlikely to fit all. The issue more specifically lies in individually assessing each child, and attempting to determine on an individual basis the likelihood of clinically manifest and subclinical epileptic activity contributing to any ongoing neurodevelopmental problems. There is no question that markers of treatment response are required, by determining individual responses as well as on the basis of group analysis. With regard to the idiopathic focal epilepsies we have little data to suggest aggressive treatment of the discharges is justified, although may need to be considered in individuals where clear outcome makers are set. In symptomatic cases, again the relative presence of an epileptic encephalopathy needs to be assessed on an individual basis and whether medication or indeed surgery is the way forward. We need to work further towards collecting data as to when, in whom and what time in the natural history of a symptomatic epilepsy surgery may be optimal, as well as in determining those where no lesion is identified, but where surgery should be actively pursued.

References

Baglietto MG, Battaglia FM, Nobili I, et al. Neuropsychological disorders relate to interictal epileptic discharges during sleep in benign epilepsy of childhood with centrotemporal or rolandic spikes. *Dev Med Child Neurol* 2001; 43: 407-12.

Bast T, Volp A, Wolf C, et al. The influence of sulthiame on EEG in children with benign childhood epilepsy with centrotemporal spikes (BECTS). *Epilepsia* 2003; 44: 215-20.

Catania S, Cross JH, de Sousa C, Boyd SG. Paradoxical reaction to Lamotrigine in a child with benign focal epilepsy of childhood with centrotemporal spikes. *Epilepsia* 1999; 40: 1657-60.

Cerminara C, Montanaro ML, Curatolo P, Seri S. Lamotrigine-induced seizure aggravation and negative myoclonus in idiopathic rolandic epilepsy. *Neurology* 2004; 63: 373-5.

Chilosi AM, Brovedani P, Moscatelli M, Bonanni P, Guerrini R. Neuropsychological findings in idiopathic occipital lobe epilepsies. *Epilepsia* 2006; 47: 76-8.

Corda D, Gelisse P, Genton P, et al. Incidence of drug induced aggravation in benign epilepsy with centrotemporal spikes. *Epilepsia* 2001; 42: 754-9.

Cormack F, Cross JH, Vargha-Khadem F, Baldeweg T. The development of intellectual abilities in temporal lobe epilepsy. *Epilepsia* 2007; 48: 201-4.

Dalla Bernardina B, Sgro V, Fejerman N. Epilepsy with centro-temporal spikes and related syndromes. In: Roger J, Bureau M, Dravet Ch, Genton P, Tassinari CA, Wolf P, ed. *Epileptic Syndromes in Infancy, Childhood and Adolescence*. John Libbey Eurotext; 2005: 203-25.

de Saint-Martin A, Massa R, Metz-Lutz MN, et al. Benign childhood epilepsy with centrotemporal spikes: is it always benign? *Neurology* 2000; 55: 1241-2.

Devlin AM, Cross JH, Harkness W, et al. Clinical outcomes of hemispherectomy for epilepsy in childhood and adolescence. *Brain* 2003; 126: 556-66.

Doring S, Cross JH, Boyd SG, Harkness WF, Neville BG. The significane of bilateral EEG abnormalties before and after hemispherectomy in children with unilateral major hemisphere lesions. *Epilepsy Res* 1999; 34: 625-30.

Elwes RD, Johnson AL, Shorvon SD, Reynolds EH. The prognosis for seizure cotrol in newly diagnosed epilepsy. *N Engl J Med* 1984; 311: 944-7.

Engel J, Jr. A proposed diagnostic scheme for people with epileptic seizures and with epilepsy: report of the ILAE Task Force on *Classification and Terminology*. *Epilepsia* 2001; 42: 796-803.

Fejerman N, Caraballo R, Tenembaum SN. Atypical evolutions of benign localisation-related epilepsies in chidren: are they predictable? *Epilepsia* 2000; 41: 380-90.

Freitag H, Tuxhorn I. Cognitive funciton in preschool children after epilepsy surgery:rationale for early intervention. *Epilepsia* 2005; 46: 561-7.

Grote CL, Van Slyke P, Hoeppner JAB. Language outcome following multiple subpial transection. *Brain* 1999; 122: 561-6.

Guerrini R, Genton P, Bureau M, et al. Multilobar polymicrogyria, intractable drop attack seizures and sleep related electrical status epilepticus. *Neurology* 1998; 51: 504-12.

Gulgonen S, Demirbilek V, Korkmaz B, et al. Neuropsychological functions in idiopathic occipital lobe epilepsy. *Epilepsia* 2000; 41: 405-11.

Harvey AS, Cross JH, Shinnar S, Mathern GW. Seizure Syndromes, Eitiologies and Procedures in Paediatric Epilepsy: A 2004 International Survey. *Epilepsia* 2008; 49: 146-55.

Irwin K, Birch V, Lees J, et al. Multiple subpial transection in Landau-Kleffner syndrome. *Dev Med Child Neurol* 2001; 43: 248-52.

Jonas R, Asarnow RF, LoPresti C, et al. Surgery for symptomatic infant-onset epileptic encephalopathy with and without infantile spasms. *Neurology* 2005; 64: 746-50.

Kahane P, Arzimanoglou A, Bureau M, Roger J. Non-idiopathic partial epilepsies of childhood. In:: Roger J, Bureau M, Dravet Ch, Genton P, Tassinari CA, Wolf P, ed. *Epileptic Syndromes in Infancy, Childhood and Adolescence*. John Libbey Eurotext; 2005: 255-75.

Kwan P, Brodie MJ. Early identification of refractory epilepsy. *New Eng J Med* 2000; 342: 314-9.

Massa R, de Saint-Martin A, Carcangiu R, et al. EEG criteria predictive of complicated evolution in idiopathic rolandic epilepsy. *Neurology* 2001; 57: 1071-9.

McLellan A, Davies S, Heyman I, et al. Psychopathology in children with epilepsy before and after temporal lobe resection. *Dev Med Child Neurol* 2005; 47: 666-72.

Metz-Lutz MN, Filippini M. Neuropsychological findings in Rolandic epilepsy and Landau-Kleffner syndrome. *Epilepsia* 2006; 47; (suppl 2): 71-5.

Metz-Lutz MN, Kleitz C, de Saint Martin A, Massa R, Hirsch E, Marescaux C. Cognitive development in benign focal epilepsies of childhood. *Dev Neurosci* 1999; 21: 182-90.

Morrell F, Whisler WW, Smith MC, et al. Landau-Kleffner syndrome; Treatment with subpial transection. *Brain* 1995; 118: 1529-46.

Neville BG, Cross H. Continous Spike Wave of Slow Sleep and Landau-Kleffner Syndrome. In: Wyllie E, Gupta A, Lachhwani D K, ed. *The Treatment of Epilpsy, Principles and Practice*. Lippincott Williams & Wilkins; 2006: 455-62.

Nicolai J, Aldenkamp AP, Arends J, Weber JW, Vles JS. Cognitive and behavioural effects of nocturnal epileptiform discharges in children with benign childhood epilepsy with centrotemporal spikes. *Epilepsy and Behaviour* 2006; 8: 56-70.

Parmeggiani L, Seri S, Bonanni P, Guerrini R. Electrophysiological characterization of spontaneous and carbamazepne-induced epileptic negative myoclonus in benign childhood epilepsy with centro-temporal spikes. *Clinical Neurophysiology* 2004; 115: 50-8.

Pulsifer M, Brandt J, Salorio CF, Vining EP, Carson B, Freeman JM. The cognitive outcome of hemispherectomy in 71 children. *Epilepsia* 2004; 243-54.

Rating D, Wolf C, Bast T, for the sulthiame study group. Sulthiame as monotherapy in children with benign childhood epilepsy with centrotemporal spikes: a 6-month randomized, double blind, placebo-controlled study. *Epilepsia* 2000; 41: 1284-8.

Rouselle C, Revol M. Relations between cognitive functions and CSWS. In: Beaumanoir A, Bureau M, Deonna T, Mira L, Tassinar CA, ed. *Continuous Spike Waves during Slow Sleep, Electrical Status Epilepticus during Slow SLeep: acqiored epileptic aphasia and related conditions*. John Libbey Eurotext; 1995: 123-33.

Saltik S, Uluduz D, Cokar O, Demirbilek V, Dervent A. A clinical and EEG study on idiopathic partial epilepsies with evolution into ESES spectrum disorders. *Epilepsia* 2005; 46: 524-33.

Semah F, Picot MC, Adam C, et al. Is the underlying cause of epilepsy a major prognostic factor for recurrence. *Neurology* 1998; 51: 1256-62.

Staden U, Isaacs E, Boyd SG, Brandl U, Neville BGR. Language dysfunction in children with Rolandic epilepsy. *Neuropediatrics* 1998; 29: 242-8.

Vargha-Khadem F, Isaacs E, van der Werf S, Robb S, Wilson J. Development of intelligence and memory in children with hemiplegic cerebral palsy. The deleterious consequences of early seizures. *Brain* 1992; 115 Pt 1: 315-29.

Vasconcellos E, Wyllie E, Sullivan S, Stanford L, Bulacio J, Kotagal P. Mental retardation in pediatric candidates for epilepsy surgery: the role of early seizure onset. *Epilepsia* 2001; 42: 268-74.

Watanabe K, Negoro T, Aso K. Benign partial epilpesy with secondarily generalised seizures in infancy. *Epilepsia* 1993; 34: 635-8.

Wirrell E, Sherman EM, Vanmastrigt R, Hamiwka L. Deterioration in cognitive function in children with benign epilepsy of childhood with central temporal spikes treated with sulthiame. *J Child Neurol* 2008; 23: 14-21.

Wyllie E, Lachhwani DK, Gupta AK, *et al*. Successful surgery for epilepsy due to early brain lesions despite generalised EEG findings. *Neurology* 2007; 69: 389-97.

Achevé d'imprimer par Corlet, Imprimeur, S.A.
14110 Condé-sur-Noireau
N° d'Imprimeur : 114380 - Dépôt légal : septembre 2008

Imprimé en France